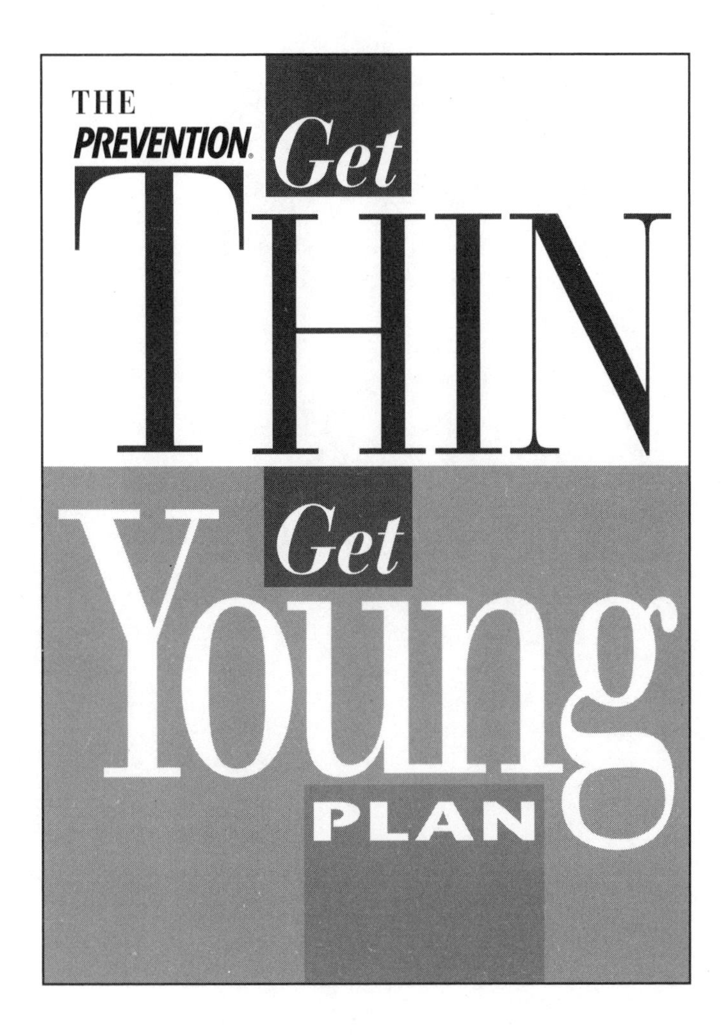
THE
PREVENTION
Get
THIN
Get
Young
PLAN

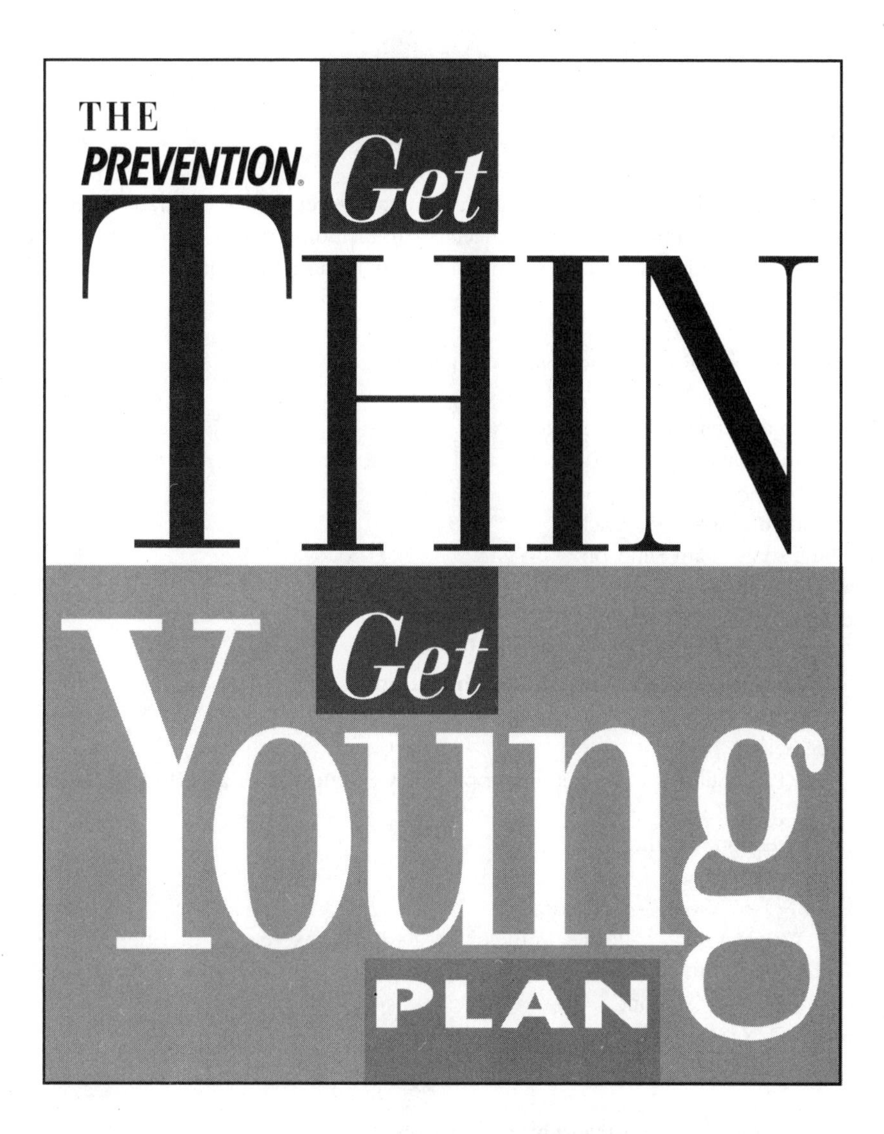

By **Selene Yeager** and **Bridget Doherty**

Foreword by Michele Stanten

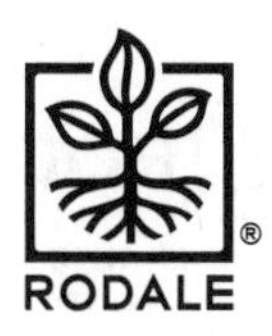

Printed in the United States of America
Rodale Inc. makes every effort to use acid-free ♾, recycled paper ♻

Hair/makeup: Coleen Kobrick
Clothing stylist: Pam Simpson
Clothing courtesy of Land's End, L.L. Bean, Reebok, Swingwear Faux Vintage Clothing, and Aardvark Sports Shop

Library of Congress Cataloging-in-Publication Data

Yeager, Selene.
The Prevention get thin get young plan / by Selene Yeager and Bridget Doherty.
p. cm.
"Prevention Health Books."
Includes index.
ISBN 1–57954–217–4 hardcover
1. Weight loss. 2. Physical fitness. 3. Reducing exercises. I. Title: Get thin get young plan. II. Doherty, Bridget. III. Prevention Health Books. IV. Prevention (Emmaus, Pa.) V. Title.
RM222.2 .Y43 2001
613.7—dc21 00-010917

Distributed to the book trade by St. Martin's Press

2 4 6 8 10 9 7 5 3 hardcover

Visit us on the Web at www.preventionbookshelf.com, or call us toll-free at (800) 848-4735.

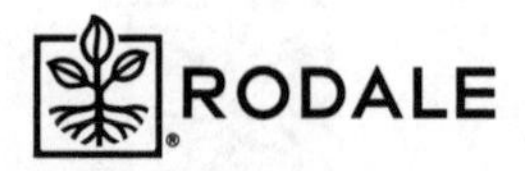

WE INSPIRE AND ENABLE PEOPLE TO IMPROVE THEIR LIVES AND THE WORLD AROUND THEM

About *Prevention* Health Books

The editors of *Prevention* Health Books are dedicated to providing you with authoritative, trustworthy, and innovative advice for a healthy, active lifestyle. In all of our books, our goal is to keep you thoroughly informed about the latest breakthroughs in natural healing, medical research, alternative health, herbs, nutrition, fitness, and weight loss. We cut through the confusion of today's conflicting health reports to deliver clear, concise, and definitive health information that you can trust. And we explain in practical terms what each new breakthrough means to you, so you can take immediate, practical steps to improve your health and well-being.

Every recommendation in *Prevention* Health Books is based upon reliable sources, including interviews with qualified health authorities. In addition, we retain top-level health practitioners who serve on the Rodale Books Board of Advisors to ensure that all of the health information is safe, practical, and up-to-date. *Prevention* Health Books are thoroughly fact-checked for accuracy, and we make every effort to verify recommendations, dosages, and cautions.

The advice in this book will help keep you well-informed about your personal choices in health care—to help you lead a happier, healthier, and longer life.

Notice

This book is intended as a reference volume only, not as a medical manual. The information given here is designed to help you make informed decisions about your health. It is not intended as a substitute for any treatment that may have been prescribed by your doctor. If you suspect that you have a medical problem, we urge you to seek competent medical help.

The Prevention *Get Thin, Get Young Plan* Staff

EDITOR: Jack Croft
CONTRIBUTING EDITOR: Matthew Hoffman
WRITERS: Selene Yeager and Bridget Doherty, with JoAnne Czarnecki, Diane Gardiner Kozak, Gale Maleskey, Karen Neely, Marie Elaina Suszynski
ART DIRECTOR: Darlene Schneck
INTERIOR DESIGNER: Lynn N. Gano
COVER DESIGNER: Christopher Rhoads
PHOTO EDITOR: James A. Gallucci
PHOTOGRAPHERS: John P. Hamel, Kurt Wilson/Rodale Images
ILLUSTRATOR: Molly Babich
ASSISTANT RESEARCH MANAGER: Sandra Salera Lloyd
PRIMARY RESEARCH EDITOR: Anita C. Small
LEAD RESEARCHER: Teresa A. Yeykal
EDITORIAL RESEARCHERS: Lori Davis, Anne Dickson, Karen Jacob, Jennifer S. Kushnier, Kathryn Piff, Joanne Policelli, Paula Rasich, Valerie Rowe, Staci Ann Sander, Terry Sutton-Kravitz, Holly Swanson, Rebecca Theodore, Barbara Thomas-Fexa, Lucille S. Uhlman
SENIOR COPY EDITORS: Karen Neely, Jane Sherman
EDITORIAL PRODUCTION MANAGER: Marilyn Hauptly
LAYOUT DESIGNER: Bethany Bodder
MANUFACTURING COORDINATORS: Brenda Miller, Jodi Schaffer, Patrick T. Smith

Rodale Healthy Living Books

Executive Editor: Tammerly Booth
Director of Series Development: Gary Krebs
Editorial Director: Michael Ward
Vice President and Marketing Director: Karen Arbegast
Product Marketing Director: Denyse Corelli
Book Manufacturing Director: Helen Clogston
Manufacturing Manager: Eileen Bauder
Research Director: Ann Gossy Yermish
Copy Manager: Lisa D. Andruscavage
Production Manager: Robert V. Anderson Jr.
Digital Processing Group Associate Manager: Thomas P. Aczel
Office Manager: Jacqueline Dornblaser
Office Staff: Susan B. Dorschutz, Julie Kehs Minnix, Tara Schrantz, Catherine E. Strouse

Contents

WEEK TWO: ON THE ROAD

WEEK THREE: TURNING BACK THE CLOCK

WEEK FOUR: A NEW YOU EACH DAY

WEEK TWELVE: MAKING IT LAST

Foreword

Most weight-loss programs are like a pair of one-size-fits-all jeans. Odds are, they won't fit you.

That's why we came up with The *Prevention* Get Thin, Get Young Plan. We don't believe that you should have to fit your life around somebody else's program. And we certainly don't believe that you have to give up the foods you love or take up some kind of exercise you hate, just because someone else tells you to.

In fact, we have this crazy notion that weight loss should be *fun*, not work. That it should be enjoyed, not endured. The only way that can happen is if the program fits around *your* life, not the other way around. And that's just what the Get Thin, Get Young Plan does. It takes you on a journey of self-discovery that will lead to a slimmer, more youthful, sexier, and more self-confident you.

Through a series of fun yet revealing quizzes, you'll figure out which activities you find most enjoyable and which best fit your personality and schedule. You'll find your own starting point, based on your personal fitness level, and discover how to keep yourself motivated after the initial thrill is gone. You'll learn which foods you can't live without and which foods you won't even miss. And you'll discover how to best show off your individual style instead of trying to conform to someone else's image of who you should be.

In just 12 weeks, taking a few simple steps at a time, you can shed unwanted pounds and turn back the clock. And the difference between the Get Thin, Get Young Plan and any other diet or exercise program you may have tried before is that our plan equips you with an exciting new lifestyle that lets you keep the weight off—forever. At the end of 12 weeks, your "diet" isn't over. Your new life has just begun.

Why am I so confident that this plan will work for you? There are three main reasons.

1. It's based on the latest scientific research. Studies have shown that everyday lifestyle activities, such as walking the stairs instead of taking the elevator at the mall, or doing gardening at home, are every bit as effective for taking weight off as traditional exercise regimens. And here's the great news: They're even *more* effective at keeping the pounds off! Throughout this book, you'll find sound, credible research supporting the program—not just some celebrity's opinion.

2. It addresses the whole person. Most diet plans focus exclusively on diet and exercise. But did you know that research has found that self-esteem is absolutely crucial for successful weight loss? Or that stress is the number one obstacle to maintaining a weight-loss program? This is the first plan that helps you boost your self-confidence and overcome stress so you can lose all the weight you want.

3. It's fun. This plan will help you learn how to play again. You'll be active for the same reasons that you were when you were a child: Because you *want* to, not because you feel that you have to.

In addition to the sound scientific foundation, we also test-drove the Get Thin, Get Young Plan with our Living Proof Panel. We had seven women and two men live the book while we wrote it to make sure that what our experts recommended really works in real life. As you'll see throughout the book, it does.

So if you're tired of fad diets and exercise gizmos that don't work, try the real thing: The *Prevention* Get Thin, Get Young Plan.

Michele Stanten
Fitness Editor, Prevention *Magazine*

A Plan That Works: Meet the Living Proof Panel

"ARE YOU SURE THIS IS GOING TO WORK?"

"I NEVER THOUGHT LOSING WEIGHT COULD BE SO EASY!"

These opposite reactions were typical of the e-mails we received within the first 2 weeks of starting nine men and women on The *Prevention* Get Thin, Get Young Plan. Half were from participants who were overjoyed that it was so easy. Half were from those who were *nervous* that it was so easy.

Where was the sweaty, exhausting exercise? Could they really lose weight on a program with no eat-cookies-and-it's-all-over dietary rules? Once the pounds started peeling away, the answer was a resounding "Yes!"

The Get Thin, Get Young Plan is based on a simple premise: Rediscover the playful, active spirit you had when you were younger, and you'll not only get younger—you'll get thinner, too. That's right, you can lower your chances for common diseases of middle age, drop clothing sizes, and feel more energized than you have in years (maybe decades) with just a few easy steps every day.

Simple Substitutions

What happens as we get older is that we gradually trade our active habits for more sedentary ones. We fall into ruts, and we put on weight, which makes us more sedentary—and that's a vicious cycle if ever there was one.

The Get Thin, Get Young Plan reverses that cycle. We ask people to start by making 30 inactive minutes in their day more active. Take a 10-minute stroll before lunch. Play Frisbee with the kids before dinner instead of watching TV. Get up and talk to a coworker face-to-face instead of sending an e-mail.

Then become a little more adventurous. Try a new activity. Build muscle with strength training. Rediscover a forgotten favorite sport. And use the same principles for your diet. Try one new recipe or food a week and break out of your food ruts.

Before you know it, you'll feel younger, look younger, and have more fun. But don't take our word for it. Take it from people just like you who tried it themselves.

Although the program's length is 12 weeks, some participants stayed on the program a few weeks longer; some stayed on a few weeks less because of conflicts in scheduling.

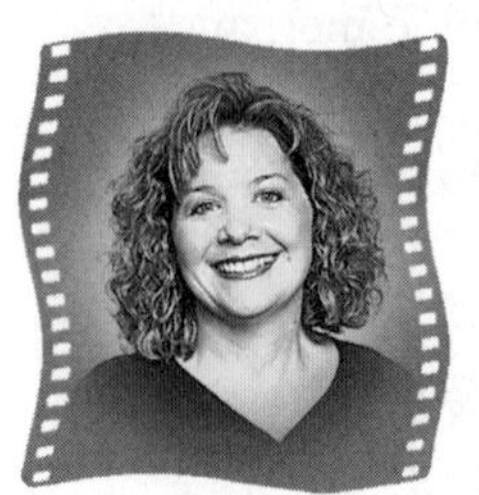

Ana Reeser, 38, bank employee

Profile: Ana is a working mom with a 4-year-old son. She struggles with low motivation and low energy levels. She often snacks at night and opts for quick meals at fast-food restaurants.

Goals: Lose 10 to 20 pounds. Increase fitness and generally feel better.

Results: Met goals—feels fabulous!

Pounds lost: 19

Body fat lost: 4 percent

Total inches lost: 15, from her arms, waist, hips, thighs, and chest

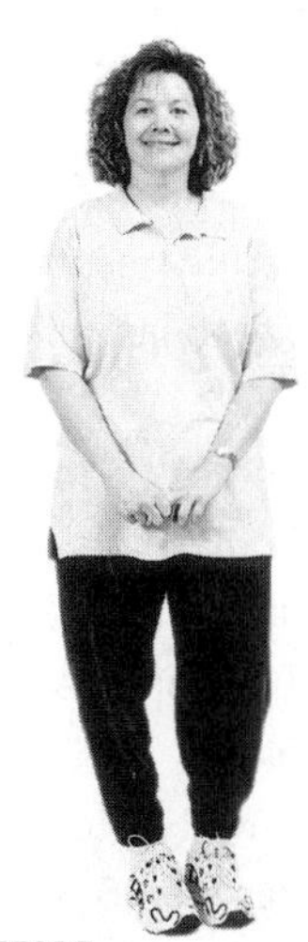
BEFORE

Ana came into the Get Thin, Get Young Plan after several failed attempts to lose the weight that she had gained from her pregnancy 4 years ago.

She had recently returned to work on a part-time basis and was enthusiastic about trying a lifestyle and weight-loss approach that could be successful for both her and her husband.

The first changes that Ana made to her lifestyle were very simple ones. She made a conscious effort to buy more fruits and vegetables during her trips to the grocery store, and she experimented with different high-fiber breakfast cereals to help satisfy her hunger during the morning hours.

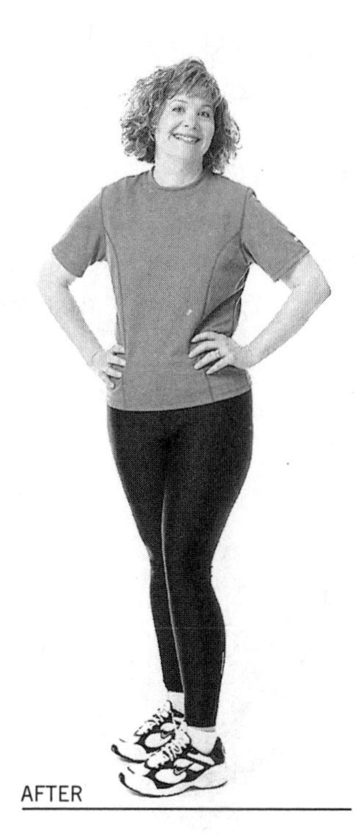
AFTER

Before work, she took a walk around her neighborhood to get her blood moving and to have some time to herself before starting her day.

Before long, the pounds started coming off, which inspired her to become even more active.

"I was so happy to finally be fitting back into my old clothes that I started walking faster and longer," she says.

There was also an unexpected bonus: Ana noticed that she and her husband, John, were saving money.

"Instead of constantly tapping the ATM machines for fast food, we ate at home more often," she says. "Not only are we saving money, but the food's a lot better!"

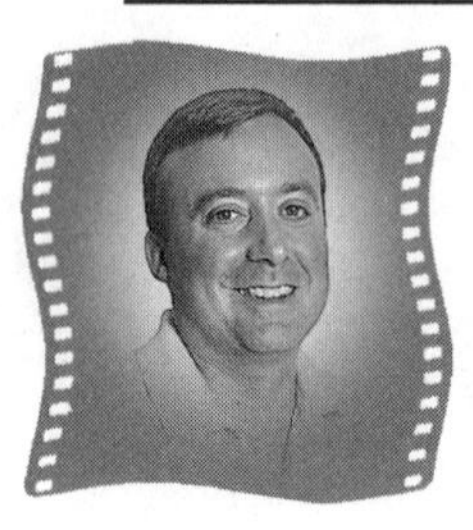

John Reeser, 38, editor and Naval Reservist

Profile: Like his wife, Ana, John struggles to balance job and family responsibilities and often lacks the motivation and energy to get active. Daily sweet cravings are his diet downfall.

Goals: Improve performance in his semiannual Naval Reserve fitness tests. Lose weight—especially from his waistline—and control his snacking habits.

Results: Big improvement
Pounds lost: 6
Body fat lost: 1 percent
Total inches lost: 6, from his hips, chest, and waist (3 inches)

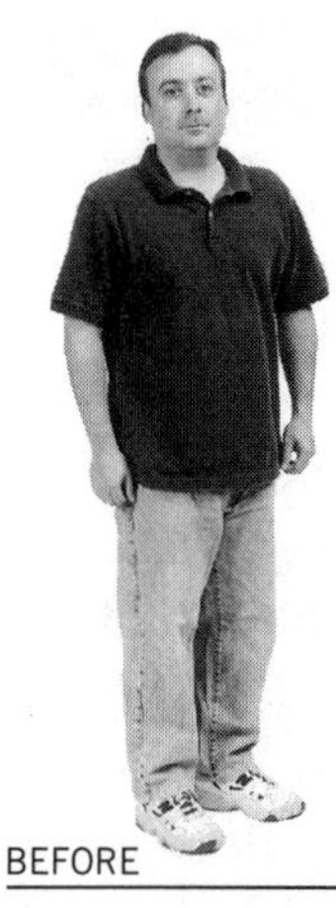

BEFORE

John joined the program realizing that he had been dissatisfied with his weight for more than 10 years and had nothing but his lifestyle to blame. "I'd been eating a lot of junk and hadn't been exercising as much as I should," he says. "But I'm not interested in making any huge changes or totally depriving myself, because I know I can't live like that on a long-term basis."

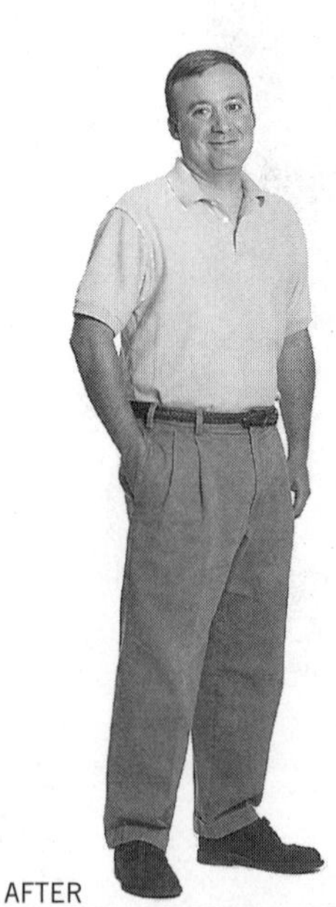

AFTER

Much to his surprise, the Get Thin, Get Young Plan was a perfect fit for him. "It's amazing how introducing just a few new foods, like high-fiber cereal and fresh fruit, into my daily diet changed my eating habits. I no longer craved sweets all the time. And when I did have a treat, I was satisfied with less."

Not an exercise zealot, John simply took a short walk in the evening after putting his son to bed and before settling in for the evening. He also parked a little farther away in the parking lot at work and took the stairs instead of the elevator. "That stuff was easy. And my pants definitely got looser soon after I started."

As John continues his progress, he hopes to lose the last few inches off his waist. Fortunately, he has a supportive exercise buddy. "Ana has been a real inspiration," he says.

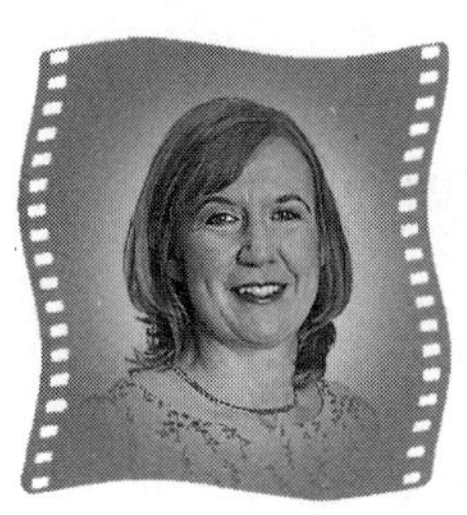

Molly Brown, 42, editorial researcher

Profile: Once very active, Molly got caught up in the rigors of raising 11- and 15-year-old daughters with her husband, while they both worked full-time. The result: 10 to 15 unwanted pounds and a lack of energy.

Goals: Lose the excess weight and firm up arms and belly.

Results: Met goals! Got the whole family active.

Pounds lost: 12½

Body fat lost: 6 percent

Total inches lost: 9¾, from her arms, waist, hips, thighs, and chest

Though she was willing to commit to making time for physical activity, Molly was not willing to sacrifice what little time she had with her husband and daughters just to lose weight. After exploring the many exercises suggested in the Get Thin, Get Young Plan, the answer dawned on her: She would find enjoyable activities that the whole family could do.

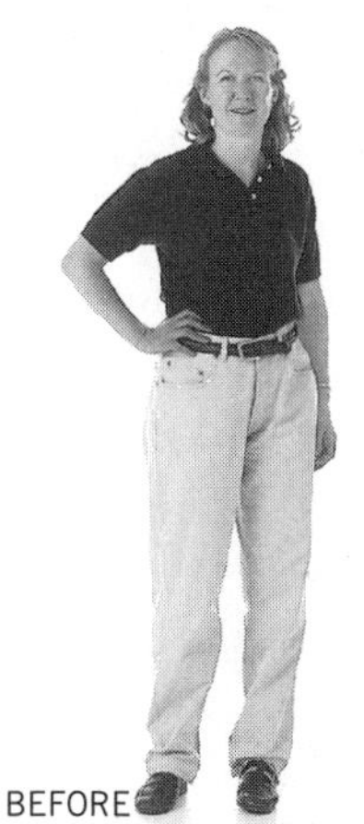

BEFORE

Molly and her younger daughter started working out with medicine balls as a fun, creative way to do strength training. They took walks and did exercise videos together. Molly even took swing dance lessons with her husband.

"The strength training has really helped me feel stronger and more energized, and I know it's so good for my daughter to build muscle and get toned, too," says Molly. "Plus, we get to have a great time together. It's so much healthier than watching television."

The best part: Though she says it's embarrassing, a few people actually have thought that the new slim and toned Molly and her older daughter were sisters. Now *that's* getting younger!

AFTER

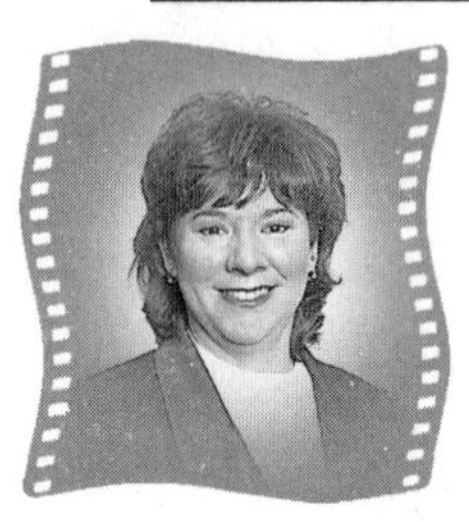

Lynn Gano, 40, designer

Profile: Lynn has battled a weight problem for much of her adult life. She fears that she's fighting "fat genes." She doesn't like the gym or traditional exercise, and she confesses to a fondness for doughnuts.

Goals: Find physical activity she can live with. Lose 10 to 15 pounds and improve mood and energy.

Results: Met goals! Feels empowered.

Pounds lost: 12

Body fat lost: 5 percent

Total inches lost: 13, from her arms, waist, hips, thighs, and chest

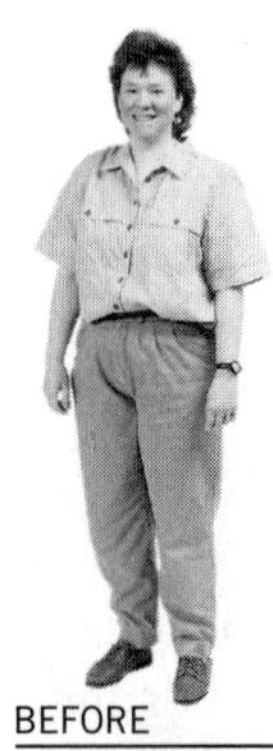
BEFORE

Like so many people today, Lynn's major barrier in her struggle with weight loss was time. As a part-time teacher and full-time designer in the high-pressure publishing business, Lynn felt constantly crunched, especially because she has an hour commute in the morning and evening.

"I often wouldn't get home till 10:00 P.M.," she says. "By then, the *last* thing I wanted to do was exercise." Making matters worse, Lynn sought high-sugar snacks like cookies and cakes for energy during the day.

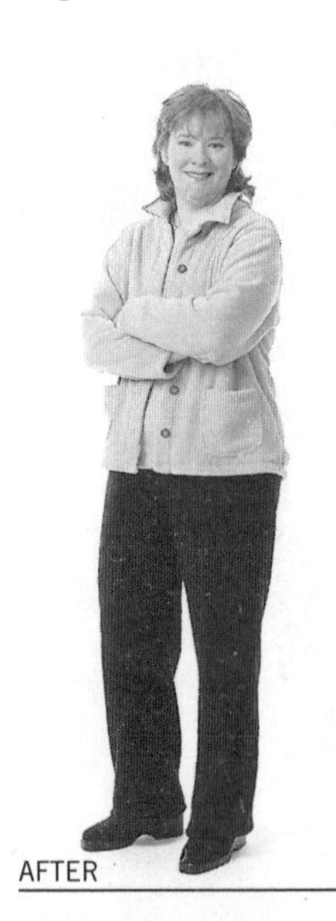
AFTER

With no time or inclination to do more, Lynn took two elements of the Get Thin, Get Young Plan and ran with them. She sneaked activity into her workday whenever she could. And she changed her high-fat snacks to high-fiber snacks. Instead of cookies, she ate fresh peaches. She parked down the street and walked farther to work. And if she felt her energy flagging during the day, she would take a 10-minute stroll.

"I am amazed how well these tiny little changes work!" says Lynn, who lost more than 7 pounds in the first month. "Plus, I feel better. I'm not tired all the time. And my back doesn't ache at the end of the day like it used to."

Lynn still indulges her sweet tooth on the weekends. And she's thrilled to have a strategy that lets her have her cake and manage her weight, too.

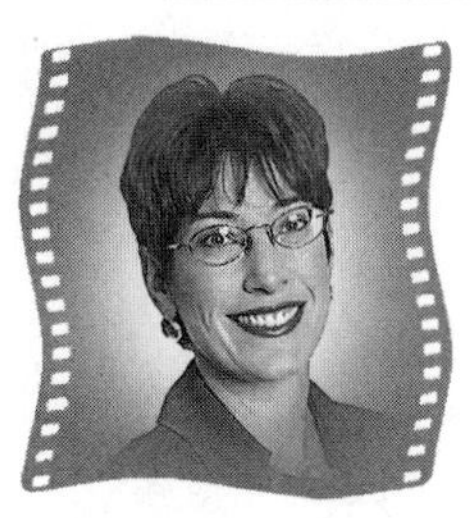

Debra Gordon, 38, writer

Profile: Deb is a working mom with three children. She has noticed creeping weight gain during the past 5 years. She suffers from frequent headaches. Time and motivation are major barriers.
Goals: Lose 10 pounds and firm up her muscles.
Results: Met goals! And no more afternoon headaches.
Pounds lost: 10
Body fat lost: 2 percent
Total inches lost: 8¼, from her arms, waist, hips, thighs, and chest

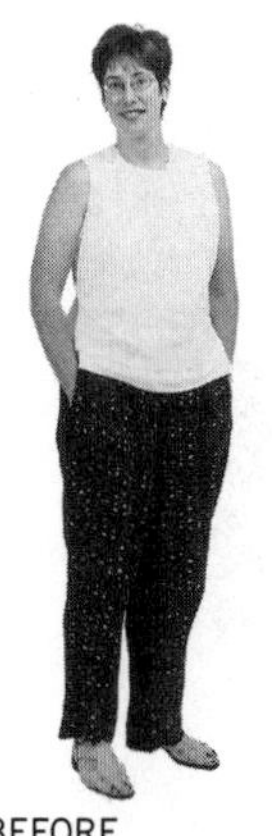

BEFORE

As a writer in the health industry, Deb knew she had to eat a healthy diet and exercise more if she wanted to shed her unwanted weight. But like so many people, she didn't know what that really meant. Did she have to cut out all sweets? Did she have to take up running? How much was enough?

Much to her relief, Deb learned that those changes were easier than she ever imagined. "All I had to do for exercise was walk and play with my kids. It was just a matter of making it happen," she says. "And the food plan made eating healthy so easy!"

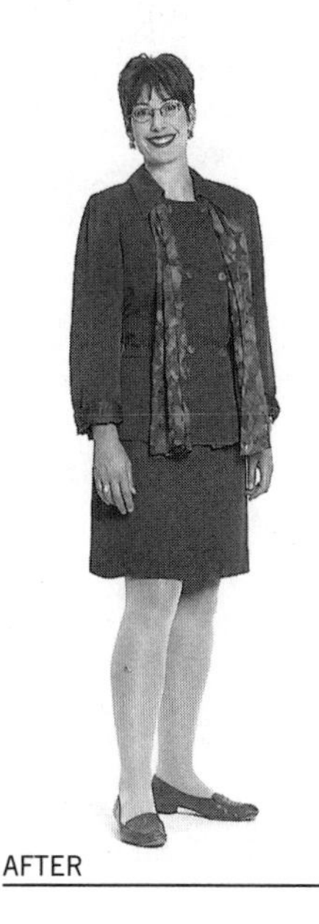

AFTER

First, she took the Get Thin, Get Young Plan recommendation to schedule daily activity in her calendar as she would any appointment. Then she applied the same principles to her eating, "scheduling" in more fruit, vegetables, and other healthful foods.

"You're so much more likely to do things when you write them down. My daily walks are in my appointment book. They're my health break," she says. Indeed. Deb dropped inches and lost her frequent headaches within a month.

"It's amazing what a big change a few small changes can make," says Deb. "You don't have to go to a gym or follow some super-restrictive diet. I really appreciate that."

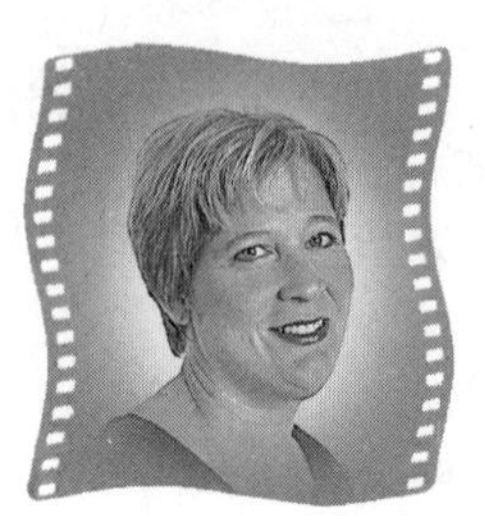

Anne Harbove, 42, full-time mother

Anne's Profile: Anne used to love going to the gym—which became an impossible luxury with four young children. Crazy schedules and finicky kids have led to a fast-food lifestyle and the pounds that inevitably follow. She is a nighttime snacker.
Goals: Ultimately lose 30-plus pounds. Tone arms and abs.
Results: Big improvement. Now managing weight *and* family.
Pounds lost: 13½
Body fat lost: 5 percent
Total inches lost: 8½, from her arms, waist, hips, thighs, and chest

Anne knew that achieving weight loss wasn't going to be easy, especially since her four children typically refused the healthy foods she tried to make at home. This time, however, Anne was armed with strategies from the Get Thin, Get Young Plan to feed her whole family right. Instead of going to Taco Bell, for instance, she learned to make her own low-fat, high-fiber wraps. She tossed the old potato chip bags and replaced them with a fruit bowl. And before she knew it, they were all on the right track.

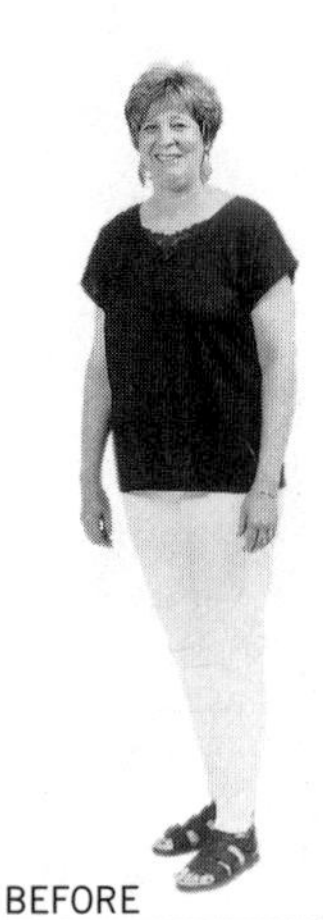
BEFORE

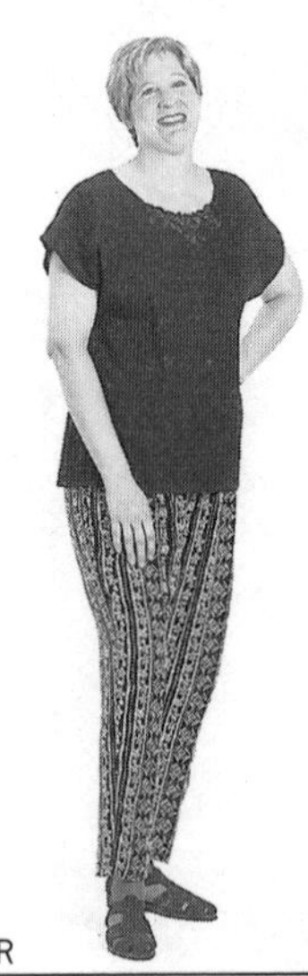
AFTER

What's more, Anne began making time for her and her husband a priority. They hired a sitter a few nights a week so they could take evening walks together through the hills around their home.

"It was more than just exercise," says Anne. "It became a time when we could talk and work through household problems without interruption." She also started weight training a couple of days a week while the kids were at school.

The changes paid off. She started losing a pound a week, while toning up and finding some much-needed time for herself.

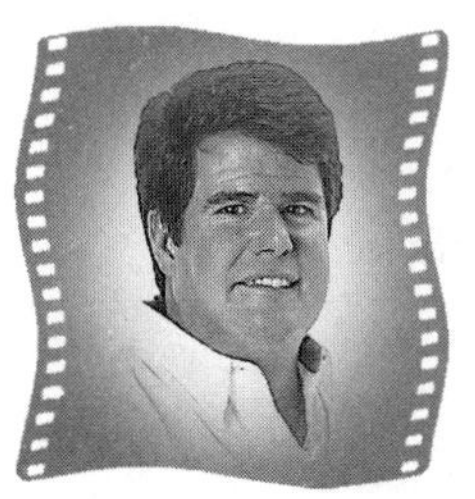

Dave Harbove, 42, sales representative

Dave's Profile: Dave's life is not conducive to living lean. His job demands hours of travel every day, and his four kids at home demand hours of attention every night. What's more, he often cleans up what his children don't eat.
Goals: Recover his waistline.
Results: Improvement. Gained muscle; lost fat.
Pounds lost: 3½
Body fat lost: 2 percent
Total inches lost: 3, from his waist and hips

With his days spent in the car, Dave knew that finding time for activity would be tough. And forget about diet. It's eat and run when you're on the road.

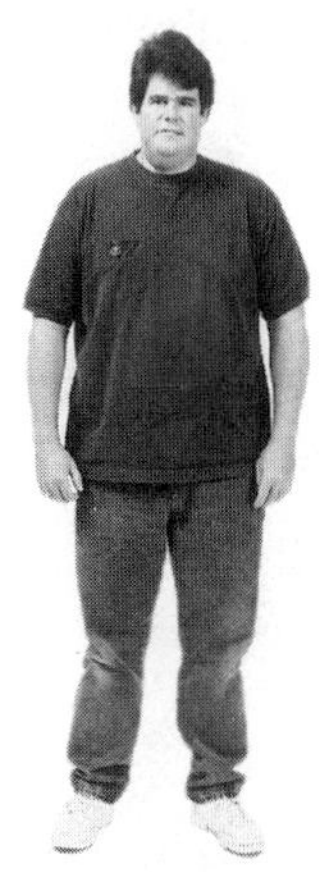

BEFORE

Though he couldn't always control where he ate during the work week, Dave learned how to make smart substitutions, even at fast-food burger joints, to cut calories and fat from his business fare. He also started walking with his wife, Anne, in the evenings as a way to unwind and energize after a long workday.

"I don't always feel like walking when I get home. But I always feel better when I do," he says.

Though Dave still has some weight to lose, he has put back the metabolism-revving lean muscle that he had lost during the past few sedentary years. His body composition analysis revealed that he had lost 6 pounds of fat while gaining 3 pounds of muscle, which left his waistline trimmer and his muscles firmer. He also decided to give his old tennis coach a call to start playing again, a move that's sure to have him feeling thinner—and younger—with every match.

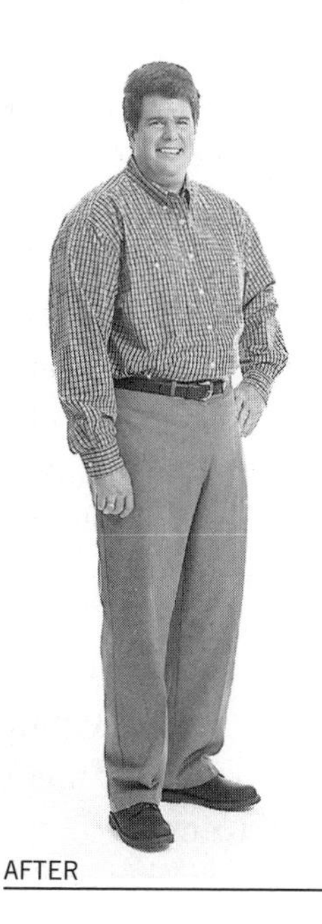

AFTER

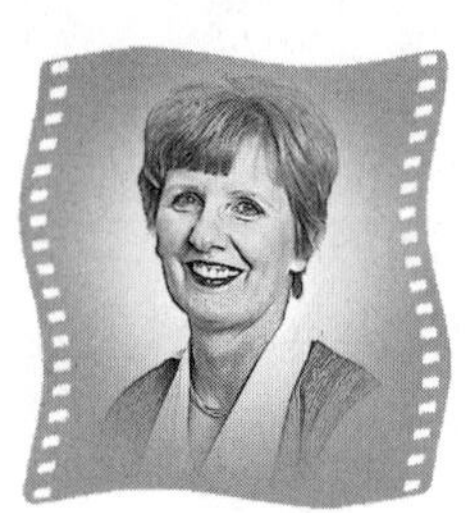

Mary Lou Stephen, 62, business support assistant

Profile: Mary Lou is a regular exerciser who loves chocolate. Recently, she has been gaining weight despite all her activity. She believes that if she could manage her eating habits, she could get back to a comfortable weight.
Goals: Lose about 10 pounds. Get comfortable in her clothes again.
Results: Met goals!
Pounds lost: 9
Body fat lost: 1 percent
Total inches lost: 7¼, from her arms, waist, hips, and thighs

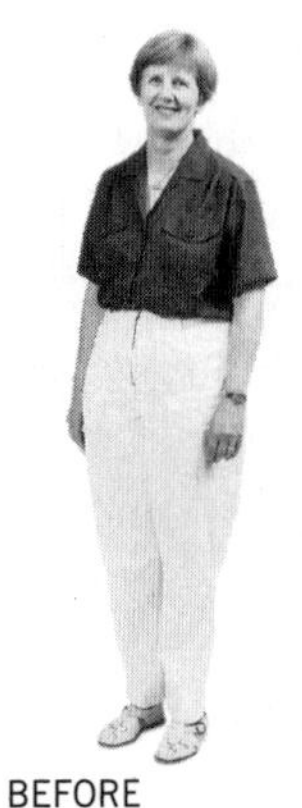
BEFORE

As a longtime avid exerciser, Mary Lou was frustrated by her recently widening waistline. Initially, she blamed it on age. But then she admitted that she probably ate more cookies and candy than she realized—especially when babysitting for her grandsons.

Like so many of us, Mary Lou thought she ate pretty well but really wasn't aware of how much her high-calorie snacking was adding up. Once Mary Lou started jotting down what she was eating and when, she began to lose weight almost immediately.

"I realized that what I remembered as a 'couple' of Oreos with my grandsons was actually six or seven!" Mary Lou says with a laugh. "By writing it down, I was more aware of what I was eating, so I'd eat only two cookies instead."

As a bonus, she started making more healthful choices on an everyday basis as well. But she freely admits that she didn't go overboard. "At my age, I'm not willing to make any huge changes!" she says. "But this program was perfect. I learned how to make simple substitutions in my diet and pay closer attention to my snacking. And I lost weight."

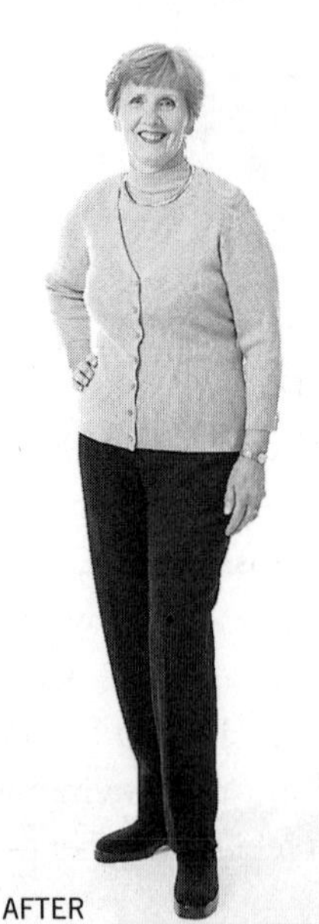
AFTER

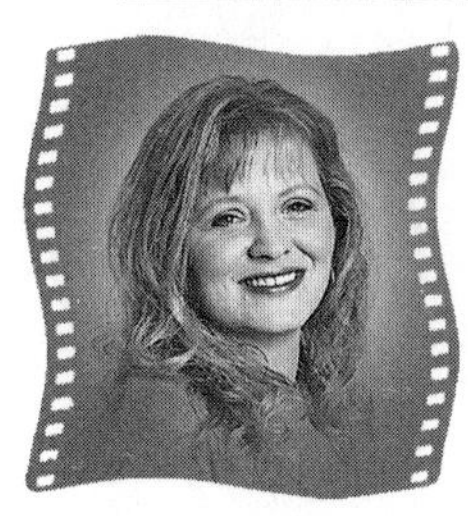

Pat Mast, 35, designer

Profile: Pat is a working mom with two sons. Though she didn't have much weight to lose, she couldn't seem to get herself moving in the right direction. She has been under considerable stress during the past year.

Goals: Lose excess weight and firm up.

Results: Big improvement!

Pounds lost: 4

Body fat lost: 0 percent

Total inches lost: 2¾, from her waist, hips, thighs, and chest

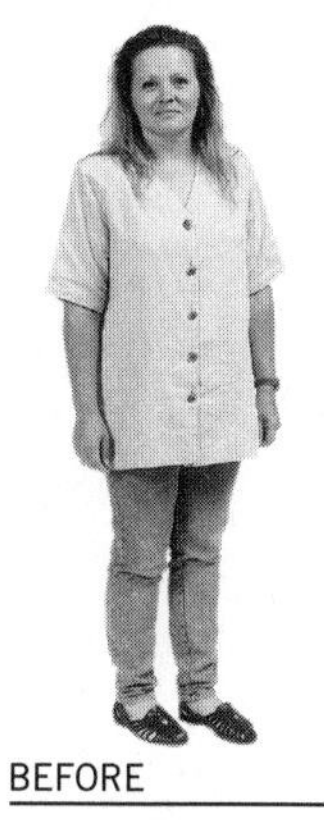

BEFORE

Pat has been an avid walker for 6 to 7 years, off and on. It used to be that she ate her regular diet, went about her day, and her weight stayed okay. Over the years, that started to change, and her weight changed, too. Unfortunately, as for many petite women, those pounds showed up quickly on her 5-foot frame.

Making matters worse, Pat's diet had fallen into a rut, and stress at work and at home was leaving her feeling run-down. Through the Get Thin, Get Young Plan, Pat learned strategies to jump-start her motivation and start managing her stress. Armed with her favorite music, Pat started taking more consistent power walks. "I'd strap on my headphones and start moving, and before I knew it, I'd forget about my stress," she says. For an added boost, she also began working in more frequent bouts of walking with a friend on a nearby nature trail on her lunch hour and during work breaks.

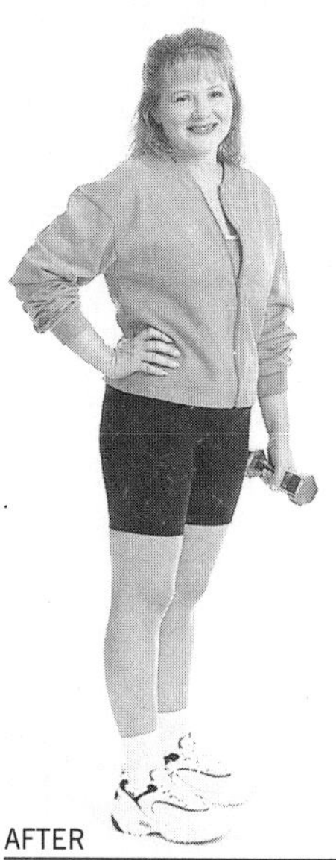

AFTER

"I felt so energized when I was finished," she says. And that energy spilled into her eating habits. "I started reading labels, trying new things, and making healthier choices."

Though she would still like to drop a few pounds, Pat feels confident with her newfound lifestyle strategies. "Now I know what I need to get moving and stay motivated."

Getting Ready

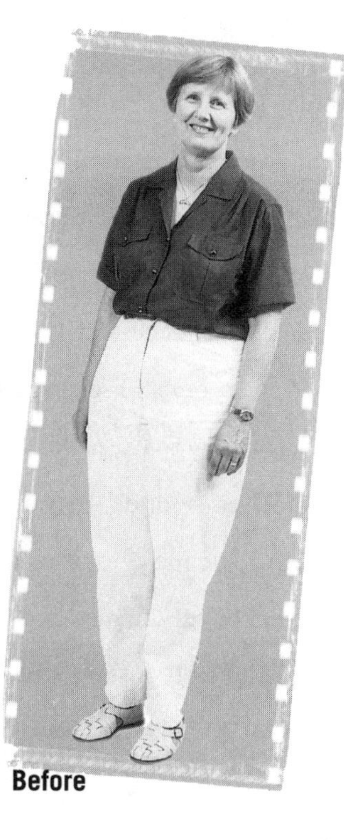
Before

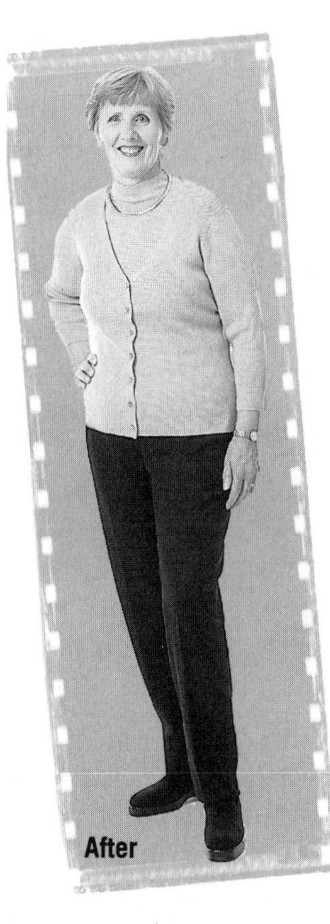
After

JUST YESTERDAY, I HAD HALF A CHOCOLATE BROWNIE, WHEREAS IN THE PAST I WOULD HAVE HAD THREE. BECAUSE OF THE FOOD DIARY, EVEN IF I DO EAT IT, I DON'T EAT THE QUANTITY I USED TO.

—Mary Lou Stephen

Getting Ready

You want to lose weight—but are you truly ready to begin? Having the desire to slim down is not enough. Without a clear action plan and commitment from you, chances are that your weight-loss efforts will fail. By following the sound advice and helpful tips in this first section, you can prepare yourself for a successful 12-week journey to weight loss.

You'll learn the secrets to setting attainable goals that will keep you motivated—and learn how to use a weight-loss diary, a tool scientifically proven to help people shed pounds. If you think all exercise is boring, the two quizzes can help you choose calorie-burning activities that you'll enjoy—and stick with—over the long haul. Plus, you'll happily discover how you can eat for pleasure and feel satisfied while you're losing weight.

The Road to a New You

FOR MANY AMERICANS, TRYING TO LOSE WEIGHT IS
A NATIONAL PASTIME. HOW'S THAT? WELL . . .

- A GALLUP POLL REPORTED THAT 52 PERCENT OF AMERICANS CURRENTLY ARE DIETING OR HAVE DIETED IN THE PAST.
- ONE OUT OF SIX AMERICANS DIET EACH YEAR.
- A SURVEY OF 629 WOMEN IN A WEIGHT-LOSS REGISTRY FOUND THAT 93 PERCENT OF THEM HAD UNSUCCESSFULLY TRIED TO LOSE WEIGHT IN THE PAST.

So chances are that you've been down this road before, too. This probably isn't the first time—it might even be the 20th time. The goal is to make it the *last* time.

How do you do that? With forethought. People often head out on the road to weight loss without first taking the time to figure out if they are ready and how they will reach their destination.

The real road to a new you starts before you take even a single step. First, take some time to prepare yourself for the journey so that the bad habits you break and the good habits you make last for a lifetime.

Weight loss—even if it involves fun and simple lifestyle changes—still requires time, dedication, and effort. You have to be ready to make these changes and to give yourself the support you need to succeed.

"In many cases, people are not geared up. And if you are really not ready to go through this, you're not going to be successful," says Ross Andersen, Ph.D., assistant professor of medicine at Johns Hopkins University School of Medicine in Baltimore and one of the nation's leading researchers on lifestyle activity and weight loss.

But how do you determine if you are ready? Try the following:

Weigh the pros and cons. Dr. Andersen asks his clients to write down the benefits and drawbacks of trying to lose weight. For example:

PROS	CONS
Will have a sleeker, healthier body.	Need to get up earlier in the morning to exercise.
Will have more energy, feel better about self.	Can't go out with the gang every Friday after work to get nachos and margaritas

"Ask yourself: 'What are the benefits of losing weight right now?' Then compare them to the sacrifices you'll have to make," Dr. Andersen says.

Most times, you'll see that the pros heavily outweigh the cons. And that means you're ready to go. But if it seems to you that the drawbacks outweigh the benefits, it may mean that this isn't a good time for you to start, he adds.

Write out your fears. What are you afraid of if you try to lose weight? Are you afraid that you won't succeed? Or that you won't be able to eat the foods you like? Put these worries on paper.

"When you start to write those things down, they don't have as much power as they did when you kept them secret. It gives you power when you put it down on paper," says Gary Ewing, M.D., director of preventive medicine at the University of South Carolina School of Medicine in Columbia. Not only will they seem less daunting, but they may even appear unfounded in black and white.

Realize that this is a lifetime plan. To be truly ready, you must come to terms with the fact that this isn't a short-term "diet." The changes you are about to make will last for the rest of your life. How do you know when you're ready for this? When you can accept that this isn't a health kick or fad, says William Smucker, M.D., designer of the Reasonable Eating and Activity to Change for Health program at Summa Health System in Akron, Ohio.

"You have to accept that this is what you eat. This is who you are. This is the way you always intend to do it. The good thing is that the longer one does it, the more likely it is to become a habit," he says.

Sign a contract. Draw up a contract that states that you are committed to giving yourself the time, resources, and energy you need to lose weight, Dr. Ewing says. Sign it, even have someone witness it, and keep it where you'll see it. That way, you'll know that you mean business. If you're willing to sign on the dotted line, you're ready.

"By signing a contract, you say to yourself: 'This is important to me, and I have every intention of following through with this,'" he adds.

Preparing for the Journey

Legendary college basketball coach Bobby Knight once said, "The will to succeed is important, but what is more important is the will to prepare." Wise words for losing weight as well. It's wonderful that you want to do it, but that desire is not enough.

After you have decided you're ready, the next step is to prepare for your journey. Just as with those long family vacations, the more you pack, plan, and anticipate those trouble spots during the long trip, the more enjoyable your travels will be.

Here's how to plot your course.

Set a start date. How many times have you decided to start a weight-loss program on Monday morning?

By Tuesday afternoon, you realize that you're not ready for this. By Wednesday night, you're off it. And by Saturday, you're saying, "I'll start again Monday." Give yourself some time to prepare. Set a start date, perhaps a week or two down the road, or maybe choose a milestone date, such as a birthday or anniversary, Dr. Ewing says. Then use the time before the start date to get ready.

But take note: Putting your start date off a few days or weeks doesn't mean that you have to eat everything in sight. "A lot of people have what we call the Last Hurrah Suppers," Dr. Andersen says. "That just sends you farther back."

Write out your goals. This road to a new you needs a clearly defined route. A road map, if you will. So write out clear-cut, attainable goals. (For more information, see Setting—And Achieving—Realistic Goals on page 21.) That way, you're saying not only that you want to lose weight but also how you intend to do so. To stay motivated, carry your goals in your wallet or post them in your kitchen or office, Dr. Smucker says.

Watch—and write down—what you eat. A week or two before your start

Living Proof
PANEL

Writing Away Her Chocolate Cravings

Mary Lou Stephen

Before I started writing in my food diary, I didn't think much about what I was eating—or how much. For instance, I am a big chocolate eater—and I know it. I'd start out with a chocolate instant breakfast and later have chocolate candy, ice cream, cake—anything. I could eat chocolate more than once a day.

Although I knew this, it took on a new meaning when I had to write it down.

In black and white, it is a *lot* different. Seeing in print just how much chocolate I've eaten makes me think twice before putting a morsel in my mouth. In fact, just yesterday I had half a chocolate brownie, whereas in the past I would have had three. Because of the food diary, even if I do eat it, I don't eat the quantity I used to.

Not only has the diary curtailed my chocolate cravings, it also has helped me to increase other good habits, such as drinking enough water. Before the diary, maybe I'd drink one glass of water a day. But having to check off my daily water goals reminds me to fill up my glass. Now I am up to three glasses a day—triple what I was doing before.

date, begin keeping a food diary. (To learn how, see Dear Diary: The Key to Self-Evaluation on page 27.) That will help you see what you need to work on before you actually start, Dr. Ewing says. It will help you anticipate potential roadblocks and cut down the odds that you'll go off course in the beginning weeks.

Plan, plan, plan. It may be a week or so before your start date, but now is the time to buy new walking shoes, collect healthy recipes that interest you, throw out the potato chips, stock up on fruits and vegetables, and clear your schedule.

"Look at all the things you have to change and start to plan out what you have to do," Dr. Smucker says.

If you wait until you start, you'll find yourself staring at an empty refrigerator on your first night wondering how you are going to make a healthy meal out of chocolate pudding, leftover pizza, and diet soda. Or you'll be inspired to take a walk but won't be able to because your sneakers barely have soles.

Learn from the Past

In 1991, Canadian explorer, adventurer, and inspirational speaker Jamie Clarke was a member of an expedition to climb Mount Everest. He and his team failed 3,000 feet from the top. Two and a half years later, he tried to scale the highest point on the planet again. When a member of his party became ill, they had to abandon the effort just two city blocks from the summit.

The two failed attempts failed to discourage him, though. On his third try, in 1997, Clarke made it to the summit. And he credits his past *failures* for his ultimate success. Clarke studied his previous two attempts and from each one learned how he would do it differently the next time up.

"You have failures, and those failures are the essence, the building blocks of future success. They are integral. Without them, you cannot have the victory. Because you learn so much from them," he says.

Losing weight can seem as daunting as climbing Everest. But like Clarke, you can use past attempts to fuel your success this time out.

Instead of chalking up previous efforts as part of a long history of unexplainable failures, study, analyze, and learn from them, Dr. Andersen suggests. "What are you going to do differently? Look at and reflect on what led to the collapse of previous attempts," he says.

Setbacks: The Key to Success

Know this scenario? You go on a diet, and you're doing just fine until you find yourself at an office party. Next thing you know, you've swallowed the caloric equivalent of what you'd normally eat in a couple of days. Feeling blue about it, you go home and sulk on the couch, eating a bag of potato chips instead of taking your usual walk. Now that you've really blown it, why bother? You give up entirely, chalking up another failed attempt at losing weight and deciding that it's useless. Then you reach for the ice cream.

The biggest mistake people make while trying to lose weight is that they don't accept their mistakes. Once they eat one morsel too many or skip one workout, they chuck the whole thing, discarding past successes and throwing aside future victories.

Setbacks aren't the end of a weight-loss effort, they are part of the process, Dr. Ewing says. When you accept this fact of life, you'll continue heading in the right direction even when you take a slight detour. The key is to make setbacks a learning tool, a mechanism that will actually increase your chances of success.

"What are you going to do when faced with these setbacks? Should you go ahead and feel guilty about them, which will cause you distress, and then you'll give up? Or are you going to accept that you will have these lapses and try to learn from each one?" Dr. Ewing says.

Consider each lapse a learning opportunity. Study it. Talk about it. Figure out what went wrong and how to avoid letting it happen again.

"Know that you will relapse. But take comfort in knowing that, and that you'll work on your reaction to these lapses. If you know this going in, it won't be so alarming when it happens. It will just be part of the process," Dr. Ewing says.

Setting—And Achieving—Realistic Goals

SCENE: THE OFFICE OF WEIGHT-LOSS EXPERT DR. ROSS ANDERSEN OF JOHNS HOPKINS UNIVERSITY SCHOOL OF MEDICINE. HE IS COUNSELING A 40-YEAR-OLD WOMAN WHO WANTS TO LOSE WEIGHT.

The conversation between Dr. Andersen and the woman goes something like this:

DR. ANDERSEN: How many pounds do you have to lose?

WOMAN: I'd love to be 112 pounds.

DR. ANDERSEN: When was the last time you weighed 112 pounds?

WOMAN: My freshman year in college.

DR. ANDERSEN: And how long did you maintain that weight?

WOMAN: I dieted down to that weight after trying to get ready for a school dance. I was there for a week, and I had a real tough time.

Dr. Andersen has had dozens of conversations like this over the years.

Let's face it, many of us dream of getting back to a weight or clothing size that we associate with a special time in our lives. It's human nature to want to aim high. "After all," the thinking goes, "I was there once, so I can get there again."

What's wrong with this reach-for-the-stars attitude? It undercuts your efforts before you even start, says Dr. Andersen.

After repeatedly setting—and missing—these pie-in-the-sky goals, you may give up on weight loss altogether. "When you fail at too many goals, then you give up setting goals," says Dana G. Cable, Ph.D., professor of psychology at Hood College in Frederick, Maryland.

The key is to set realistic weight-loss goals, ones that provide inspiration and a road map to success. With an attainable goal constantly on your horizon, you're always motivated to better yourself. "Goals give us something that is a little out of reach, where we have to commit ourselves," Dr. Cable says.

Goal setting also is a key to staying young, Dr. Cable says. When you know that new benchmarks and successes await you in the future, you'll continue to strive, learn new things, accomplish new goals, and see yourself with a lot more to do in life—no matter how old you are.

Realistic goal setting takes the dreaded failure cycle and turns it completely on its ear. You set short-term, within-reach goals. You achieve those goals, and you feel good about yourself, so you set new goals. Next thing you know, you're tackling goal after goal. And losing pound after pound.

The Gold Standard of Goals

Anyone can dream up an arbitrary goal, but good goals require thought, planning, and creativity. Properly set goals map out the road to get there as well as the final destination.

"A goal without a plan is likely to fail," says Raymond C. Baker, Ph.D., a clinical psychologist and director of the Center for Wellness and Counseling at Bradley University in Peoria, Illinois. So when establishing your weight-loss goals, they should contain the following vital characteristics.

They are specific, yet flexible. A goal of "I will exercise this week" is too nebulous. It doesn't give you parameters of how or when you will accomplish it, Dr. Baker says. Instead, be as specific as possible so that you give yourself a plan as well. For example, a good goal would be: "I will walk for 30 minutes, 5 days this week during my lunch hour or right after work."

Just be sure to allow yourself some flexibility. If you could walk only 20 minutes or you had to skip a day, don't feel that you have failed, Dr. Baker adds. Just because you don't always meet your exact goal doesn't mean that you should abandon the effort.

They are reasonable and attainable. If you haven't been exercising lately,

Living Proof
PANEL

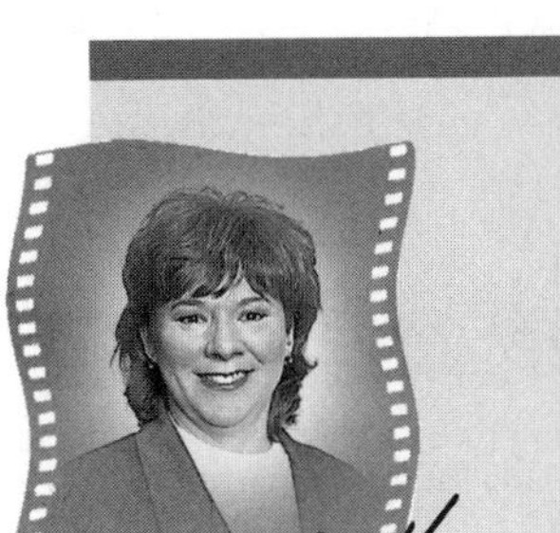

One Goal at a Time

When I set my goal at the beginning of the program, I didn't think about weight. My goal was to go down one dress size. That's it.

I also had to keep telling myself that it took me years to put this weight on and that I'd have to accept the fact that it was going to be a slow process to take it off. I think that's why weight loss hadn't worked for me in the past. I'd starve myself and work out like crazy, but then get upset that the weight wasn't coming off fast enough. So I'd get frustrated and stop.

By setting such a reasonable and simple goal, I made it! Because of that, I feel great and want to continue. My next goal is focused more on my exercise. I want to go 10 minutes longer during my walk each day. What is another 10 minutes? By doing that, I'd like to see how much more weight and how many inches I can shed.

a goal of walking 10 miles a day every day of the week is not realistic. If you can't picture yourself doing it, chances are that you can't do it, Dr. Baker says. That's not to say that you can't work up to it, but to go for it right off the bat will doom you to failure. Set goals such as "I'll walk a mile 4 days this week." Once you've mastered this goal, then step it up a notch.

They are measurable. Here's a commonly heard goal: "I'll eat healthier." But just how do you know if you have met that goal? You must be able to evaluate and quantify your success. Set goals that you can count or mark off as you accomplish them, such as getting 30 grams of fiber every day, eating nine servings of fruits and vegetables, walking for 30 minutes, or trying one new food every week, says Dr. Baker.

They can be tracked for progress. By recording your development, you'll see how you are improving and changing. That in itself provides positive feedback and reinforcement, giving you the encouragement you need to keep going, Dr. Baker says. Writing down your progress also allows you to see when you've accomplished one goal and when it is time to reevaluate and move on to others.

Playing the Numbers Game

When measuring your weight-loss goals, the scale should not be your only guide. Use other criteria for success, such as how your clothing fits, how you feel, and what your fitness level is. The scale places too much emphasis on a number, experts say.

A slow, steady weight loss is healthier and easier to keep off.

While that all certainly is sound advice, the reality is that most of us who are trying to lose weight consider the scale to be the ultimate measure. Based on this fact of life, chances are that you have—or want to set—a goal weight. So if you are going to do it, do it right.

When picking a goal weight, people tend to make one of two mistakes. Either they pick a weight they have to torture themselves to get to, or they have a lot of weight to lose, so they pick a daunting, long-term weight-loss goal—such as 50 pounds or more.

In the first case, Dr. Andersen says, even those who make it to their target weight find that they can't stay there. "It's one thing to diet down to a certain weight. Some people, however, can't keep it there, but they still think that is their ideal weight," he says. In the second case, setting a goal that seems so far away can overwhelm people before they even begin. "That's part of a big problem. They say, 'I have so much to lose—I don't know how to get started.'"

That's why Dr. Andersen has developed a strategy for choosing a weight-loss goal. It takes into account both common mistakes. It allows you to lose a reasonable amount of weight that you'll be able to maintain. Also, it breaks a major weight-loss goal down into smaller pieces, making it seem much less daunting. Here's how to choose a weight-loss goal that you can reach—and maintain.

Go to the 5 and 10. Reaching a weight-loss goal of 5 to 10 percent of your total weight is considered a huge success. Even if you want to lose much more, start with this goal, Dr. Andersen says. With this percentage, you'll see health and appearance differences, but it isn't so drastic a goal that it is unattainable or unmanageable. So if you are 160 pounds, your initial goal will be between 8 and 16 pounds.

Strive for 1 to 2 pounds a week on average. A slow, steady weight loss is not only healthier but also easier to keep off, Dr. Andersen says. Rapid weight loss, on the other hand, is usually done through drastic measures, so once you go back to your old habits, the weight returns as quickly as you lost it.

Make the lifestyle changes recommended in this book, and you should shed 1 to 2 pounds a week. Just keep this in mind, he advises: Think about it on average over the course of time, instead of worrying about how many pounds you lost in one particular week. One week, you may only lose 1 pound, but the next week, you could lose 3.

Keep it off for a while. Once you reach your 5 to 10 percent goal, your next goal should be maintaining your new weight, Dr. Andersen says. For many, keeping the weight off is the real challenge. By spending a few weeks or months simply staying at your new weight, you give your body and yourself a breather from the mental and physical rigors of trying to lose weight.

This maintenance period also allows you to make sure that lifestyle changes become just that—permanent changes that you'll carry with you for the rest of your life, not just changes you made for short-term weight loss.

Reevaluate your goal. As you stay in your maintenance phase, think about your next goal. After achieving your initial weight loss, your ideas about how much weight you want to lose and can lose may change. Also, think about what is going on in your life. If it is a hectic time, maintaining your weight for a longer period of time may be more realistic than trying to lose more, Dr. Andersen says.

Strive for another 5 to 10 percent. If you decide to lose more weight, stick to another 5 to 10 percent, Dr. Andersen says. Breaking it down into 5 to 10 percent chunks is more effective than trying to lose a large amount in one shot. "Most people who have significant weight loss do it in chunks. They slice it up a bit."

Making Change

You don't lose 20 pounds just because you want to. "You must exhibit certain attitudes, beliefs, and behaviors that will lead to weight loss," Dr. Baker says.

To do that, you have to set what Dr. Baker calls process goals. These are things you do that lead to weight loss. "You want goals on how to reduce the fat in your diet, increase the amount of fruits and vegetables. These aren't even weight related. But if you accomplish them, the weight will come off."

Homing in on behavioral goals will help you keep the weight off. And the best way to do that is to focus on specific lifestyle changes. "Try not to make weight loss the goal. Make the behavioral changes the goal. I tell my clients that the weight loss is a fringe benefit," says Lisa Tartamella, R.D., a nutrition specialist at Yale–New Haven Hospital in Connecticut.

Process goals differ from one person to the next—it depends on what you need to work on. To get a good idea of what your behavioral goals should be, keep and study a weight-loss diary, Dr. Baker says. But here are some ideas of process goals that you could set.

■ Walk for 30 minutes, five times a week.

■ Read a book instead of eating when bored.

■ Use your food diary every day this week.

■ Bring fruit to work for a snack.

■ Try one new fruit, vegetable, or grain each week.

■ Schedule 15 minutes each day to just sit and relax.

■ Try a new sport or activity once every 2 weeks.

■ If you did not meet your goals today, start fresh again tomorrow instead of calling it quits.

Dear Diary: The Key to Self-Evaluation

YOU PROBABLY ALREADY KNOW ABOUT THE TWO CORNERSTONES OF WEIGHT LOSS: EATING RIGHT AND EXERCISING. BUT NOW YOU NEED TO ADD A THIRD COMPONENT THAT IS SCIENTIFICALLY PROVEN TO TAKE OFF THE POUNDS: WRITING.

When I get a new person in my program, I show them the data on weight-loss diaries, and I just tell them right up front, 'You need to be willing to do this.' Every good weight-control program stresses the importance of self-monitoring. It causes the changes that lead to weight loss and control," says Dr. Raymond C. Baker of the Center for Wellness and Counseling at Bradley University.

Study after study has shown that keeping track of eating and exercise is the key to losing weight and keeping it off. Here are some of the highlights.

- A group that kept detailed food diaries during a 10-week study lost 64 percent more weight than a group that didn't.
- Out of 10 ways to alter eating habits, self-monitoring was the only one that allowed people to keep the weight off for up to 1½ years, one study found.
- In another study group, 89 percent of the people who maintained their weight loss relied on record keeping.

The Secret to Holiday Weight-Loss Success

For even the strongest-willed person, the holidays can prove to be an unforgiving weight-loss nemesis. Surrounded by good food, good drink, good fun, and not much time to exercise, many throw their hands up in defeat and concede that they'll pack on 5 to 10 pounds between Thanksgiving and New Year's Day. If only there was some secret to ward off those unwanted pounds.

Well, now there is. And it's something you should already be doing: Stick with your weight-loss journal.

Dr. Raymond C. Baker of the Center for Wellness and Counseling at Bradley University asked people in a weight-loss program to keep diaries during the holidays.

Those who stayed on track and kept extremely diligent food and activity journals actually lost weight between Thanksgiving and New Year's Day.

"It keeps people focused on their goals and improves their decision making," Dr. Baker says.

■ Two studies have shown that people who self-monitored consistently lost more weight than those who only kept track less than half the time. Only those who self-monitored consistently lost a significant amount of weight.

The reason for this phenomenal success is that people often are unaware of their own behaviors. They get so wrapped up in their day-to-day lives that they don't notice the little things or habits they develop that hamper weight-loss efforts. Because they never identify these problems, they never get the opportunity to fix them.

A weight-loss diary acts as a mirror. Through it, you get a true picture of yourself, your eating patterns, and your exercise routines. You clearly see what you do right, what you need to modify, what works, and what doesn't, Dr. Baker says. It awakens people to their own habits and behaviors and gives them the power to make positive changes.

"It puts you in charge. It gives you the information you need to figure out what works for you. Through self-monitoring, you hit upon a successful eating and exercise plan," Dr. Baker says.

More Than Just Record Keeping

Your weight-loss journal can be more than just the nuts and bolts of your eating and exercise routine. If you want, it can be a source of inspiration, comfort, and relief. Writing may help you unleash what's on your mind, enabling you to lose weight as well as what might be weighing you down. By doing so, it can help you feel younger both physically and mentally, says Howard J. Rankin, Ph.D., psychological advisor to the TOPS (Take Off Pounds Sensibly) Club and author of *Seven Steps to Wellness*. Here are just a few of the other benefits of keeping a weight-loss journal.

Increases accuracy. There's an old Chinese proverb that says, "The palest ink is better than the best memory." With all you have to remember during the day, it's easy to forget the cookies you ate at 3:00 P.M. or the fact that you didn't take your daily walk.

And it's those little things you forget that add up and often make the most difference in your weight-loss efforts. Writing it down guarantees an accurate record, says Dr. Rankin.

Provides clarity and resolution. Some of you may decide that you want your diary to be a daily journal as well. Writing out stressful events or problems often allows you to work through them.

"Writing is thinking. When you start to write something down, you are really crystallizing thoughts and feelings," Dr. Rankin says.

Reminds you of your goals. Not only should your daily diary chronicle what you have done, it should also contain what you want to do. Write down daily, weekly, and long-term goals, says John P. Foreyt, Ph.D., director of the Behavioral Medicine Research Center at Baylor College of Medicine in Houston and coauthor of *Living without Dieting*. Each time you open it, you'll be reminded of what you are striving for.

Motivates you. Your diary will map out your progress. You'll see how far you've come in changing your eating habits, how you've increased your exercise, and how you've met certain goals. It's tangible evidence of your success that you can revisit for inspiration.

"It can be self-rewarding and reinforce what you are doing," Dr. Foreyt explains.

The Write Stuff

There are all kinds of ways to keep a weight-loss diary: Write it down in a notebook, buy a published food and activity log, jot down notes on paper and then transcribe them into a computer file. It doesn't matter how you do it, as long as it works for you, Dr. Baker says.

However you choose to do it, here are some guidelines to ensure that your journal contributes to your weight-loss success.

Make it your constant companion. When Dr. Baker sees food and coffee stains all over someone's diary, he knows that person is doing it right.

"I want that diary to be out there in the battlefield. I don't want a nice, clean diary," he says.

Your journal should be compact enough that you can carry it with you at all times. Look for a notebook or journal that will easily fit in your handbag or jacket pocket. If it isn't with you, you're more likely to forget important details or not maintain the diary at all.

Write it down immediately. Whip out your diary after each meal and after exercising. Why? Because recording your actions immediately helps you plan for the rest of the day, Dr. Baker says.

For instance, say you've had a high-fat meal for lunch. By writing it down soon after, you note that you'll have to plan a healthier dinner to offset your lunch. "It allows people to problem-solve and make changes that will help their behaviors," Dr. Baker says.

Remember the little things. That pat of butter on your bread, the nibbling you do while making dinner, the three or four cookies you grabbed during your coffee break—these little things add up to pounds over time, Dr. Baker says. And it's these little things that are sometimes the most important to record.

A study at a clinical nutrition center in Cambridge, England, found that people who didn't accurately record their daily intakes of food in their food diaries were overlooking snacks eaten between meals. To get a true picture of your eating habits, you must write everything down, Dr. Baker says.

Be honest. "What I most keenly wish is not to forget that I am writing for myself alone. Thus I shall always tell the truth, I hope, and thus I shall improve myself," said French artist Eugène Delacroix in the opening page of his diary back in 1822. Take the painter's words to heart. This diary is for your eyes only, so don't feel that you have to fudge or hide something you

Keeping Track

Based on his published studies and clinical experience, Dr. Raymond C. Baker of the Center for Wellness and Counseling at Bradley University has identified specific details that people need to write down in order to develop a successful weight-loss plan. These questions will construct your weight-loss diary and allow you to discover what you need to do to become thinner and younger. They make you think about much more than what you eat—they address when you eat, why you eat, how you feel when you exercise.

Depending on how you decide to keep your weight-loss diary, write these questions in your journal or photocopy this page and tuck it away in your diary.

Food

- What did you eat?
- How much? (Record portion sizes)
- How many calories?
- How many grams of fat?
- What did you drink?
- What time did you eat?
- How fast did you eat?
- Were you hungry? If you weren't, why did you eat?
- Where were you? What were you doing?
- What emotions were you feeling?
- Did something other than hunger trigger your eating?
- Did you snack?
- What are your dietary goals—and were they met? (For example, amount of fiber, number of servings of fruits and vegetables, glasses of water per day)
- Did you try new foods or ways of preparing foods? Did you like them?

Exercise

- What activity?
- Was it a new activity? Did you enjoy it?
- How long (minutes, hours) or how many repetitions and sets?
- At what intensity did you exercise? (High, medium, low)
- How did you feel afterward?
- If you skipped exercise, why?

did. There's no reason to be embarrassed by your actions. By being honest and writing them down, you're taking the first step toward making a positive and successful change.

Time to Review

What to do with the mountain of information that you're recording in your diary? Study it, Dr. Baker says. For inside the pages of your diary lies the map to your weight-loss goals. Your evaluation will reveal your own personal weight-loss strategy—a program for you, by you.

Here's how to transform your writing into action.

Analyze weekly. Pick a day—maybe each Sunday—when you look over your diary.

"A week's time is more meaningful, and you'll get a general idea of the trends," Dr. Baker says. Study your goals and results as a weekly measure.

For instance, don't study how much fiber you ate by the day. If you had a bad day, you could get discouraged. Yet if you add up your grams of fiber over the course of the week and divide by 7, you may realize that you did very well on average.

Look for triggers. Scan your diary and look for trends. Did you overeat every time you felt stressed-out? Do you always blow off exercise because you feel tired? Does watching TV automatically send you to the refrigerator? Do you always eat on the run, barely tasting your food? These are the connections you want to discover, Dr. Baker says.

Search for successes, too. A weight-loss diary chronicles what works as well as what doesn't, Dr. Baker says. If you notice that you lost weight the week you tried a new exercise or changed an eating habit, you have discovered an effective weight-loss tool for you.

"Losing weight is very individualized, and this will help identify what works for you," he says.

Change your criteria periodically. The goal of this weight-loss diary is to help eliminate bad habits and develop good ones, Dr. Baker says. If you've mastered a behavior such as drinking enough water or walking every day, drop it from your diary. Then concentrate on new goals or other habits that you'd like to break.

Quiz

Child's Play

Like all of us, Molly Brown used to like to run, bike, and dance when she was a kid. She even kept it up into her young adult years. Then marriage, career, and family moved in where her running, jumping, and playing used to be. A few years later, something else moved in, too—extra weight.

"I just got out of the habit of being active," she recalls. "With everything else going on, I guess I forgot about it, or it didn't seem as important. But when I started to feel unhealthy and out of shape, I knew I had to get back into the swing of things."

With the help of her 11-year-old daughter and her eager-to-be-active husband, Molly now embraces a life full of activity, including aerobic dance, brisk walking, and strength training with her daughter and swing dancing with her husband.

"Getting back into shape can be as easy as getting in touch with the things you liked to do when you were young," says Paul Konstanty, clinical supervisor and exercise therapist at the University of California OrthoMed Spine and Joint Conditioning Center in San Diego. "Adults just need to remember that—like when they were kids—fitness doesn't have to be confined within four walls of a gym. It's a big wide world, and there are all kinds of activities that you can do and sports you can play outside to have fun and keep fit."

Not sure what you'd like to play now that your freeze-tag buddies have grown up and moved away? The following quiz, developed by Selene Yeager, a certified fitness trainer and health writer in Allentown, Pennsylvania, can help you find new activities for your old playful self.

Circle the answer that most describes you. (You can choose more than one if it's a tie. You just have more activities to choose from as an adult!)

1. My favorite playground game was:

a. Tag
b. HORSE
c. Jump rope
d. Hopscotch
e. Four-square

(continued)

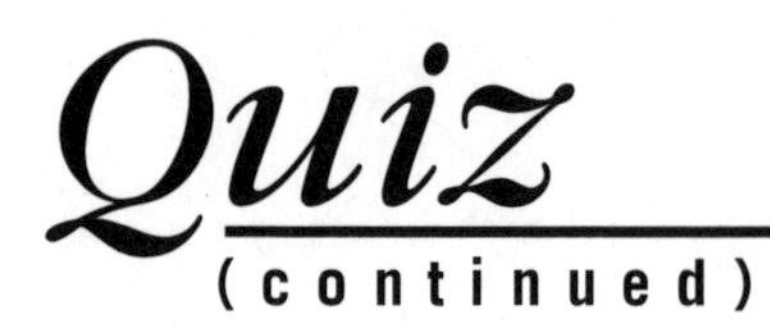

(continued)

2. My favorite sport in school was:
  a. Basketball
  b. Soccer
  c. Softball
  d. Gymnastics
  e. Cheerleading

3. My favorite picnic game was:
  a. Horseshoes
  b. Croquet
  c. Bean-bag toss
  d. Lawn darts
  e. Volleyball

4. My favorite activity was:
  a. Dancing
  b. Bicycling
  c. Swimming
  d. Sledding
  e. Roller-skating

Score Yourself

1. IF YOU CIRCLED . . .

a. Try joining a jogging, bicycling, or day-hiking group. There's a playful spirit of chase in these groups that you'll love.

b. Buy a ball and shoot some hoops. You can even put up a net in your own driveway.

c. or d. Try rebounding (aerobics on a mini-tramp) for a nonimpact, fun jump-around workout. Or try skipping rope again. You can even pick up videos for workout ideas.

e. Take up tennis or racquetball. You still have to hit the balls where you want them, only now you have racquets.

2. IF YOU CIRCLED . . .

a. Can't find adult hoopsters to share a game with? Join an adult volleyball league for ball-jumping fun or call your local recreation center for information on adult basketball or volleyball leagues.

b. or c. Most communities have adult soccer and softball leagues filled with people just like you who haven't played for years but miss the game.

d. or e. Check out one of the new-generation aerobics classes. Many feature energetic Latin, urban, and salsa dance that will get you moving again.

3. IF YOU CIRCLED . . .

a., b., c., or d. Golf is a great adult game that you can play almost all year-round, and it is good exercise, too, if you don't use a cart. Intimidated by the game? Go to a chip-and-putt course first. All the holes are short and most folks are at the beginner skill level. Or try bowling, another eye-hand coordination game.

e. Check the paper for adult volleyball leagues and go play.

4. IF YOU CIRCLED . . .

a. You can always put on music and dance yourself silly in the living room. But it's more fun to grab a partner and take classes in swing, ballroom, or country line-dancing.

b. Stop in at your local bike shop and ask about group rides in your area. There are usually regular rides for all fitness levels.

c. Most local recreation centers and health clubs have masters' swim programs that meet regularly and help water-loving adults get back into the swim of things.

d. Try out some winter sports for adults, like snowshoeing and cross-country skiing. You can play in the powder, and you don't have to worry about skidding into the trees.

e. Inline skating is a whole lot easier than old four-wheel roller-skating. And it's a great workout. Check with your local sports shops that sell skates. They may also offer free lessons.

The Play Principle: All Workout and No Play Makes Fitness Dull

START PLAYING TENNIS A COUPLE OF TIMES A WEEK, AND A YEAR LATER, YOU COULD BE ALMOST 20 POUNDS LIGHTER. YOU'LL ALSO HAVE MADE SOME GREAT NEW FRIENDS. HAD A TON OF FUN. AND FELT YOUNGER THAN YOU HAVE SINCE HIGH SCHOOL.

Plus, you'll have younger, stronger bones and muscles, including your heart.

Tennis not your game? Try taking a walk, starting a garden, or skating. Adding a little play to your life each day can help you knock off weight and keep it off *even better* than a structured exercise program does.

In a groundbreaking study from Johns Hopkins University, a group of overweight women who simply started walking, gardening, or generally being more active for about 30 minutes a day lost as much weight—around 18 pounds—as a similar group who did step aerobics three times a week.

Even better: A year later, the women doing the less rigorous activity regained less than ½ pound on average. The exercise-program women gained back 3½ pounds.

That's right. You don't have to join a gym, purchase expensive equipment, strap on a heart-rate monitor, figure your max VO_2, or do any of the other exercise-discouraging jazz that so-called fitness gurus have been trying to get you to buy into for the last 20 years.

All you have to do is have some fun.

No Pain—All Play!

It's hard to believe that fitness is so simple after years of hearing (and feeling!) how hard it was. "No pain, no gain" was the credo we were taught to live by.

And if we didn't work out at our target heart rate for at least 20 minutes, 3 days a week, we were told that we weren't doing any good. No wonder so many folks quit!

Today, fitness experts know better, says exercise physiologist Robert Brosmer, vice president of health and wellness at the Central Florida YMCA in Orlando and coauthor of *Health and High Performance.*

"In the beginning, fitness experts weren't being taken seriously, so they responded by making exercise a very serious business," Brosmer says. "And while we were running around talking about target heart rates, a lot of people quit exercising. Now we know that what really matters is getting off the couch and getting a little active—even if it's just for 10 minutes at lunch and 10 minutes in the evening on a regular basis."

The best part is that you can get fit by doing things you love, says exercise therapist Paul Konstanty of the University of California OrthoMed Spine and Joint Conditioning Center.

"Throw out the notion that it's too tough to exercise," he says. "It's easy. It's fun. And it doesn't have to be a huge time commitment."

Turning Back the Clock

The easiest way to tap into the new exercise attitude is to remember what you liked to do as a child, or even as a younger adult, and take up similar activities, Konstanty says.

"Maybe you liked to play in the woods and ride your bicycle. Or maybe you just ran around town with your friends," he says. "Whatever it was, you

Having Fun Can Whittle Your Waistline

Find a game you like to play. Or pick up a new active hobby. Then watch the pounds peel away. The chart below lists different activities you can enjoy and the number of calories they burn per hour (based on a 150-pound person).

Play a little harder sometimes, and you'll burn even more.

ACTIVITY	CALORIES BURNED PER HOUR
Jumping rope	680
Swimming (breaststroke)	680
Aerobics, high-impact	476
Canoeing (4 mph—moderate)	476
Kickball	476
Racquetball	476
Roller-skating	476
Sledding	476
Soccer	476
Tennis	476
Dancing	420

can re-create that today. You can go hiking. Ride a bike in a local park. Or pair up with a friend and make weekly dates to go for an energizing walk around town or in the park."

Right now is one of the best times in history to take up a fun, youthful activity, because there are more activities to choose from than ever, says John Yetter, M.D., medical director at SSM Rehab Sports Medicine in St. Louis.

"People have been ingenious at blending the fun parts of sports with exercise classes," he says. "You can try anything from kickboxing to jumping rope in a fun, instructional setting."

Or you can join an active group and go hiking, biking, swimming, or fitness walking. "There are groups for all activities at all levels," says Dr. Yetter. The key is recapturing some of the spirit of your youth.

ACTIVITY	CALORIES BURNED PER HOUR
Tag	374
Aerobics, low-impact	340
Softball	340
Golf	324
Badminton	306
Gardening (weeding)	306
Hopscotch	272
Volleyball	272
Bicycling (6 mph—leisurely)	240
Walking (3 mph—moderate pace)	238
Body surfing	204
Frisbee	204
Horseshoes	204
Croquet	170
Lawn darts	170
Swinging on a swing	136
Walking (2 mph—shopping pace or stroll)	136
Tubing on a river	102

Having trouble getting your adult brain thinking like a kid? No sweat. These fail-proof steps will have you back to your carefree, active self in no time.

Skip your chores. Acting like a kid again has one benefit that you're sure to love, says Laura Senft, a registered physical therapist at the Kessler Institute for Rehabilitation in West Orange, New Jersey: You get to ditch the housework.

"When we're young, we beg to go out and play and clean our rooms later. The only reason we don't play is that our parents won't let us," Senft says. "Now you're the adult. So, ditch the dishes and go have some fun. Having time to be active is much more important for your well-being than doing any housework.

Living Proof
PANEL

Taking the "Work" Out of Workouts

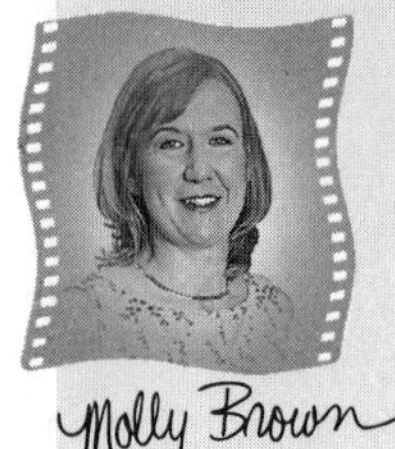

I have decided that fitness should be fun and interesting for the whole family, not just some workout I do by myself. My 11-year-old daughter and I do aerobic dance tapes together. She rides her bike while I take my walks. And when we get bored, we figure out new, fun things to do together.

I've taken the same approach with my husband. We signed up for swing dance classes on Thursday evenings just because we thought it would be fun to get out there and laugh at ourselves while we get some exercise.

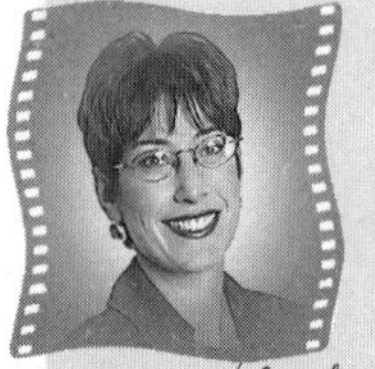

A few nights during the summer, I've taken my kids to the pool to play. While we're there, I play with them, and I try to do some water exercises for fun when they're off doing their own thing. It's a nice way to spend a summer evening. And if I can shape up while I'm having fun, that's great, too.

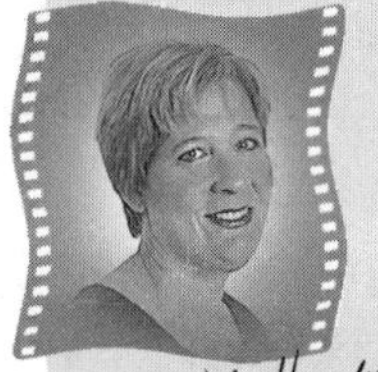

Horseback riding is the thing I love most. It really works all those thigh muscles that people exercise in the gym, but it's a whole lot more fun!

"The laundry will always be there. Make a date to do it on a rainy day or during the evening," she says.

Swapping some of those boring adult responsibilities for fun activities with friends will not only make you thinner and healthier, it'll make you feel younger, too.

Try something new. Lots of adults don't exercise because they don't know what they like to do, says certified international lifestyle fitness expert Lynne Brick, owner of Brick Bodies Health Clubs in Baltimore.

"We didn't know what we liked to do as kids, either. The difference is that we went out and tried tons of stuff," Brick says. "You don't have to stop trying new things just because you're a little taller and few years older. Make a list of three to five activities that look fun to you, then go try them."

You won't even have to make much of an investment. Most health clubs will let you sample classes for free or at a minimal charge. And sporting goods stores often rent bikes, inline skates, and hiking equipment—as well as offer free clinics—for people to get a taste of different activities.

Reconnect with your body. When you're a kid, you *live* through your body, says Michael Gilewski, Ph.D., a clinical psychologist for post-acute care services at Cedars-Sinai Medical Center in Los Angeles.

"But as we grow up, we become more brain-centered and start living above our necks," he says. "There needs to be a healthy balance for us to feel and function at our best. To feel healthy and young again, you need to reconnect with your body, which means moving just for the sake of moving."

"You don't have to start by running around the block," he adds. "Just take one evening this week to sit outside after dinner and feel the air on your face. Maybe go for a stroll the next morning. Gradually start spending some time enjoying the world through your body again."

Play outside. Check out the local park, and you'll see that it's swarming with kids. Chances are, when you were a kid, you couldn't wait to get out of the house and play outside, too.

"Too often, as adults with jobs, we forget about the outside completely, as we walk from the house to the car to the office and back again," Konstanty says. "The best cure for that is to look up the parks and hiking trails in the areas near you, take an hour on a Saturday morning, and go for a nature walk.

"Once you're reminded of how refreshing and beautiful the outdoors can be, you'll be looking for excuses to go play outside," he says.

Find a friend. Just as children often grow bored when there's no one to play with, adults can get bored if they don't have someone to exercise with, says Deborah Saint-Phard, M.D., an exercise physiatrist for the Women's Sports Medicine Center at the Hospital for Special Surgery in New York City.

"Getting together with a buddy three times a week to walk or work out is one of the best things women can do for their health," she says. "They not

Vacation Yourself Thin

A good vacation can make you not only feel like a new woman but also look like one. Though some women fret about widening their waistlines while on vacation, dietitians find that some folks actually come back from time-off a few pounds lighter.

"Time away from your routine means you're not eating out of habit or boredom," says exercise physiologist Joyce A. Hanna of Stanford University. "If you're seeing new places, you also tend to walk a lot more and be more active."

So next time you're feeling in a rut, pick a fun, new destination and send yourself and your extra pounds packing.

only can lose weight and lower their blood pressures, but they can keep in touch with friends, chat, share some laughs, and reduce their stress."

Join the kids. One surefire way to exercise like a kid again is to exercise with your kids, says Brick.

"Instead of sitting in front of the TV, grab your boots and go for a hike. Take a day trip to the shore. Or just pick up a basketball and play HORSE in the driveway," she says. "Every little action counts to make a big difference!"

Dance, dance, dance. The quickest, easiest way to put some youthful spring in your step even when you aren't "exercising" is to keep upbeat, jazzy music playing in the background of your house all day long, says Joyce A. Hanna, associate director of the health improvement program at Stanford University and an exercise physiologist in Palo Alto, California.

"You'll find yourself tapping your feet, swinging your hips, and bopping around without even thinking about it," Hanna says.

Quiz

Choosing the Right Exercise for You

Most people spend more time picking out a pair of shoes than they do their exercise programs. And that's probably the number one reason why most folks quit their exercise programs within 6 months of starting them. Like a bad pair of shoes, they don't fit, they're not comfortable, and hey, they're just not "you."

"The real trick to sticking with an exercise program is finding something you honestly love to do," says exercise therapist Paul Konstanty of the University of California OrthoMed Spine and Joint Conditioning Center. "Some people love competitive sports and the energy of a group setting. For other folks, that's their worst nightmare. To be successful, you have to choose what's right for you."

The problem is, if you've never worked out, you might have no idea which exercises, sports, or activities go best with your unique personality. Fortunately, there's an easy answer. It's a fitness-personality quiz, developed by Charles Yokomoto, Ph.D., a consultant who has studied personality types and sports for years.

Simply answer the following 10 questions, then match your personality type with the exercises that work for you.

What's your fitness personality?

The following list of questions may help you find a workout that you can stick with. Each question has four descriptions that may or may not apply to you. Using the numbers 4 to 1, rate these descriptions from the one that describes you the most (4), to the one that describes you the least (1). Remember: Each description gets a number, and you can use each number only once per question.

Most like me	**4**	**Hardly like me**	**2**
Somewhat like me	**3**	**Least like me**	**1**

1. When contemplating my weekend activities, I prefer to:

___ a. Plan several days in advance.

___ b. Keep my options open until Friday.

___ c. Select activities that are intellectually stimulating.

___ d. Select activities that help my personal growth.

(continued)

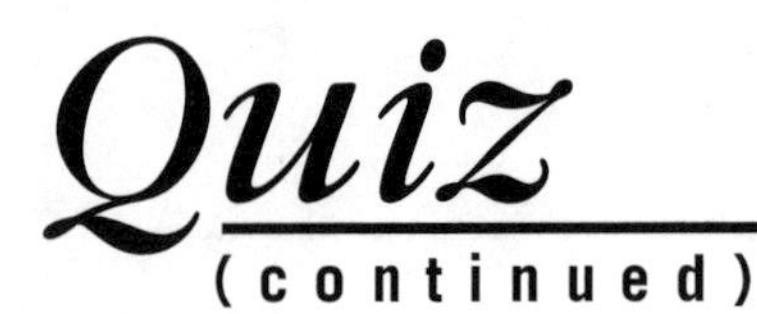

(continued)

2. If I were a team leader, my style would be to:

___ a. Inspire people to develop their potential.
___ b. Resolve crises and conflicts after they arise.
___ c. Develop clear procedures and practices.
___ d. Study principles of good leadership and incorporate them into my leadership style.

3. If I could choose a particular office function to be in charge of, I would like to be responsible for:

___ a. Making the office a fun place to work.
___ b. Compiling a reading list of books that I feel people should read.
___ c. Developing personal-growth workshops.
___ d. Developing a training guide that describes office procedures.

4. In relationships with others:

___ a. I am considered idealistic.
___ b. I am sometimes late for appointments because I get involved in something fun and forget the time.
___ c. I am known to get impatient when I'm not understood.
___ d. I have expectations of how others should behave.

5. When I take part in activities such as games and sports:

___ a. I tend to focus more on emotion and inspiration than strategies.
___ b. I tend to use conservative, conventional strategies that have been proved to be successful by others.
___ c. I like to create my own strategies.
___ d. I basically just try to have fun.

6. Those who know me well say:

___ a. I am empathetic and inspirational.
___ b. I am reliable and dependable.
___ c. I am intelligent and clever.
___ d. I am fun to have around when things become dull.

7. When it comes to taking part in planning activities at work or at home:

___ a. I like to see the big picture.

___ b. I like to get it done quickly and go on to something more enjoyable.

___ c. I like to inspire others to contribute their good taste.

___ d. I like to be methodical and not miss any important details.

8. When a supervisor wants to compliment me for something done well:

___ a. I like to hear how cleverly I reacted to a crisis.

___ b. I usually already know.

___ c. I like to hear how valuable I am.

___ d. I like to hear how responsible I am.

9. When trying to resolve a problem at work or at home:

___ a. I am good at coming up with an intuitive solution.

___ b. I am patient with complicated problems.

___ c. I prefer tried-and-true solutions.

___ d. I tend to select a quick fix and not dwell on it.

10. If my close friends were to be honest, they would say that:

___ a. I hold firm to my opinions.

___ b. I am flexible to the point that I change my mind a lot.

___ c. I am intellectually curious.

___ d. I am a good listener.

Score Yourself

Transfer your answers to the table below. (Note that the spaces aren't always in a-b-c-d order.) After filling in your answers, total your points in each column. The column with the highest number indicates your preferred workout style. If your two highest totals are nearly equal, it may mean that you adapt well to both workout styles. Read the descriptions of both types to see which fits you best.

(continued)

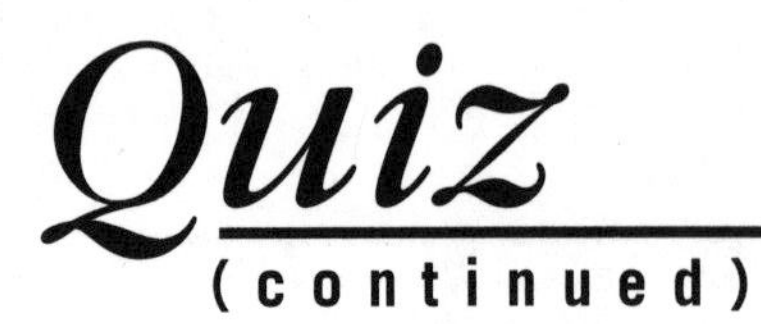

Quiz (continued)

1.	a.____	b.____	c.____	d.____
2.	c.____	b.____	d.____	a.____
3.	d.____	a.____	b.____	c.____
4.	d.____	b.____	c.____	a.____
5.	b.____	d.____	c.____	a.____
6.	b.____	d.____	c.____	a.____
7.	d.____	b.____	a.____	c.____
8.	d.____	a.____	b.____	c.____
9.	c.____	d.____	b.____	a.____
10.	a.____	b.____	c.____	d.____
TOTAL	___	___	___	___
	O	S	A	I

O **Organized** **A** **Analytical**
S **Spontaneous** **I** **Inspirational**

WHAT YOUR TYPE MEANS

Organized

You feel best when life is orderly. In your home, there's a place for everything, and you like to keep it that way. You're punctual and dutiful, and once you agree to something, you're likely to follow through. You like rules and routine.

Your exercise Rx: Result-oriented workout. You like a schedule. It's no problem for you to set aside a block of time each day for exercise or even to stick with an activity that's repetitious. But to keep your interest, you need feedback. That's why cardio machines, which let you methodically monitor your progress, might be just the ticket. Most have computers that track your heart rate, calories burned, and distance traveled. Or keep a fitness log to monitor your progress.

Spontaneous

Life is a game, and your strategy is always changing. Doing the same thing over and over again is boring. You're good at handling crises, partly because you often find yourself in the middle of one of your own creation. While you aren't much for rules, you'll follow them if they're simple and help you have fun.

Overcoming Obstacles

To smooth the transition while testing out a new activity, fitness-personality expert Dr. Charles Yokomoto suggests a few ways to help battle specific problems that your fitness personality type may face.

Organized. Since you like things to run smoothly, glitches perpetrated by others can trip you up. If, for instance, you decide to try out an exercise class, but the teacher is disorganized and lackadaisical, you're likely to drop it like a hot potato.

Solution: Stick with workouts that you control.

Spontaneous. Your biggest enemy is an idle mind. Even short workouts can turn torturous if there's nothing to occupy your brain.

Solution: Watch TV or listen to music while exercising, or grab a workout partner to chat with.

Analytical. Even a varied routine can become, well, too routine for you. If there's no challenge to your exercise, you're likely to turn into a no-show. But there are bound to be times when even the most diversified exercise regimen will seem more simplistic than you like; it's inescapable.

Solution: Make a list of your reasons for exercising (your motivators) and refer to it when the going gets tough. Then, when you push past those times, reward yourself with a small, sweet treat; a massage; or a nice dinner out.

Inspirational. Because you may often engage in activities that involve instructors or coaches, you run the risk of being turned off by corrections or criticism aimed at you—or anyone else in your group.

Solution: Remind yourself that the teacher or coach is only trying to help you. If that doesn't work, look for a class or team that focuses more on teamwork or for a teacher or coach whose style you prefer.

(continued)

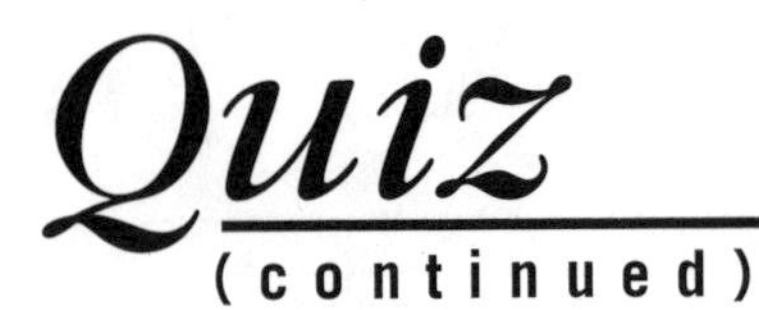

(continued)

Your exercise Rx: Short-but-sweet activities. Lifestyle activities that allow you to accumulate exercise time throughout the day may be a good choice, according to fitness experts.

Walk for 15 minutes after lunch, then for another 15 minutes after dinner. Park as far away from your destination as possible and expend energy taking the stairs. Ride your bike on the weekends or go for hikes.

Analytical

You don't mind complexity. In fact, you enjoy working out problems and puzzles and learning the theories and principles behind them. Your goal is to be competent at whatever you do. If an activity is too simple, you may drop out in search of something more challenging. You are also imaginative, but you like things to make sense.

Your exercise Rx: Diversity training. Since analytical types fare best with challenge and variety, cross-training may be the perfect option. You have the challenge of developing your own program but keep potentially tedious activities fresh by mixing them up. Try a schedule that works something like this: Monday, 20 minutes on the stairclimber, 20 minutes on the stationary bike; Wednesday, aerobics class; Friday, 20 minutes on the cross-country ski machine, 20 minutes on the rowing machine. On alternate days, take up an activity that requires you to develop new skills.

You don't like "to do for the sake of doing." Instead, you appreciate why your heart rate should reach 120 beats a minute during aerobic exercise or which muscles you're stretching when you do a lunge. Read up on whatever activity you choose to help keep your interest and improve your skills.

Inspirational

You're the type who catalyzes other people into action. You know how to say all the right things, which is why people gravitate toward you, tell you their problems, and look to you for inspiration. You're creative and are concerned about achieving personal growth.

Your exercise Rx: Dual-purpose exercise. To you, working out is engaging only when it's about more than just your body. You are more apt to enjoy it if it's about being part of a community—the reason that group social activities such as exercise classes and team sports are a natural selection for you—or about exploring your inner self. The cre-

The Best Choices

ORGANIZED

Cycling
Running
Stairclimbers
Stationary bikes
Swimming
Treadmills
Walking

SPONTANEOUS

Basketball
Bike riding
Frisbee
Hiking
Racquetball
Short walks throughout the day
Squash
Taking the stairs
Tennis

ANALYTICAL

Cross-training
Golf
Racquetball
Rock climbing
Sailing
Tennis
Training for a 5-K, 10-K, or triathlon

INSPIRATIONAL

Dance class
Softball
Swimming
Tai chi and other martial arts
Trail running
Volleyball
Water aerobics
Yoga

ative side of you can appreciate the elaborate movements required in dance classes and water aerobics. The spiritual side of you may like the mind-body aspects of martial arts or the serenity of swimming laps. To enhance your spiritual side, try listening to music to set the mood for a peaceful workout.

The $100 Home Gym

HERE'S A WEIGHT-LOSS SECRET YOU'LL NEVER HEAR AT THE BIG, EXPENSIVE HEALTH SPAS: BY EXERCISING IN THE PRIVACY OF YOUR OWN HOME, YOU CAN LOSE MORE WEIGHT THAN YOU WOULD BY WORKING OUT IN A CLUB OR A GYM. THAT'S RIGHT. IN A STUDY AT THE UNIVERSITY OF FLORIDA IN GAINESVILLE, RESEARCHERS HAD 49 OVERWEIGHT WOMEN WORK OUT EITHER AT A LOCAL GYM OR AT HOME. THE HOME-BASED EXERCISERS LOST 10 MORE POUNDS THAN THOSE WHO WENT TO THE GYM.

"If a woman is more comfortable exercising in the privacy of her home, where she doesn't feel self-conscious or inconvenienced, that is where she will be most successful," says Elena Ramirez, Ph.D., a clinical psychologist and weight-management researcher at the University of Vermont in Burlington. "There's no rule that says you have to join a club to lose weight."

Still, many women overlook this option because they think they need to invest in expensive equipment to do it right. Not so. Smart fitness shoppers can get everything they need for a total-body workout for about $100.

"The most important thing is that you choose equipment that provides an aerobic workout as well as one that strengthens your muscles," says certified fitness instructor Kelly Bridgman, wellness director for the Peggy and Philip B. Crosby Wellness Center of the YMCA in Winter Park, Florida.

Equipment You'll Actually Use

We all have at least one fitness gizmo or gadget that seems to make a better coatrack than a fat burner. Partly, this has to do with quality: Far too much equipment designed for home use is flimsy, unstable, or clunky. To make sure that you get the right gear, consider these guidelines from the American Council on Exercise. And be sure to test equipment that you're thinking about buying before handing over your hard-earned money.

- Does your body move in a safe, natural manner when you use the equipment?
- Is the equipment comfortable, easy to use, and adjustable? Or does it come in the right size for your specific height and body type?
- Is it space efficient?
- Is it made from high-quality materials?
- Does it look and feel safe and sturdy to use?

There's one more thing you need to think about when you're looking for equipment, and this is actually the most important: Will you enjoy using it? says James Rippe, M.D., associate professor of medicine at Tufts University School of Medicine in Boston; director of the Center for Clinical and Lifestyle Research in Shrewsbury, Massachusetts; and author of *Fit over Forty*. "If you can't see yourself still using it in a year, don't buy it."

If you're serious about setting up a home gym, here are a few tips you'll want to consider. Simply choose among the different categories to assemble what you need for a personalized fitness routine.

Aerobic Alternatives

The only thing that you really need to do to burn calories is to move your body at a brisk pace, says exercise physiologist Joyce A. Hanna of Stanford University. Treadmills are the most popular pieces of fitness equipment for folks hoping to shed pounds and make bones stronger, but you can get the same benefits, spend less money, and have more fun working out by investing in a few less expensive items.

Aerobic step. Stairclimbing is a great exercise for burning calories. If you weigh 150 pounds, for example, 1 hour of stairclimbing burns more than 400 calories. Plus, it makes your bones stronger, says Hanna. You can walk up and down your steps at home for free, but you'll do a little better if you buy a nonskid adjustable-height aerobic step. It costs about $50. You'll spend a little more if you decide to add a step-aerobic video.

Jump rope. "If I were to buy only a few items for a home gym, one of them would definitely be a jump rope," says certified personal trainer Jana Angelakis, founder of PEx Personalized Exercise in New York City. "Jumping rope is great for improving cardiovascular fitness. It's low impact, so it promotes healthy bones; it enhances balance and coordination; and you can do it anywhere." It also burns a lot of calories—170 in 15 minutes at moderate intensity.

Get a rope that is as thin as a string of licorice with ball bearing handles, which makes twirling it easier. It costs less than $20. Be sure to skip rope on a surface that has some give, like a wood or carpeted floor. If you're going to skip on cement, use an exercise mat to minimize impact and prevent injury.

Videos. "There are tons of exercise videos to choose from these days," says Angelakis. "You can choose any kind of music, from salsa to country. You can choose an aerobic-dancing tape or one with sports-inspired moves. And you can pick the kind of workout you like, depending on your goals and your present fitness level." Most exercise videos are pretty inexpensive—less than $20 a tape.

Aerobic shoes. High-quality shoes made for aerobics are ideal, says Bridgman. You can get a pair of cushioned, supportive shoes for about $70—and for quite a bit less on sale. "A good pair of shoes will let you exercise longer without your tiring or getting sore. And you can pack them for a business trip or vacation so you can sneak out for a quick walk," Bridgman says.

Easy Toning

There's simply no reason to buy an enormous weight set just to tone your muscles. You can strengthen your muscles and bones just as well, if not better, with compact balls and stretchable bands and tubes, says Michael Romatowski, director of personal training at Athletic Express Health Club in

Gaithersburg, Maryland, and author of *Secrets of Medicine Ball Training*. "I actually prefer some of these products to traditional weights because the exerciser learns how to move like a human being is supposed to move."

Resistance bands. For about $10, you can buy a pack of three resistance bands, providing light, moderate, and heavy resistance. "These bands are great for working your upper and lower body—and they are extremely portable," says Angelakis. No matter what your fitness level, there are countless safe and effective ways you can use resistance bands—for arm curls and leg lifts, for example. When you buy a pack, make sure it includes an instructional poster or booklet that shows proper technique and form.

A woman can do just about all the strength training she needs with dumbbells.

Medicine balls. These are softball- to basketball-size weighted balls that can be used as substitutes for dumbbells and barbells. They also allow you to do exercises that don't work well with other weights, says Romatowski. You can do bending and twisting exercises with medicine balls to strengthen your buttocks, hips, abdomen, middle and upper back, neck, and head, all of which make up the body's core, he says. Prices range from $20 to $90. You'll also want to invest in a book that shows proper form and technique, probably for about $12.

Tubing. Like resistance bands, stretchy rubber tubing attached to handgrips is portable and great for resistance training. "The handgrips make them super easy to use, and you can do the same strengthening exercises with them as you would with dumbbells," says Bridgman. Resistance tubing comes in varying degrees of resistance, with each tube costing between $4 and $6. As always, be sure the tubing you buy comes with an instructional guide.

Body bars. Used in body-sculpting aerobics classes, body bars are rubber-covered, weighted bars that are perfect for traditional strength-training exercises, like arm curls and squats, says Bridgman. They come in a variety of weights, from 1 to 18 pounds. Prices range from $12 to $33.

Dumbbells. Though bands, balls, and tubes are fun and effective, some folks love the classics, and there's nothing wrong with that, says Romatowski. "A woman can do just about all the strength training she needs with a pair of 5- and 10-pound dumbbells." And they're inexpensive. Two sets of metal dumbbells will cost about $20.

Homemade gear. "You don't have to spend a dime on strength-training equipment if you don't want to," says Michael Bourque, certified personal trainer and personal training coordinator for the Center for Health and Wellness of the Central Florida YMCA in Oviedo. "Rinse and save old plastic milk jugs. You can fill them partway with sand and use them as hand weights for lower-body exercises, such as lunges and wall squats," he says. "Want something to do arm curls with? Grab a can of beans from the shelf. If you're inventive, everything you need is in your home."

Great Abs at Home

There's no shortage of home equipment designed to work the abdominal muscles and give you a strong, firm tummy. But many of these devices are expensive, unnecessary, and "just plain silly," says Romatowski. "All you really need to work your abdominals is a carpeted floor to do crunches on. But there is one piece of equipment that makes crunches even better—a stability ball."

Stability balls are big, inflatable balls that you can use for a variety of exercises. They're particularly useful for abdominal work. When you lie back on a stability ball, your abdominals are extended farther than if you were just lying on the floor, explains Romatowski. "So, those muscles have to work harder to bring your shoulders up into a crunch." Stability balls are available in different sizes according to your height. They cost about $20.

Since the floor may be too hard or uncomfortable on your back to exercise on, especially for doing abdominal work, you'll probably want to invest in a mat, says Angelakis. "A basic exercise mat is really a must. It gives you a cushioned surface for exercising and stretching comfortably," she says. "It also creates a designated 'exercise spot.' Some people find that their home workouts just feel more legitimate when they use a mat." A basic mat will cost about $15.

The Pleasure Principle

Do not bite at the bait of pleasure, till you know there is no hook beneath it.

—Thomas Jefferson

So much for "the pursuit of happiness." Jefferson's skeptical admonition pretty well sums up the way many of us feel about eating for pleasure. We can't help feeling that if it tastes good, there must be a hook. It must be fattening or bad for us in some other way.

Deprivation, dieting, and sacrifice are seen as the path to weight loss. Pleasure is viewed as the problem. But it's not: It's the solution. In fact, feel free to consider it an inalienable right.

Wait a minute. This is America. Land of pie-eating contests, super-size fries, all-you-can-eat buffets, and butter-drenched popcorn served by the bucket. Seems like we're fulfilling our pleasure quota quite nicely.

But pleasure isn't measured by the quantity of food that we eat. What matters most is the *quality* of our eating experience, says Julie Waltz Kembel, a behavioral counselor at Canyon Ranch spa in Tucson and author of *Winning the Weight and Wellness Game.*

Deep down, we don't think we can enjoy eating *and* lose weight. Sensible diets aren't fun, are they? In fact, a survey of nearly 3,400 overweight men and women, conducted by *Consumer Reports* in conjunction with researchers from Wesleyan University and Yale University, showed that next to lack of exercise, most believed they'd gained weight simply because they enjoy eating.

A World of Pleasure

Whatever your tastes, there is one universal principle for healthy eating that's often overlooked: Eating should be a pleasurable experience, one to truly be savored. Sometimes that's hard to remember when you're calculating grams of fat and measuring portions.

Here's how it's said around the world.

- Enjoy your food. —*First dietary guideline, United Kingdom*
- Food + Joy = Health. —*National Nutrition Council, Norway*
- Happy eating makes for a happy family life. —*Japan*
- A happy family is one whose members eat together, enjoy treasured family tastes and good home cooking. —*Thailand*
- Eating is one of life's greatest pleasures. —*Introduction to Dietary Guidelines for Americans*

So to lose weight we deny our innate desire for pleasure and follow a laundry list of diet no-no's. We banish sweets. Say no to snacking. Forsake our favorite foods. We force ourselves to eat steamed vegetables and plain broiled chicken night after night.

"We're so focused on getting rid of the fat that we forget the positive and pleasurable aspects of eating. And that can lead to overeating," says Kembel.

It also sets us up for disappointment because the simple fact is this: Diets that deny our basic need for pleasure inevitably fail.

Eating for Pleasure

"I'm a big believer in approaching every day with joy," says John La Puma, M.D., a Chicago physician who is the founder and medical director of the CHEF (Cooking, Healthy Eating, and Fitness) Clinic, which uses a cutting-edge approach to weight loss based on putting flavor first and making exercise fun. "People simply will not stick with a weight-loss plan that is not pleasurable."

So if you want to lose weight, don't waste calories on food that doesn't taste good, says Dr. La Puma. To start eating for pleasure, follow these principles.

Think first. Before you take the first bite, ask yourself: "What do I want to eat?"

"Foods need to feel good," Kembel says. "If we can heighten the experience by pleasing our palate with exactly what we want, then we diminish the volume that we need to eat."

If a side of mashed potatoes is what feels right to you, plan around it, advises Kembel. Have a salad, more vegetables, and less meat. And then savor every comforting, creamy bite.

Feed all of your senses. Eating involves more than good-tasting food. To make each meal a pleasure, stimulate all of your senses, says David Sobel, M.D., in his book *The Healthy Mind, Healthy Body Handbook.* Play some soothing background music during meals. Arrange the table and your plate attractively.

Long before food crosses your lips, you *taste* with your eyes. And you can bet that a plate of white cauliflower, white rice, and white chicken breast is as boring to your tastebuds as it is to your eyes.

Sensory pleasure and the positive feelings it creates are nature's way of letting us know that we're doing something that's good for our health, according to Dr. Sobel, who is regional director of patient education and director of the regional health education department at Kaiser Permanente Medical Center in Los Angeles.

Satisfy your taste for variety. We instinctively love variety and crave new taste sensations—two of the keys to eating a healthy diet, says James J. Kenney, R.D., Ph.D., a nutrition research specialist at the Pritikin Longevity Center in Santa Monica, California.

But sometimes we get stuck in a routine of eating the same foods week after week. The result? Boredom, which can lead to overeating.

So just what is variety? Ten foods a day? Twenty? Research has shown that people who eat the most varied diets—in one study, that meant 71 to 83 different foods over a 15-day period—consume fewer calories, less sodium, a little less saturated fat, and more antiaging antioxidants than people who eat the same-old, same-old.

But just in case you're wondering, that doesn't mean you can consume a large variety of sweets, snacks, condiments, and carbohydrates. If you do,

Chocolate Ecstasy

To fully enjoy food, you need to fully engage all of your senses. Take a piece of dark, rich chocolate. Really—take a piece of dark, rich chocolate. Now. (Belgian chocolate is best for this experiment.)

Savor every aspect of it, following these steps outlined by Kaiser Permanente Medical Center's Dr. David Sobel in his book *The Healthy Mind, Healthy Body Handbook.*

- Appreciate the beautiful, dark color of the chocolate before you put it in your mouth.
- Feel the weight and smooth texture as you gently toss it in your hand.
- Slowly inhale the rich aroma.
- Take the smallest bite that you can and extract as much taste as possible. This first bite coats the palate.
- Now take a larger bite. Feel how it melts from a solid to a liquid in your mouth.
- Savor the creamy feel of the chocolate and the intense flavor as it melts at precisely body temperature.
- Swallow and enjoy the lingering aftertaste.
- Prolong the pleasure by slowly sipping a cup of warm water. It fills you up and cleanses the palate so you will not want to eat more.

research shows that you're more likely to be overweight than if your diet contains a big variety of fruits and vegetables.

Plan indulgences. Whether your passion is chocolate or cheesecake, give yourself permission to eat simply for pleasure. And do it without guilt. Kembel suggests allotting 300 calories per day for a special treat that satisfies your cravings.

"We all want something special," Kembel says. "The tricky but essential part of this strategy is to be scrupulously honest in buying no more than 300-calorie portions of that food, one portion at a time."

Once you understand that almost every day, you really can have a food that pleases and satisfies you, some of your excessive cravings for that food will subside.

Don't use food as a substitute. The next time you feel hungry, consider whether it's food that you really want. Eating is a fast, easy way to feel good. Perhaps you're feeling emotionally hungry, and another type of sensory pleasure would be more satisfying—having companionship, going for a scenic walk, listening to relaxing music, taking a soothing bath, or getting a massage.

"Food is an expedient comfort. It's the only touch that we may get," Kembel says. "We have to learn ways to hug and hold ourselves without using food. If we could suck our thumbs and hold our blankets, we'd be better off."

The Physiology of Pleasure: Why Food Tastes So Good

LONG BEFORE HUMAN BEINGS KNEW A THING ABOUT GRAMS OF FAT AND CALORIES, FOOD PYRAMIDS AND WEEKLY SUPERMARKET SPECIALS, OUR HIGHLY EVOLVED SENSES OF TASTE AND SMELL TOLD US WHAT TO EAT.

"How good something tasted was a pretty good indication of whether it was good for you," says Dr. James J. Kenney of the Pritikin Longevity Center.

A sweet tooth guided our ancestors to ripe fruit, a steady source of nutrients and energy. A taste for fatty foods, like nuts, seeds, and salmon—a rich source of calories and vitamins—helped tide them over in winter.

Considered by some to be the most pleasurable of the five senses, taste still determines what we choose to eat and drink. And if broccoli tasted as good as ice cream, maybe we could rely on our innate appetite for pleasure to guide us to a healthy diet.

But we live in a world of overabundant, ready-made food that's formulated specifically to titillate our lust for sweets and fat. That simple rule—if it tastes good, eat it—simply doesn't apply anymore.

How can we turn nature around in our favor? "Paradoxically, by paying more attention to the flavor of what we eat," says Kaiser Permanente Medical Center's Dr. David Sobel in his book *The Healthy Mind, Healthy Body Handbook.* "If we really savor every bite, we're likely to eat less but enjoy it more."

A Taste of Pleasure

What we think of as taste is really a combination of taste and smell. Located mostly on the tongue, tastebuds are sensitive to four basic qualities in food: salt, bitter, sour, and sweet. Some experts also add a fifth that the Japanese call *unami,* which roughly translates into "wonderful taste." It elicits a sensation often described as brothy, meaty, or savory.

Most of what we perceive as the actual flavor of food comes from the aroma—the result of volatile food molecules wafting back up to our nasal passageway while we're chewing and swallowing.

Researchers estimate that our sense of smell is 4,000 times more sensitive than our sense of taste. In fact, 80 percent of a particular flavor depends on information from the olfactory receptors located in the top of our noses.

Not convinced? Take three different flavors of jelly beans and eat them one at a time while you're pinching your nostrils shut, says Marcia Pelchat, Ph.D., a sensory psychologist at Monell Chemical Senses Center in Philadelphia. With air flow to the nose blocked, all of the jelly beans will taste the same—sweet.

"Then let go of your nostrils, and all of a sudden, you get a huge burst of flavor," says Dr. Pelchat. "The brain combines the taste and smell information, and you have flavor."

When asked the secret of how you can add pleasure to your diet while still losing weight, Dr. John La Puma of the CHEF (Cooking, Healthy Eating, and Fitness) Clinic, replied emphatically: "Flavor. Flavor. Flavor. Cook new and familiar foods with little fat but a lot of flavor."

So if you've always thought that losing weight meant giving up great-tasting foods, cheer up. The truth is that great taste is actually one of the secrets to successful weight loss.

Your best bet for foods that are low in calories but high in flavor are low-fat, simple versions of soups, stews, chili, pasta and rice dishes, stir-fries, baked potatoes, fruits, steamed vegetables, and salads.

But doesn't tasty food cause you to overeat? "No," says Dr. Kenney. "Research in both animals and people clearly shows that they don't eat more calories simply because their food tastes better."

Five Fascinating Olfactory Facts

1. A person with a healthy sense of smell can detect as many as 10,000 different odors.

2. Women tend to have a keener sense of smell than men, and it's more acute during ovulation.

3. Your sense of smell is heightened when you're hungry.

4. Odor perception peaks around age 40.

5. You have a dominant nostril, just as you have a dominant hand. If you're right-handed, your right nostril will be more sensitive because of greater nerve sensitivity on that side.

Here's how to punch up flavor without adding calories or fat.

Expand your tastebuds. Approach food with a sense of adventure, says Dr. La Puma. Compared to our ancestors, we actually eat fewer foods—only about 50 animal and 600 plant species out of the thousands that hunter-gatherers are believed to have hunted and gathered.

Add more flavor and fun to your meals by trying a variety of never-before-tasted foods. Every time you go to the grocery store, buy a vegetable, fruit, or seasoning that you've never tried before.

Add taste, not fat. Cook new foods and old favorites with little fat but lots of flavor, says Dr. La Puma. Toss a few spicy peppers into soups and sauces. Chop fresh herbs for pasta and pizza. Splash balsamic or fruit-flavored vinegars over salads and vegetables. Mix concentrated anchovy, sun-dried tomato, onion, or wasabi paste into stir-fries or marinades.

Warm up to your food. Not too hot and not too cold—Baby Bear's porridge tasted just right. Warm food transmits more vapors to the smell-sensing cells in the back of the nose, making it easier to taste, Dr. Pelchat says.

Also, the tongue's sensitivity to some flavors is affected by the temperature of the food. Heat will increase the intensity of sweet or bitter flavors, while cold will reduce it. On the other hand, salt flavor can intensify in a food that is seasoned when warm and then served cold.

Ride in the fat-mobile. Fat is the carrier of flavor. So get the most out of oils and cheeses by choosing the highest-flavor, highest-quality ones, such as sesame and olive oils and Greek or Bulgarian feta cheese. You'll need less and won't feel deprived.

"Fat is the transportation, but I discovered flavor doesn't have to ride on an 18-wheeler," says Don Mauer, author of *Lean and Lovin' It* and *The Guy's Guide to Great Eating.*

Prepare a feast for the eyes. Food that looks better seems to taste better, says Karen Teff, Ph.D., a researcher at Monell Chemical Senses Center in Philadelphia. Studies suggest that attractively presented food may also trigger physiological responses that increase the number of calories you burn.

Decorate your plate by serving a palette of colors, textures, and flavors. And switch from one dish to another often, alternating sweet and sour or crunchy and smooth.

Take a hands-on approach. Pick up your food and eat it. Having food right under your nose draws more odor molecules up to smell receptors, intensifying flavor.

"Also, it's just more fun to hold food in your hands and eat it," Dr. Pelchat says. "Maybe that's why we love cheeseburgers so much."

Take Your Time

We approach meals at the same breathless pace at which we go through life. Thoughtlessly and automatically, we wolf down food while we're working at our desks, driving our cars, watching television, or talking on the phone.

"Eating is the most sensual experience next to sex. Why are so many of us in such a hurry to get it over with?" asks behavioral counselor Julie Waltz Kembel of Canyon Ranch spa. "We rush through dinner, and our fangs are still hanging down to our toenails when we're done. So we go to the refrigerator. We're looking for something—pleasure. The problem is, we're out of pleasure too fast."

To eat less and enjoy it more, first you have to slow down. Think of how you eat an ice cream cone. Each lick is pleasurable. A cone lasts twice as long as a dish, and it's more fun to eat.

"It's not the volume of food you eat but the length of time you take to eat it that satisfies your innate appetite for pleasure," says Kembel.

Pause for a moment and switch gears before you take your first bite. Take a deep breath, then think for a moment or just settle yourself. And follow these tips.

Chew slowly and thoroughly. People who overeat chew their food less, says Dr. Teff. And by hurriedly gulping their food, they also get less flavor and fewer nutrients. Chewing releases flavor molecules and forces odors into the nasal cavity. The longer the food is in your mouth, the more flavor you'll experience.

Downsize your spoon. Use smaller, baby-size utensils to take smaller bites. Smaller mouthfuls make your meal last longer, says Kembel. If you don't have small utensils, just dip the tip of your spoon into the food. If you're eating a sandwich, hold your fingers very close to the edge. You'll be forced to take smaller bites or run the risk of chomping on your own finger.

Put it down and back away slowly. Put down your fork, your sandwich, your chicken leg—whatever—until you have completely chewed and swallowed the food in your mouth, advises Kembel. If you have to pick the food up before you take another bite, you won't eat as fast.

Dive in. Choose foods that require effort to eat, says Kembel. Shellfish (still in their shells), artichokes, and corn on the cob take longer to eat simply because you have to work a little harder to get a bite of food.

When you order Asian food, be adventurous and learn how to use the chopsticks that come with the meal. Order entrées that require some type of assembly, such as fajitas, but leave off the high-fat sour cream and cheese.

Take a break. Once or twice during the meal, stop eating. This will help you break your eating rhythm and slow down your pace, says Kembel.

Dim the lights. Lower lighting promotes relaxation and helps to slow eating. "Just look at the bright lights in a fast-food restaurant, where the pace is hurried, and contrast that with the atmosphere of a more formal restaurant, where dim lighting and leisurely eating enhance pleasure," observes Kembel.

Heat it up. Eat hot soup, hot potatoes, hot tea or coffee. Whether you have to sip it slowly or blow on each bite before you pop it in your mouth, hot food slows you down, Kembel says.

Mind Your Mouth

You've jazzed up your plate with flavorful food. And you've taken time to savor each bite. But you're wondering: "How is this going to help me lose weight?" By taking it one step further and letting your tastebuds, not your stomach, tell you when it's time to stop eating.

You may have heard weight-loss experts recommend that you wait 20

It's a Bird . . . It's a Plane . . . It's Supertaster

Grapefruit juice make you gag? Rather starve than eat even one Brussels sprout? You may be a supertaster. Some people inherit an enhanced sensitivity to certain bitter compounds. If so, you may tend to avoid strong-tasting foods such as broccoli, spinach, and kale.

To find out if you're a supertaster, do this test, suggests Adam Drewnowski, Ph.D., a researcher at the University of Michigan in Ann Arbor. Dip a cotton swab in blue food coloring and paint the surface of your tongue. Check your tongue in the mirror. If it's mostly blue with occasional pink dots, you probably have normal tasting ability. If you see many pink tastebuds grouped closely together, chances are that you're a supertaster, he explains.

About a quarter of the population are supertasters, most of them women. Another quarter, called nontasters, have fewer tastebuds than average.

"Being a supertaster is a normal genetic variation, like blue eyes," says Dr. Marcia Pelchat of Monell Chemical Senses Center. "You shouldn't view being a nontaster as a tastebud deficit. We don't say people with blue eyes have a pigment deficit."

If you're a supertaster who can't stand to eat your vegetables, Dr. Pelchat recommends a pinch of salt. The sodium ion in salt is a potent suppressor of many bitter taste components.

minutes after eating your prescribed portions for your stomach to tell your brain that it's satisfied. Sounds reasonable, in theory.

But when you're feeling famished, it's easy to consume way too many calories before your brain and your stomach decide to talk to each other. You need a faster way to know when you've had enough.

"Satiety starts at the point of entry—the mouth," says John Poothullil, M.D., a physician at the Brazo Sport Memorial Hospital in Lake Jackson, Texas, who is researching the role of taste and smell in weight maintenance.

Hunger is linked to our need for nutrients, not our need for energy, theorizes Dr. Poothullil. As you eat, receptors in the mouth and nasal cavity not only tell you how good something tastes but also register the intake of nutrients. Our signal that we have had enough of a good thing is the moment when food starts to lose its flavor.

It happens to all of us every time we eat more than one bite of food. Flavor is most intense when you first start eating, and then it begins to fade. You can taste the chocolate and the cream filling on the first Oreo. By the third, all you taste is sweet.

"This is nature's way of telling you that you have had enough. Do not wait until a food is unpleasant," Dr. Poothullil says.

When Dr. Poothullil tested his innovative idea on a group of women with elevated cholesterol levels, all of the women lost significant amounts of weight in the first month, and most were able to maintain the loss for at least a year. The group was told to eat what they desired when they were hungry. Then they were instructed to eat slowly, chew thoroughly, and stop eating as soon as the pleasantness of flavor subsided.

"The study shows that taste and smell sensations can help you regulate food intake," he says. "But we still don't have a complete picture of what normal-weight people are doing right."

You can use the same three-step technique to enhance your own weight-loss efforts. It's an easy-to-learn skill that you can use whether you're eating out in an elegant restaurant, picking up some burgers for a quick lunch, or sitting down to Thanksgiving dinner.

- Eat slowly.
- Chew thoroughly.
- When the pleasantness of the flavor subsides, stop eating.

Eating and Emotions: The Link between Food and Mood

YOU'VE NO DOUBT NOTICED IT. YOU SIT DOWN, FINALLY, TO DO YOUR INCOME TAXES, AND SUDDENLY, YOU'VE REMATERIALIZED IN THE KITCHEN AND INHALED A HANDFUL OF M&M'S. OR YOU'RE AT HOME AT NIGHT CHANNEL SURFING, WHEN THAT BOWL OF SALTED NUTS ON THE COFFEE TABLE JUMPS RIGHT DOWN YOUR THROAT.

Or you're making a mandatory appearance at some family function, nodding politely as Aunt Agatha tells you about her arthritis. What you really want to do is scream. Instead, you bulldoze your way down the buffet table.

All of us turn to food at least once in a while to satisfy emotional needs. We eat as a comforting distraction when we're anxious, bored, lonely, angry, or caught up in a whole mix of confusing feelings, says Edward Abramson, Ph.D., professor of psychology at California State University in Chico and author of *Emotional Eating: What You Need to Know Before Starting Another Diet.*

"Eating can improve your mood, although why that's so is open to some speculation," he says. "Whether it's entirely physical or it's psychological with a physical component is not entirely clear, but eating does tend to soothe emotional upsets for a lot of folks."

One theory states that an overeater who craves carbohydrate-rich foods when depressed or anxious, for instance, may be attempting to increase brain levels of serotonin, a naturally occurring substance that regulates mood, notes Richard Atkinson, M.D., professor of medicine and nutritional sciences at the University of Wisconsin at Madison.

Through a series of natural chemical reactions in the body, carbohydrates allow more of the amino acid tryptophan to enter the brain, causing more serotonin to be released and thus relieving negative moods. Some antidepressants work in the same way.

Research also suggests that, in animals at least, stress hormones fuel the consumption of sugar.

But most emotional eating doesn't involve craving a specific food. "Emotion provokes an undifferentiated food craving, and any palatable food will do," says Dr. Abramson. Unfortunately, *palatable* usually translates into *sugary* or *fatty*.

Emotional eating is far more likely to occur as snacking, nibbling, or binge eating rather than as a full meal. It's also more likely to occur from midafternoon on, when your energy level is low if you haven't eaten since lunch. Morning and early afternoon are "safer" periods if you're an emotional eater, Dr. Abramson says, since you have breakfast and lunch to sustain you.

Emotional eating is okay to do once in a while. We all do it. It has a big downside, though, if it becomes your modus operandi. You can gain weight because you are overeating. You can feel guilt and shame about enjoying food.

And you can develop an empty, never-satisfied feeling because you are not experiencing your true feelings. Your needs for love, passion, independence, self-confidence, achievement, freedom, or a sense of belonging are not being truly satisfied, Dr. Abramson says.

Plus, if you're trying to lose weight, sooner or later you're going to have to learn to deal with emotional upsets without using food, says Madelyn H. Fernstrom, Ph.D., director of the Weight Management Center at the University of Pittsburgh Medical Center.

"If you don't, the inevitable emotional upsets will also upset your diet," she warns. One study of dieters in a University of Pittsburgh Medical Center weight-loss program found that almost half of the relapses happened while

Why Antidepressants Help Some People Lose Weight

Get happy! Lose weight!

In studies, two popular antidepressants, fluoxetine (Prozac) and sertraline (Zoloft), have been shown to help some people lose weight. Both are selective serotonin reuptake inhibitors (SSRIs). That means they help brighten your mood by keeping more of the neurotransmitter serotonin available in your brain.

Serotonin also apparently plays a role in regulating food intake, body weight, and energy expenditure, says Dr. Richard Atkinson of the University of Wisconsin.

Both of these drugs can help people lose weight, at least initially, probably by reducing appetite and enhancing a sense of satiety, he says. "At 6 months, the weight loss looks good for many people."

But after that, something happens. "How it works is not at all clear, but people obviously develop a tolerance to these drugs. So by the end of a year, most have regained their lost weight," he adds.

A doctor may use Prozac in combination with phentermine (the "safe" part of the old fen-phen combination), hoping to overcome this tolerance problem. But not enough research has been done with this combination to know yet whether it is safe or effective in the long term, Dr. Atkinson says.

"This use is very experimental, and patients need to be followed very closely if they are using it," he says. "There's still no magic bullet for weight loss."

the dieter was experiencing a negative emotion—most often anxiety, followed by feelings of depression or anger.

Seeing the role that negative emotions can play in weight-loss failures, and realizing that weight loss itself can cause emotional arousal, can help you devise strategies to get around this major roadblock. Here's how.

Take 10—better yet, 20. Next time you feel an irresistible craving, pause for a few minutes. If you can ride out the initial urgency, you may be able to resist the craving, since it usually lasts less than 20 minutes, Dr. Abramson says. If not, the food will still be there.

And while you're waiting, ask yourself what you are feeling. "What emotions did you feel before you started craving the food? Are you tense or stressed? Bored? Angry? Lonely? Sad? See if you can find the feeling beneath the craving," Dr. Abramson says. "Don't worry if you can't define it exactly, just get a general sense of how you are feeling."

Then try to figure out why you feel this way. Did someone do something to hurt your feelings? Are you alone? Are you anticipating something in the near future that has you worried? Did someone treat you unfairly? Once the source of the feeling is clarified, the craving usually becomes less urgent.

Eating something about every 4 hours works for a lot of people.

Chart it. This is yet another reason to keep a food diary that notes when and where you ate something and your mood. Answer the question "What was I feeling when I decided to eat this?" Write it down when it happens—your memory can trick you.

Keep a food diary for at least a week, and then, see if you can discern patterns in times, places, and feelings that trigger eating, Dr. Abramson says. This will help you make sense of your own food-mood connections.

Slow down and savor the experience. When you eat, ask yourself: "Am I hungry?" If you can't answer yes, chances are pretty good that you're experiencing emotional eating, Dr. Fernstrom says.

"People tend to eat until they're stuffed, until they can't eat another bite," she says. "We need to learn to tune in to the earlier signals of satiety—contentment and satisfaction." Eating more slowly and savoring food helps this process.

Create the mood without the food. Find other ways besides food to reward yourself, Dr. Fernstrom recommends. Certainly, the self-esteem you gain by learning more about yourself as you explore the food-mood connection is one reward.

But you can also use creative and spiritual endeavors, relationships, and other stress-relieving, pleasurable activities to help you feel good without food, she says. Aerobic exercise, especially, can be a potent ally in this regard, since it triggers a release of feel-good neurotransmitters.

Eat early and often. People in the midst of changing the way they eat are more likely to be highly emotional and to lapse into emotional eating than people who aren't trying to lose weight. One way to get around this is to avoid getting so hungry that your brain's cognitive control is short-circuited, Dr. Fernstrom says.

Don't eat so little at breakfast and lunch, for instance, that you pig out at night. "Eating something about every 4 hours—three meals and one planned snack—works for a lot of people," she says.

Plan ahead. If it's not in the refrigerator or the house when you want it, are you willing to go out for it? Lots of us don't want it that badly, or at least, having to make the decision gives us some time to reconsider, Dr. Fernstrom says.

Keep healthier alternatives handy, such as V8 or tomato juice, broths, low-fat popcorn, graham crackers, frozen bananas, and ice pops. If you're going out for dinner, have some idea in mind of what you'll order before you get there. If you can't stick with the program, don't go there.

Are Some Foods Really Addictive?

Remember that "bet you can't eat just one" commercial? The food in question was a particular brand of potato chip—thin, crisp, salty. Just hearing the crunch was enough to send TV viewers scurrying to the kitchen cupboard.

Many of us are "dietetically challenged" by particular foods—chocolate, ice cream, pizza, chips, you name it. We might believe that we are better off avoiding these foods altogether rather than trying to "eat just one."

Dietitians call these trigger foods—foods that seem to have the power to set us off on an eating frenzy that doesn't stop until the bag is empty or we pass out.

But are any foods truly addictive? Besides alcohol, which everyone agrees can be addictive, there's no consensus. A few foods do contain substances that have the potential for addiction. Coffee and cola, for example, contain caffeine. And chocolate contains small amounts of mood-altering chemicals, including phenylethylamine, which has a chemical structure similar to a well-known addictive substance: amphetamine.

But it's possible that some other foods not normally considered addictive may affect our brain chemistry in a manner similar to addictive substances such as amphetamine or cocaine, says Seema Bhatnagar, Ph.D., assistant professor of psychology at the University of Michigan in Ann Arbor. This has not been demonstrated, however.

Take sugar, for instance. In animals, sugar helps to reduce high levels of stress hormones, so it helps them cope better with stressful situations. What's more, high levels of stress hormones induce animals to eat more sugar than normal, which makes them fat. "Whether the same is true in humans has yet to be proven, but it's common knowledge that lots of people say that they

Living Proof
PANEL

How Sweet It Is

John Reeser

Just recognizing that I'm not really hungry, that I don't need it, and that I will feel worse in an hour or so if I eat it now makes a big difference in resisting it.

I'm talking about sweets, my major dietary weakness. My tendency is to head for the cookies and candy bars after lunch at work and after dinner at home, especially if I've had a stressful day.

Now I've learned to stop and think before I eat. Just that act of taking a moment to ask 'Am I hungry? Do I really want to eat this?' is often enough for me to back away from unnecessary eating.

I drink a lot of water now, and it really does fill me up and reduce my cravings.

crave sugar when they are under stress," says Elizabeth Bell, Ph.D., a postdoctoral researcher at the University of California at San Francisco.

People who belong to Overeaters Anonymous, for instance, list sugar and refined carbohydrates as the foods they are most likely to find necessary to avoid altogether. And a whole slew of books aim to cure the weight woes of carbohydrate "addicts."

Still, cravings—even so-called addictions—don't necessarily have to leave us powerless over food.

"Even most people addicted to alcohol can learn ways to control their intake," says Dr. Fernstrom. "Don't be a food victim. Don't think, 'My brain made me do it. My metabolism made me do it.' That is not correct thinking."

Instead, learn to exercise conscious control around your own personal trigger foods. Here are some strategies that can help.

Avoid a "sugar cycle." If you eat a lot of refined sugar at one time, your blood sugar levels first go high, then plummet, perhaps lower than they were before you ate. And that's bad because low blood sugar levels can trigger more eating.

You're better off eating a snack with a mix of protein, some carbohydrates, and perhaps a bit of fat, like low-fat yogurt or low-fat cheese and wheat crackers. Unrefined carbohydrates—those with a high percentage of fiber, both soluble and insoluble, such as fruit or oatmeal—also stabilize blood sugar better than white sugar or white bread. The fiber slows down the rate of absorption of carbohydrates, which keeps blood sugar and insulin levels from spiking.

Moderate fat. Researchers have found that the body's level of galanin, a chemical produced by the brain that has been linked to a craving for fat, is actually increased by fat intake. So, if you eat a fatty lunch, you will be more tempted to eat more fat throughout the day.

When it comes to alcohol, know thyself. Alcohol tends to loosen inhibitions and can make you overeat. Some people can fit one drink into a meal with no problems. Others will find, however, that sticking with club soda helps them stay in control better, says Dr. Fernstrom.

Figure out what you need to get your fix. Trigger foods are best avoided altogether, Dr. Fernstrom says. But instead of depriving yourself, experiment to come up with a "safe" food that will satisfy the same craving. If you have a chocolate craving, for instance, a Tootsie Pop or frozen fudge bar might suffice. "It's very individual," she says. "One person's Hershey's Kiss can be a real lifesaver, and for someone else it can mean they will eat the whole bag."

Week One

Getting Started

Before

After

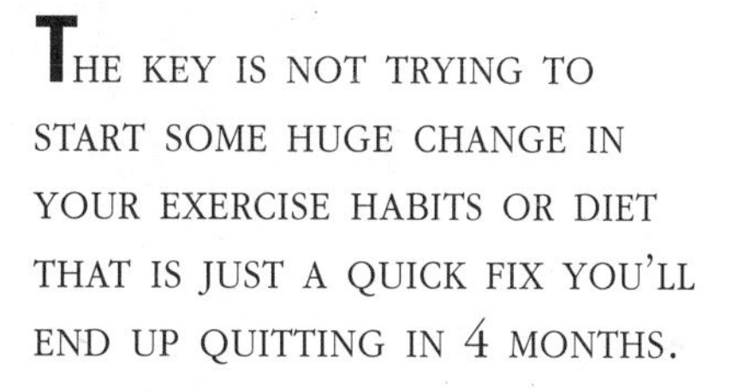

THE KEY IS NOT TRYING TO START SOME HUGE CHANGE IN YOUR EXERCISE HABITS OR DIET THAT IS JUST A QUICK FIX YOU'LL END UP QUITTING IN 4 MONTHS.

—John Reeser

Week One

You've written down your goals in your weight-loss diary. You've been collecting some healthy yet appetizing recipes and are making an effort to buy more fresh fruits and vegetables. And your exercise clothes are folded on the chair, ready for action. Finally, the date you set to embark on your weight-loss plan has arrived. But how do you begin?

The best way to start a weight-loss program is to ease into it, literally taking one step at a time. Chances are, you've been away from regular physical activity for a while. So first take the fitness test in this section to determine what shape you're in. Then read on and discover how you can quickly and easily strengthen your muscles by walking a few days a week and doing some stretches. Plus, you'll be introduced to the first goal in The *Prevention* Get Thin, Get Young Plan: mastering portion control.

Three Simple Steps to Starting a Fitness Program

FOR MOST FOLKS, THE HARDEST PART ABOUT STARTING A FITNESS PROGRAM IS SIMPLY GETTING STARTED. THAT'S BECAUSE THEY GO INTO IT AS THOUGH IT WERE AN ARRANGED MARRIAGE. THEY DREAD THE THOUGHT OF DRAGGING THEMSELVES THROUGH ACTIVITIES THAT THEY DON'T REALLY ENJOY—DAY IN AND DAY OUT FOR THE REST OF THEIR LIVES.

The truth is, if you start out right, your exercise program can be a longtime love affair that keeps you glowing for years to come. But first, forget almost everything you've learned about exercise.

"In the past, we've made starting to exercise a daunting task," says Joyce A. Hanna, associate director of the health improvement program at Stanford University and an exercise physiologist in Palo Alto, California. "We made people get medical signatures, monitor their heart rates, take fitness tests, and so on. No wonder no one wanted to get started."

Do You Need a Doc's Okay?

Most healthy folks can roll right into a gentle fitness plan without checking with their doctors, says exercise physiologist Joyce A. Hanna of Stanford University. But if you've had health problems, you really should talk to your doctor before starting. You can use the following list as a guide, marking the items that apply to you.

__You have a heart condition and have been advised to do only medically supervised physical activities.

__During or right after exercise, you frequently have pains or pressure in the left side of your chest or neck or in your left shoulder or arm.

__You have developed chest pain within the past month.

__You sometimes lose consciousness or fall over because you're dizzy.

__You feel unusually breathless after mild exertion.

__You're taking medication for your blood pressure or a heart condition, or you have other physical problems, such as insulin-dependent diabetes.

__You have bone or joint problems that may get worse from physical activity.

__You are middle-aged or older and have not been physically active before, and you're planning a relatively vigorous exercise program.

If you've checked one or more items, see your doctor before you start. If none of these apply to you, then you can get started.

Courtesy of the American Heart Association, the British Columbia Ministry of Health, and the Department of National Health and Welfare in Canada.

Though some people should see their doctors before starting any kind of physical activity (see "Do You Need a Doc's Okay?"), for the most part, starting to exercise is no more difficult than putting down this book for 10 minutes and taking a quick walk around the block.

"Exercise doesn't have to be this big, long commitment that people think it is," says John Yetter, M.D., medical director at SSM Rehab Sports Medicine in St. Louis. "It should be about having some fun, like playing Frisbee with your kids or walking your dog through the park. We get to a point as adults where we get so tied up with the responsibilities of education, family, and career that we don't do these fun, active things anymore. Then we wake up one day and find that we can't button our pants, and we feel out of shape and old. It doesn't take more than 10 to 15 minutes—today—to break that cycle and start feeling younger and fitter again."

And it's never too late to start. Even people in their nineties can get stronger, improve their moods, and reduce their risk for serious illnesses by putting more activity into their daily lives.

Here are three simple ways to put your mind, body, and spirit in motion today.

Step 1: Jump-Start Your Mind

The biggest obstacle to a fit body is an unfit mindset. People often think that they are too old, too busy, or too out of shape to ever enjoy regular physical activity. So before working your body, you have to train your brain, says certified international lifestyle fitness expert Lynne Brick, owner of Brick Bodies Health Clubs in Baltimore. "Once your thoughts start moving in a younger, more energetic direction, your body will quickly follow."

Treat yourself like a friend. Your brain can be your best ally or your worst enemy when it comes to getting active. "Make a decision to make it your friend," says Brick. "Whenever you start thinking, 'I'm old, I'm uncoordinated, I'm out of shape,' stop and ask yourself if you would tolerate a friend talking to you that way. Chances are that you wouldn't. Well, don't tolerate it from yourself either. Be encouraging, as a friend should be. Tell yourself, 'Okay, I'm not where I want to be, but I have the ability to make myself better.'"

Don't make it a project. Once we become responsible adults, there is a tendency to become project-oriented—to make everything seem like a big deal, says Michael Gilewski, Ph.D., a clinical psychologist for post-acute care services at Cedars-Sinai Medical Center in Los Angeles. "We make all these big decisions, like buying a car, switching jobs, or moving to a new home, that take detailed planning. Exercise isn't like that, yet many folks treat it the same way," he says. "Instead of making exercise yet another project, look at it as a *break* from your projects. Don't wait for the right time. You don't have to have all the right information or the right clothes. Just take a break right now and go do something."

Make Your Goals REAL

Setting goals is a great way to kick off a new fitness program. But many people choose goals that are somewhat fuzzy, like "I want to get in shape." This type of goal is tough to measure, so you'll never be sure if you're succeeding, says fitness expert Lynne Brick of Brick Bodies Health Clubs.

When you're setting goals, she recommends using a mental checklist called REAL. This means making goals that are:

R*ealistic.* If you're just getting started, don't expect to run 5 miles tomorrow. Instead, make it your goal to walk briskly for 20 minutes, 4 days a week, followed by longer sessions the following week.

E*xplicit.* Be very specific about the goals you want to achieve. Tell yourself, for example, "I want to lower my body fat 5 percent by the end of the year." This is much more explicit—and motivating—than just telling yourself, "I want to lose weight."

A*ctionable.* Big goals are daunting. That's why it's often best to break down your "real" goal into smaller, actionable parts. For example, if your goal is to run a 5-K (about 3 miles), mentally break it down into ½- or ¼-mile increments. Achieving the parts makes it much easier to stay motivated for the whole.

L*ivable.* Exercise is something you'll spend the rest of your life doing. So your goals should make you feel good, not miserable. Don't waste time forcing yourself to do things you don't enjoy. Find activities that you truly like. That way, you'll always be motivated to keep doing them.

Stop "working" out. Exercise will never be fun if you think of it as work, says Laura Senft, a registered physical therapist at the Kessler Institute for Rehabilitation in West Orange, New Jersey. "Exercise shouldn't be work or drudgery. It should be fun and invigorating, more like play. So think of it as a play break for your mind, not a punishment session for your body."

Turn off the TV. The number one reason people give for not starting an exercise program is that they don't have the time. Don't believe it. "We all have the time—it all depends on how we use it," says Michael Bourque, certified personal trainer and personal training coordinator for the Center for Health and Wellness of the Central Florida YMCA in Oviedo.

"Sit down and figure out all that you do in a day," he says. "That includes eating, sleeping, working, and miscellaneous activities. Inevitably, you'll find 2 to 3 hours that are unaccounted for. You can use that time to start an exercise program."

Promise yourself just 15 seconds. For some people, the idea of doing something physical for 45 minutes—or even 15 minutes—feels overwhelming. If that's the case, then promise yourself that you'll take just 15 seconds, says Al Secunda, author of *Ultimate Tennis* and *The 15-Second Principle*. "You can do anything for 15 seconds. Promise yourself you'll do just 15 seconds' worth of abdominal crunches or 15 seconds' worth of squats," he says. "Some days that may be all you do, and that's great. But most days, once you move for that 15 seconds, you'll find yourself revved up enough to do more."

Step 2: Ready . . . Set . . . Go Slow!

One sure way to burn out on physical activity and end up feeling older rather than younger is to start out of the gate too quickly. It's important to ease into any activity. This allows your muscles to feel energized rather than wiped out and your mind to be invigorated rather than fatigued.

Rebuild your mind-body connection. Within your body, there are physical "memories"—of running around, riding a bike, or playing hopscotch. But for most of us, these memories get buried beneath years of inactivity. "You can tap into them again by building up your activity level day by day," says Dr. Gilewski. "Today, go for a simple walk or ride around the neighborhood. It might feel a little awkward at first, but your body will start to remember what to do—and you'll be feeling great. Stop there, then go a little farther tomorrow. By the end of the month, you'll be back into the swing of things," he says. "In a few months, your body will think of exercise as a normal part of the day, and you'll start to crave it."

Warm up, cool down. Diving into any activity full blast puts undue strain on your muscles and tendons, and this almost guarantees that you'll stop your fitness program before it really gets going. Even if you're in the mood for a brisk jaunt around the park, start at a moderate pace for a few minutes, then pick up your speed, says Brick. Likewise, don't stop dead in your tracks when you're done. Slow to an easy walk and cool down before you stop.

Get comfortable. "You won't stay active very long if your feet hurt, you're overheated, or you're too cold," Dr. Gilewski says. "Try your new activity once or twice, then figure out what you need to be comfortable. If you're

Living Proof
PANEL

Changes We Can Live With

John Reeser

Getting started on this program hasn't been as hard for me as I thought it would be. And I think it's because my wife, Ana, and I have committed ourselves to making small changes that we can live with for the rest of our lives.

I got a large bottle to keep on my desk, so I would remember to drink water during the day. We've been buying more fruits and vegetables to include in our dinners and eating high-fiber cereals for breakfast so that we get more fiber into our diets.

Little changes like parking the car farther away from work, taking the stairs, and getting up a few minutes earlier in the morning to take a walk have been easy because they're not overwhelming commitments.

The best part is that it's working. Ana has lost weight, and my clothes are definitely looser. The key is not trying to start some huge change in your exercise habits or diet that is just a quick fix you'll end up quitting in 4 months, but rather making small adjustments in your daily habits that you can continue for a lifetime.

walking, for example, you should have comfortable walking shoes and clothes that keep you warm while letting your body breathe."

Step 3: Boost Your Spirit

No matter how psyched up you feel about an exciting new physical activity, you are bound to hit some lulls soon after starting. It's just human nature, says Paul Konstanty, clinical supervisor and exercise therapist at the University of California OrthoMed Spine and Joint Conditioning Center in San Diego. You can avoid hitting a serious exercise slump by planning some rewards to acknowledge your efforts, boost your spirits, and keep your activity fresh.

Treat yourself well. One of the best ways to stay motivated is to establish a reward system right off the bat, says Konstanty. "Promise yourself that if you are active so many days out of the upcoming month, you'll treat yourself to something nice. It could be a new pair of shoes or a night on the town," he says. "It'll give you something fun to look forward to, which is something we overlook all too often."

Plan some do-nothing days. Odd as it sounds, your fitness program will go longer and stronger if you occasionally blow it off and do nothing, says Dr. Gilewski. "Your muscles need days off now and then to recover," he says. "Giving yourself permission to take a day to lounge around will make your fitness program seem less like a job, and this will leave you feeling even more energized to go back to it the next day."

Shoot for something. Kids play games and sports for a reason—they're not only fun but also rewarding and motivating. You can tap into that same spirit by giving yourself a little goal to shoot for, says Brick. "Even something as simple as planning to walk in a 5-K for charity can be all the motivation you need to get out there and keep going."

Build yourself up. The fear of failure can be a huge barrier to your success in a fitness program. It's something we all face, no matter how old or young or confident we are, says exercise physiologist Robert Brosmer, vice president of health and wellness at the Central Florida YMCA in Orlando and coauthor of *Health and High Performance.*

"Fear of failing is especially daunting in the beginning, when maybe you don't feel as sure of your abilities as you'd like," he says. "A good way to beat down that fear is to build up your confidence. Make a list of all the difficult tasks in your life that you've accomplished—raising children, buying a home, getting a degree, and so on. Then, when you start to feel your confidence flagging, tell yourself, 'If I could accomplish those things, I'm sure I can accomplish this.'"

Fitness Test

How Fit Are You?

Being in shape means being able to enjoy daily life to the fullest. It means bounding up stairs, hustling down the block, and hoisting groceries without feeling tired or weak. What's the best way to get back in youthful shape? Exercise, of course. But it's a whole lot easier to reach your fitness goals if you know where to begin.

That's where fitness testing comes in. By taking a few simple fitness tests, you can find out where you've maintained your fitness over the years and what's fallen by the wayside. That way, you can tailor your fitness program to maintain what you have, improve what you don't, and start stepping confidently toward a fitter, stronger you.

Intimidated by the thought of taking a fitness test? Don't be. Unlike the ones you took in phys ed class, no one is watching or judging you. And the truth is, you're probably in better shape than you think.

"People often assume that because they're heavier than the models they see in magazines, they must be in terrible shape, but that's not usually true," says exercise physiologist Joyce A. Hanna of Stanford University. "Usually, folks find that they're a little weak in a couple of areas but pretty well off in others. It's very empowering to know where you rank against the norm and that with just a little effort, you can really improve."

The following tests will check important aspects of fitness such as flexibility, stamina, strength, and balance. Some of these are a little tough. Some are just fun. Take them all and see where you rank. Then try the suggestions for improvement and come back again in a month or two to try them again.

We bet that you will not only score higher the second time around but also start enjoying life a little more as everyday tasks get easier to do and you find yourself with energy to burn.

Fitness testing requires some exertion, but it should be fun, not taxing, says Carla Sottovia, a certified exercise physiologist at the Cooper Fitness Center in Dallas. Use common sense. As you would before starting a new exercise program, check with your doctor before trying these tests if you have health problems. If you've been inactive lately, don't try to do all of them at once. Rather, spread them out over a day or two. And don't push yourself past the point where you feel comfortable.

Can You Take a Bow?

Few of us think of flexibility when we think of fitness, but we should, says Michelle Edwards, a certified personal trainer and a health educator for the Cooper Institute for Aerobics Research in Dallas. "Tight, inflexible muscles make daily living harder. We stop being able to tie our shoes without sitting down. We're more likely to pull muscles and get injured. Flexible muscles just make you feel better."

THE TOE-TOUCH TEST

Stand with your feet shoulder-width apart.

Keep your legs straight (but don't lock your knees), bend over from your waist, and reach toward the floor.

Note how close your fingertips get to the ground.

Score Yourself

IF YOU REACHED . . .	YOUR SCORE IS . . .
The floor, palms down	Excellent
Your toes	Good
Your ankles	Fair
Above your ankles	Too tight

BEND BETTER

It takes only about 10 minutes a day to improve flexibility and make those muscles long and limber. Try the full-body stretch routine in Stretching Made Easy on page 93, and you'll be touching those toes in no time.

(continued)

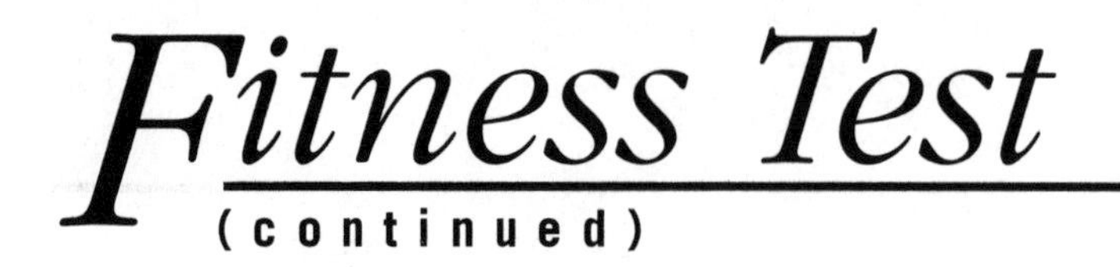

Fitness Test (continued)

Are You Strong to the Core?

Strong trunk, or "core," muscles such as your abdominals make everyday tasks easier to do, from vacuuming the floor to working long hours at a desk job, because they can support your body better. "Strong abdominal muscles are also important for helping prevent back pain," says Edwards. Here's how to test yours.

THE CURLUP TEST

Lie on your back with your knees bent and have someone hold your feet flat on the floor. Fully extend your arms down by your sides, with your palms down.

Set a timer or have someone time you for 1 minute.

Do as many curlups as you can. For a curlup to count, you have to move both hands forward 3 inches along the floor by flexing your torso, then lower yourself back down so that your shoulders touch the floor. Keep your head in line with your back throughout the exercise.

Score Yourself

MEN

RATING	NUMBER OF CURLUPS				
	Age				
	18–29	**30–39**	**40–49**	**50–59**	**60+**
Excellent	>50	>45	>40	>35	>30
Good	30–50	22–45	21–40	18–35	15–30
Fair	<30	<22	<21	<18	<15

WOMEN

RATING	**Age**				
	18–29	**30–39**	**40–49**	**50–59**	**60+**
Excellent	>45	>40	>35	>30	>25
Good	25–45	20–40	18–35	12–30	11–25
Fair	<25	<20	<18	<12	<11

Source: Medicine and Science in Sports and Exercise, vol. 13, 1981.

BUILD A STRONGER CORE

The recipe for building a strong core starts with strong abdominal muscles. You can improve yours quickly and easily with a few of the exercises in Goal: A Taut Tummy on page 335. As a bonus, your tummy will feel thinner, too!

(continued)

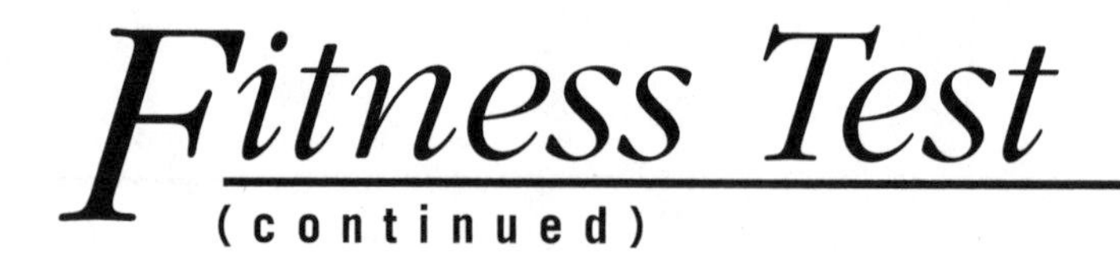

Your Upper-Body Oomph

"Americans are getting very, very weak in their upper bodies," says Hanna. Good upper-body strength makes all the fun stuff in life, like gardening and home projects, a whole lot easier, she says. "And it's particularly important for women to help prevent osteoporosis," she notes. Here's a quick way to check yours.

THE PUSHUP TEST

Get in a pushup position, with your legs bent so that you're supporting your weight with your hands and your knees. Your body should form a straight line from your head to your knees. (This is a modified pushup position for women, since they are built with less upper-body mass than men. Men can do pushups off their toes instead.)

Keeping your back straight, lower your chest until it's about 3 inches (the size of a fist) off the floor. Push back up. That's one pushup.

Set a timer or have someone time you, and do as many pushups as you can in 1 minute. (You can rest between repetitions if you need to, but only in the "up" position, not on the floor.)

Score Yourself

MEN

RATING	NUMBER OF PUSHUPS				
	Age				
	20–29	**30–39**	**40–49**	**50–59**	**60+**
Excellent	47–61	39–51	30–39	25–38	23–27
Good	37–46	30–38	24–29	19–24	18–22
Fair	29–36	24–29	18–23	13–18	10–17
Poor	22–28	17–23	11–17	9–12	6–9

WOMEN

	Age				
	20–29	**30–39**	**40–49**	**50–59**	**60+**
Excellent	36–44	31–38	24–32	21–30	15–19
Good	30–35	24–30	18–23	17–20	12–14
Fair	23–29	19–23	13–17	12–16	5–11
Poor	17–22	11–18	6–12	6–11	2–4

Source: The Fitness Specialist Manual. *© The Cooper Institute, Dallas. Revised 2000. Reprinted with permission.*

BUILD A BETTER UPPER BODY

The exercise you just did, pushups, is one of the best for building upper-body strength, says exercise physiologist and certified personal trainer Ann Marie Miller, fitness director of the New York Sports Clubs in Manhattan. Try doing two sets of 8 to 12 repetitions twice a week. For even stronger, shapelier arms, check out the exercises in Goal: Firm Arms on page 366.

(continued)

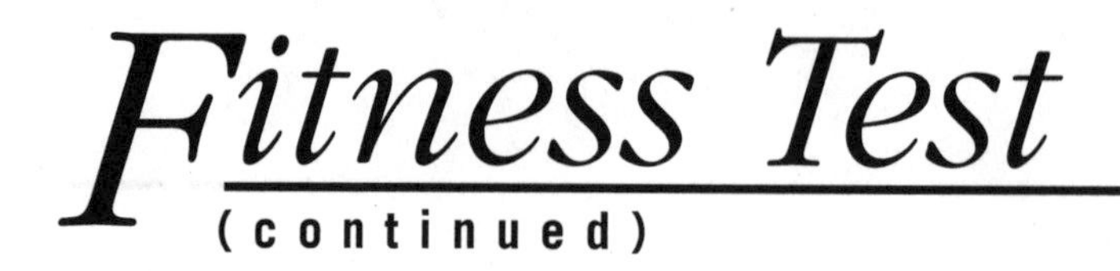

Your Best Balancing Act

Our balance often gets shakier as we get older, mostly because we stop using it, says Dr. John Yetter of SSM Rehab Sports Medicine. "All the running and jumping we do as kids requires a lot of balance. Staying active as adults can help us keep it. And that means fewer falls as we get older."

THE SINGLE-LEG STAND

Stand on your strongest leg (usually on the same side as your dominant hand).

Raise the opposite leg so that the knee is out in front of you, while keeping the knee of the supporting leg slightly bent. You can flex the raised knee about 30 degrees if that's more comfortable.

Keep your arms down by your sides and see how long you can balance.

Score Yourself

IF YOU BALANCED . . .	YOUR SCORE IS . . .
More than 30 seconds	Excellent
21–30 seconds	Good
11–20 seconds	Fair
10 or fewer seconds	Poor

BE BETTER BALANCED

Strong muscles build better balance, says Edwards. "Basic weight training to strengthen your legs, back, and torso can sharpen your balance and improve your strength dramatically." Try the 10 easy exercises in The Joy of Strength Training on page 135.

How's That Tiger in Your Tank?

With all the elevators and escalators, it's easy to lose those little bursts of power for bounding up stairs or striding up steep hills. But good anaerobic fitness (the kind of fitness you use for short bursts of speed and power) means that you can sprint for a bus and run up a flight of stairs without heaving for breath and feeling ready to drop.

"When you improve in this category, you really start feeling younger. You have spring in your step again," says Dr. Yetter.

THE STAIRCLIMB TEST

Walk up 30 to 40 steps (or walk up and run down a small flight of fewer steps several times) without stopping. You can hold the handrail if you need to.

Wait 60 seconds, then take your pulse for 10 seconds and multiply that number by 6. (It's easiest to take your pulse by lightly placing two fingers on the side of your neck.)

Score Yourself

IF YOUR PULSE WAS . . .	YOUR SCORE IS . . .
Less than 90	Excellent
90–100	Good
101–120	Fair
Above 120	Poor

POWER UP

Building stronger legs will help put more stride in your step. The step-ups exercise in Goal: Thinner Thighs on page 359 is a great place to start. Then add the other leg exercises from that chapter as you see fit.

(continued)

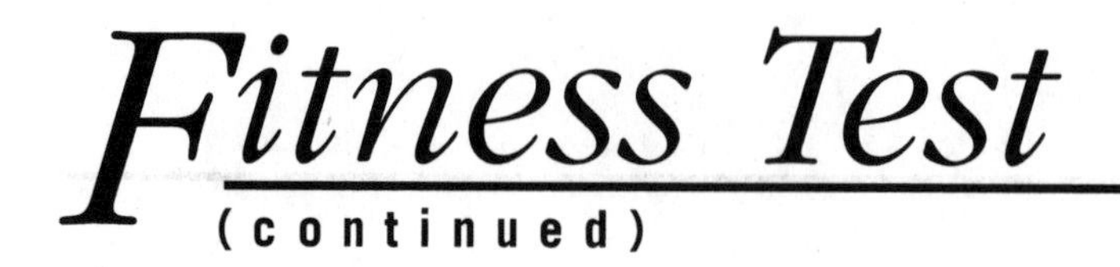

Can You Shop Till You Drop?

The walking test is one of the best tests of your aerobic fitness for everyday life. "You have to be able to walk to enjoy things like shopping and sightseeing," says Sottovia.

1-MILE WALK TEST

Map out a flat 1-mile course. (A ¼-mile walking track is ideal.) Warm up by walking leisurely for 3 to 5 minutes, then stretch gently. Note the time and begin walking quickly, without running, at a pace you can sustain for the entire course. Check the time at the finish, cool down, and stretch.

Score Yourself

MEN

RATING	TIME TO FINISH (min) Under 40	Over 40
Excellent	13:00 or less	14:00 or less
Good	13:01–15:30	14:01–16:30
Average	15:31–18:00	16:31–19:00
Below Average	18:01–19:30	19:01–21:30
Low	19:31 or more	21:31 or more

WOMEN

RATING	Under 40	Over 40
Excellent	13:30 or less	14:30 or less
Good	13:31–16:00	14:31–17:00
Average	16:01–18:30	17:01–19:30
Below Average	18:31–20:00	19:31–22:00
Low	20:01 or more	22:01 or more

Source: One Mile Walk Study conducted by William E. Oddon, Ph.D. Reprinted by permission of StayWell Health Management, Saint Paul, Minn.

DO THE WALK OF LIFE

For tips on walking, check out The Joy of Walking on page 104.

Stretching Made Easy

OF ALL THE EXERCISES YOU CAN DO TO STRENGTHEN MUSCLES, LOOK FIT, AND FEEL YOUNGER, STRETCHING IS BY FAR THE QUICKEST AND EASIEST. UNFORTUNATELY, IT'S ALSO THE MOST OVERLOOKED—AND THAT'S A SERIOUS MISTAKE.

Maybe we don't think about stretching because we never had to do it when we were kids. We just cartwheeled through life, never worrying about sore muscles or achy joints. But flexibility was one of the first things we lost when we traded in those cartwheels for car wheels. And losing that can make us look and feel older long before we should.

Some loss of flexibility is natural as we age, but the main cause of stiffness is simply a lack of movement, says Majid Ali, a certified fitness instructor in Los Angeles. "Our muscles become more calcified with disuse, so they're less pliable and not as responsive when we do try to move them," he explains.

Making matters worse is our sit-down society, says physical therapist Laura Senft of the Kessler Institute for Rehabilitation in West Orange, New Jersey. "Sitting all day in cars, at desks, at computers, and in front of the TV not only makes us overweight but also shortens our hip flexor muscles and rounds our shoulders, so we become stiff and hunched over."

Thankfully, we can reverse this process simply by stretching, says Joy Lynn Freeman, D.C., a chiropractor and stretching instructor in Prescott, Arizona, and author of *Express Yourself*. "Stretching makes your body more beautiful. You stand taller, appear slimmer, and move more freely when you stretch regularly. The more limber you are, the younger you feel. It's like a youth capsule."

Wringing Out the Waste

Of course, it isn't just the inactive among us who need to stretch. It's equally important when you're active and getting in shape. Exercising your muscles without stretching can actually make them tighter. And the tighter your muscles, the more prone they are to injury. You'll be much less likely to get hurt when you stretch regularly. As a bonus, stretching muscles after a good workout will help make them stronger and help prevent that postexercise soreness.

You stand taller and appear slimmer when you stretch regularly.

"A good postexercise stretch is like wringing out your muscles," says Dr. Freeman. Lactic acid and other cellular waste—the stuff that makes your muscles tender the day after a tough workout—are normal by-products of muscle use. "Stretching helps increase circulation through the muscles and flushes out those lingering waste materials," she explains.

Because stretching increases your range of motion, it also gives you a stronger stride when you walk, a more powerful swing when you play tennis, and more strength for everyday hobbies and activities, says Ali.

As if that weren't enough, stretching does more than make your muscles act and feel younger. They will look younger, too, giving you a taller, leaner appearance, says fitness expert Lynne Brick of Brick Bodies Health Clubs. In addition, the more you elongate them, the more elastic they become.

"Your muscles have memory," says Brick. "If the last thing you do is contract them with exercise, they'll stay shorter and tighter, which can potentially lead to injury the next time you exercise. But if you stretch after exercise, your lengthened muscles will help you begin your next exercise session with greater ease."

The Best Ways to Stretch

As with any exercise, it's important to stretch properly to get maximum benefits and to avoid injuring yourself. "Ironically, most people's biggest mistake is to make stretching harder than it has to be," says Dr. Freeman. Here are some guidelines for safe, healthy stretching.

Warm up. Always warm up for 5 to 10 minutes before stretching. Walk around and move your muscles a bit. Stretching muscles when they're "cold" can lead to strains and tears. "Think of your muscles as rubber bands," says Marti Currey, an exercise physiologist at the Methodist Healthcare Systems Institute for Preventive Medicine in Houston. "If you take a rubber band out of the refrigerator and try to stretch it, it'll probably crack. But if you warm it up, it will stretch nicely."

Breathe in rhythm. "Holding your breath while you stretch, as many people do, will tense you up and make the stretch more difficult," Ali says. "Stretching should be relaxing." He recommends taking a deep breath, then exhaling as you bend into your stretch. If you hold a stretch for more than 10 seconds, your breathing should be a cycle of slowly inhaling and exhaling.

Stretch slow and steady. People used to stretch with way too much exuberance—bobbing up and down and trying go a little bit farther with each bounce. You'll get the best results when you make your stretches slow and steady, says Currey. "Slowly stretch to the point of mild discomfort. Hold it there until the discomfort subsides. Then stretch a little farther if you are able."

Count to 30. It takes a little time for muscles to elongate and for blood to flow through the muscle tissue and the joints. You'll want to hold each stretch for 15 to 30 seconds, which is more than enough time to bring in nutrients and flush out wastes.

Always stretch after exercise. The best time to stretch is after you've finished exercising. "Your muscles are completely warmed up," says Brick. "And you need to take some time to cool down anyway. Stretching will help prevent blood from pooling in your extremities, which gives you that lightheaded feeling. And it'll help prevent muscle soreness."

A 10-Minute Plan for Total-Body Stretching

It won't take more than about 10 minutes a day to keep your muscles loose and limber. Here's a full-body routine that hits the major muscle groups most prone to tightening. If you have a favorite activity like golfing or bike riding, you may want to spend more time stretching the muscles you use in that particular sport. For the best results, try doing each stretch twice on the days that you exercise.

Neck Stretches

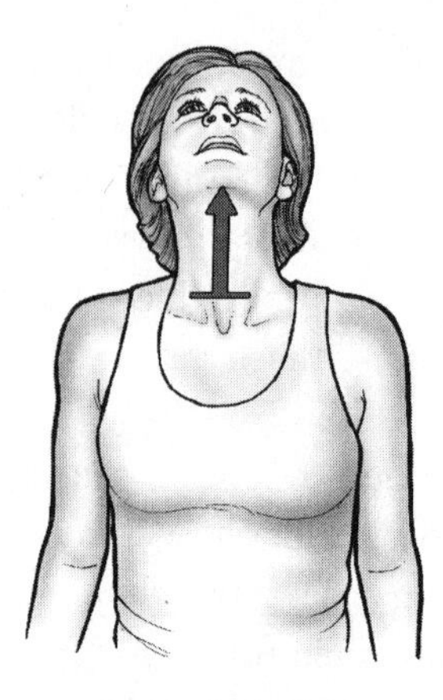

Sit or stand with your head facing forward. Slowly turn your head to the right as far as it will comfortably go. Hold for about 10 seconds. Then turn it to the left and hold. Return to the starting position.

Next, keeping your upper body straight, slowly drop your head, tucking your chin into your chest until you feel a mild pull. Hold for about 10 seconds. Then slowly tilt your head upward until you are looking straight up. (Do not rest the back of your head against your shoulders.) Hold for 10 seconds, then return to the starting position.

Shoulder Stretches

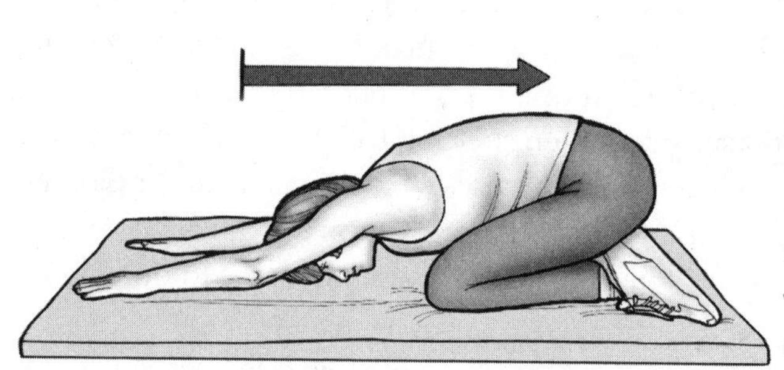

Get down on your hands and knees. Keep your back flat, your neck straight, and your eyes on the floor. Slowly shift your weight backward until your butt is resting on your heels. Straighten your arms in front of you. You should feel a stretch in your arms, shoulders, and hips.

Arm Stretches

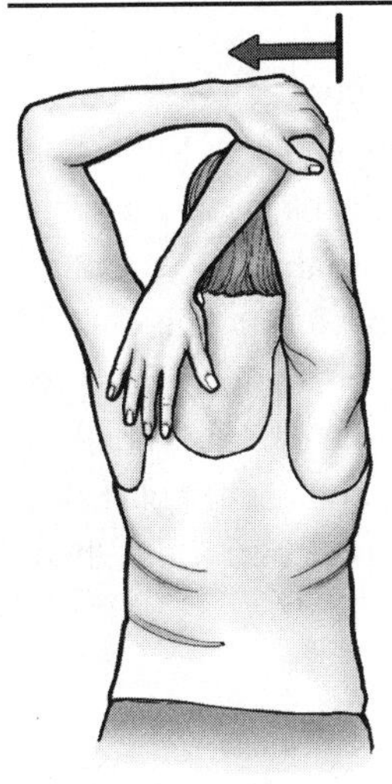

Stand or sit with your head facing forward. Raise both arms over your head. Grip your right elbow with your left hand (you can bend your arms if that's more comfortable). Gently pull your right elbow toward your left arm. You should feel the stretch in your upper arm and shoulder. Hold for a moment, then relax. Repeat with your other arm.

Chest Stretches

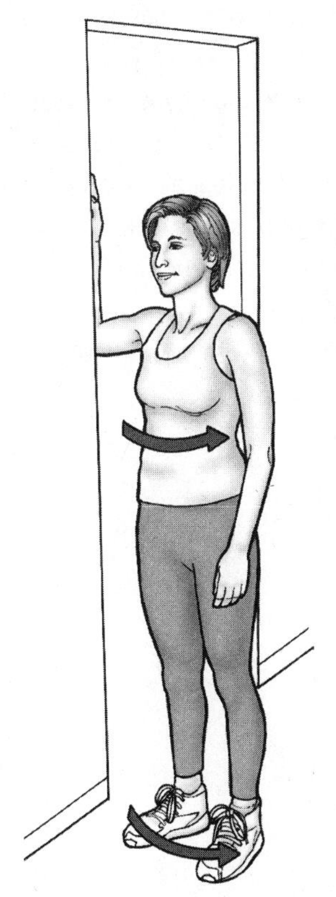

Stand in front of a doorway with your feet shoulder-width apart and parallel to the doorway. Lift your right arm and bend your elbow so that your upper arm is parallel to the floor. Press your hand and forearm against the inside of the doorway. Your fingers will be pointed at the ceiling. Slowly rotate your body toward the opposite shoulder, so that the arm against the doorway is pulled back. You should feel the stretch across your chest and shoulder. Switch sides and repeat with your other arm.

Back Stretches

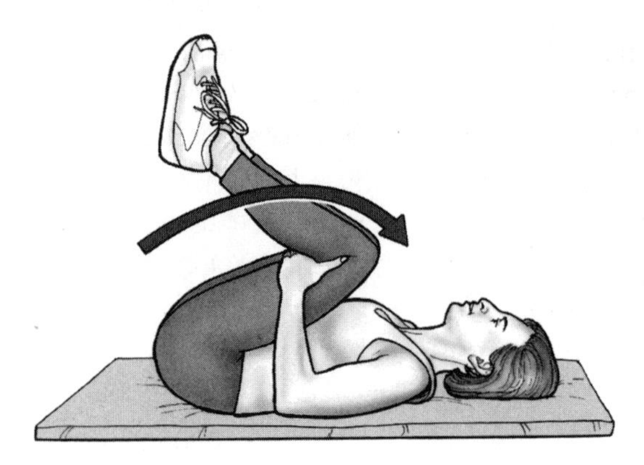

Lie on your back with your knees bent and your feet flat on the floor. Keeping your head and shoulders on the floor, lift your legs and bend your knees up toward your chest. To increase the stretch, grip both legs behind the knees and gently pull them closer to your chest. Hold, then relax.

Quad Stretches

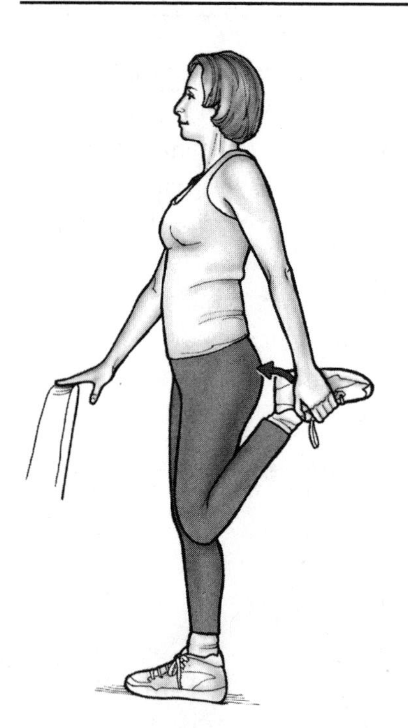

Stand with your right hand resting on a chair or a table for support. Bend your left leg behind you. Grip the top of your left foot with your left hand and slowly pull your heel toward your butt until you feel a stretch in your quadriceps (front of thighs). Be sure to keep your hips and knees aligned, and don't lock the knee of your supporting leg. Hold, then relax. Repeat with your other leg.

Hamstring Stretches

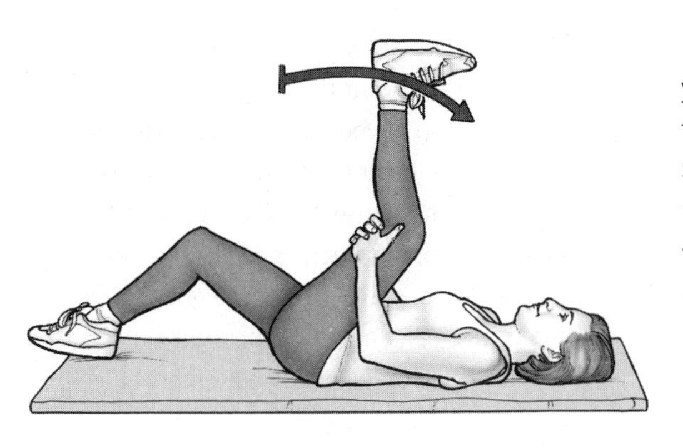

Lie on your back with your knees bent and your feet flat on the floor. Straighten your left knee and lift your leg straight toward the ceiling. Keep both hips on the floor. Grip your left leg below the knee and pull gently to increase the stretch in your hamstrings (back of thighs). Return to start, then repeat with your right leg.

To make this stretch more difficult, begin with both legs fully extended on the floor. Then bend your right knee up toward your chest and slowly straighten it toward the ceiling.

Groin Stretches

Lie on your back with your knees bent and your feet flat on the floor. Slowly let your knees separate and fall toward the floor, rotating your feet so that the soles are touching. You should feel a stretch in your inner thighs.

For a stronger stretch, sit up in a "butterfly" position with your back straight, your knees open to the sides, and the soles of your feet touching. Place your hands on the insides of your thighs close to your knees and gently push downward.

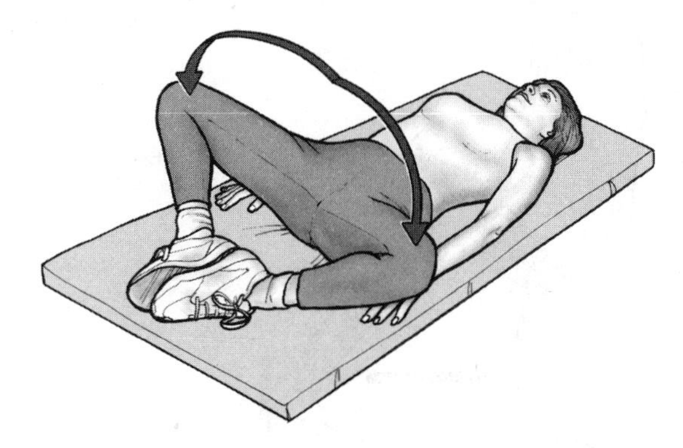

Hip Stretches

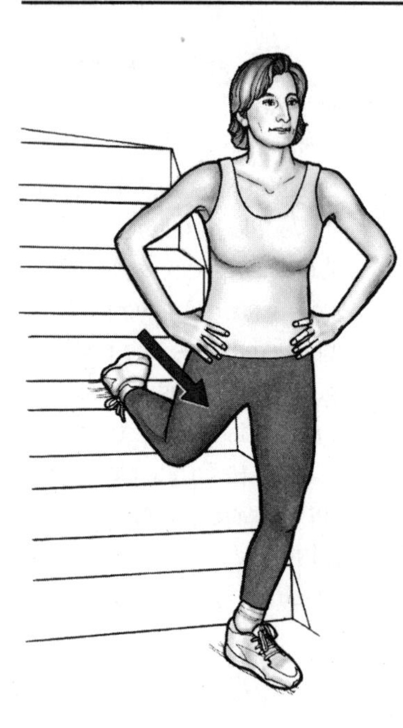

Stand facing away from a staircase or a chair. Carefully extend your right leg behind you, placing the top of your foot on the third step of the flight of stairs or on the chair. Place your hands on your hips—or hold on to a wall or table—for support. Keeping your right foot securely in place, gently pull your right thigh forward. You'll feel a mild pull through your right hip and thigh. Repeat with your other leg.

Calf Stretches

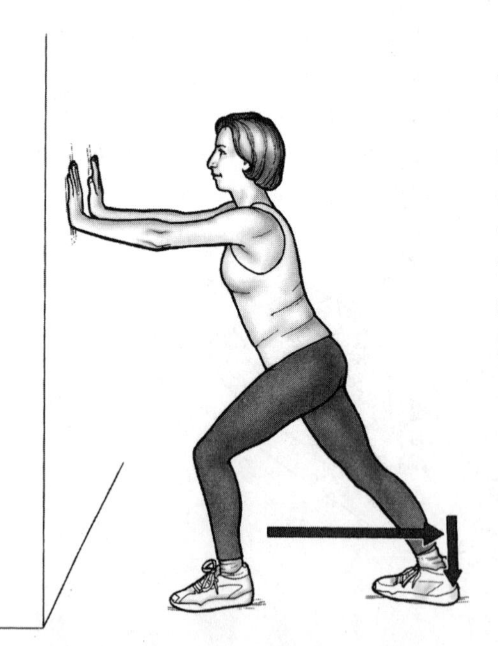

Stand an arm's length away from a wall and place your palms flat against the wall. Extend your right leg 2 to 3 feet behind you and press your right heel to the floor. (Your left knee will bend as you extend back.) Keep both heels flat against the floor. Hold, then relax. Repeat with your other leg.

Quiz

What Motivates You?

Nobody had to prod you to go out and play when you were 10. It was something you did naturally. Why then is it so hard for so many of us to force ourselves out for a daily walk? Why do we join gyms, go once, and then never go back?

It's simple. Unlike when we were 10 and going out to play because we wanted to, now we often go out and exercise because we feel as though we *have* to. And that's just no fun.

"The motivation simply isn't there for a lot of folks," says running coach Dr. Michael Gilewski of Cedars-Sinai Medical Center. "When we're young, we naturally gravitate toward the activities that are satisfying to us. If we like the thrill of competition, we play sports. If we like blowing off steam and playing, we jump rope or play Frisbee.

"We tend to lose touch with that side of ourselves when we get older and are doing so many things because we have to," he adds. "Sure, for some folks, the health benefits of exercise are enough motivation for them to stick with almost any activity. But for others, that just isn't enough to keep them going."

And that's why so many new exercisers quit after just a week or two, says Ross Andersen, Ph.D., assistant professor of medicine at Johns Hopkins University School of Medicine in Baltimore and one of the nation's leading researchers on lifestyle activity and weight loss. "One of the biggest mistakes people make when they start exercising is forcing themselves to do activities that aren't well-suited for them. It's little wonder they don't continue. They don't know why they're doing them. They don't even like them."

Not sure what activities would make you tick? The following quiz will help you match your personal motivations to the right exercises.

Circle one answer per question.

1. In my life, I wish I had more:
  a. Quiet time
  b. Time with friends or to meet new people
  c. Time outside
  d. Fun "toys"
  e. Freedom

(continued)

Quiz
(continued)

2. At a party, I'm most likely to:
- a. Talk mostly to my spouse or date
- b. Cut loose and mingle
- c. Take a tour of the house and check out the furnishings and artwork
- d. Go out shopping days before for just the right dress and accessories
- e. Sample everything at the buffet table

3. My dream car is a(n):
- a. Convertible
- b. Minivan
- c. SUV
- d. Sports car
- e. Luxury automobile

4. I feel happiest when I'm:
- a. Curled up with a book
- b. Out dancing
- c. Outside
- d. Spending the day shopping
- e. At a new restaurant

5. My friends would describe me as:
- a. Thoughtful
- b. Gregarious
- c. Outdoorsy
- d. A collector
- e. Pleasure loving

Score Yourself

Tally up the number of times you circled each letter. The one circled most is your predominant motivator. If you have a fairly even split (i.e., two *b*s and two *d*s), try the activities in both of those categories. If you have one of each, you have some experimenting to do, but that's half the fun!

IF YOU CIRCLED . . .

Mostly *a*s

You are motivated by: Time for yourself. You appreciate relaxing with your own thoughts and having quiet, stress-free time to enjoy and contemplate life.

For exercise: Try stress-reducing, solitary exercises such as yoga, walking, running, swimming, hiking, or strength training with home exercise equipment.

Mostly *b*s

You are motivated by: Social interaction. You thrive when you're in large groups. And you love to meet new people and try new things—the more the merrier!

For exercise: Try fun social activities such as working out at a large neighborhood gym, taking group exercise classes, or participating in walking/hiking clubs, tennis, or team sports like volleyball.

Mostly *c*s

You are motivated by: The great outdoors. You love the beauty of nature, seeing new places, and taking in the world at large. You're in your glory when tending your garden or strolling through a new park.

For exercise: Try outdoor sporting activities such as hiking, sea kayaking or canoeing, mountain biking, walking, or snowshoeing.

Mostly *d*s

You are motivated by: New fun gear to try. You're like a kid on Christmas morning every time you get a new "toy" to try out. You love to shop and check out all the interesting stuff there is to buy.

For exercise: Try gear-oriented activities such as golf, bicycling, cross-country skiing, home exercise equipment, or racquet sports like tennis or squash.

Mostly *e*s

You are motivated by: Pleasure and rewards. You want palpable results for your efforts. You enjoy dining out and treating yourself to nights on the town.

For exercise: Try quick-result calorie-burning activities such as strength training, stairclimbing, jumping rope, power walking, or jogging.

The Joy of Walking

IT'S AS SIMPLE AS PUTTING ONE FOOT IN FRONT OF THE OTHER. BUT IF YOU DO IT EVERY DAY, YOU CAN LOSE WEIGHT, BURN MORE CALORIES, GET MORE ENERGY, LOWER YOUR RISK FOR CHRONIC DISEASE, REDUCE YOUR NEED FOR MEDICATION, BOOST YOUR BRAINPOWER, CALM YOUR NERVES, IMPROVE YOUR MOOD, AND LIVE LONGER.

Walking is not only something we can—and should—do every day. Every extra bit we do goes a long way toward improving our health. In a study of nearly 16,000 twins, Finnish researchers found that those who took about six ½-hour walks a month were 30 percent less likely to die of natural causes, such as heart disease and cancer, during the study than their more sedentary siblings.

"There is no better exercise than walking," says Dr. John Yetter of SSM Rehab Sports Medicine. "It takes you out into the world where you can be alone with your thoughts and appreciate the beauty of nature. It makes you feel younger, more fit, and energized. If I can get people out walking for about 20 minutes, 3 or 4 days a week, I know they will be hooked."

Walking Away from Illness

Many of the conditions that we call age-related aren't all that age-related at all. Rather, they are caused by inactivity, says James Rippe, M.D., associate professor at Tufts University School of Medicine in Boston; director of the

A Simple Shape-Up Plan

Even though walking just comes naturally, when you're trying to get in shape, you should treat it like any other exercise. This means not overdoing it. Start slowly and work your way up. This simple 12-week program can help get you started. Try to walk 3 to 5 days a week, following the recommended times and intensities.

WEEK	WARMUP	TARGET ZONE EXERCISING	COOLDOWN	TOTAL TIME
1	Walk 5 min	Walk briskly 5 min	Walk more slowly 5 min	15 min
2	Walk 5 min	Walk briskly 7 min	Walk 5 min	17 min
3	Walk 5 min	Walk briskly 9 min	Walk 5 min	19 min
4	Walk 5 min	Walk briskly 11 min	Walk 5 min	21 min
5	Walk 5 min	Walk briskly 13 min	Walk 5 min	23 min
6	Walk 5 min	Walk briskly 15 min	Walk 5 min	25 min
7	Walk 5 min	Walk briskly 18 min	Walk 5 min	28 min
8	Walk 5 min	Walk briskly 20 min	Walk 5 min	30 min
9	Walk 5 min	Walk briskly 23 min	Walk 5 min	33 min
10	Walk 5 min	Walk briskly 26 min	Walk 5 min	36 min
11	Walk 5 min	Walk briskly 28 min	Walk 5 min	38 min
12	Walk 5 min	Walk briskly 30 min	Walk 5 min	40 min

Source: Reproduced with permission from Exercise and Your Heart, *1993. © American Heart Association.*

Center of Clinical and Lifestyle Research in Shrewsbury, Massachusetts; and author of *Fit over Forty*. "People have this mistaken notion that getting older means getting out of shape and getting sick. What really happens is that they become less active, and their bad health habits catch up with them."

The weight that accumulates with the passing years is also related to activity—or the lack of it, says Dr. Rippe. "Instead of buying some 'miracle' weight-loss gimmick, all that people really need to do is walk." The benefits are so dramatic that it's worth taking a look at them one by one.

A youthful waistline. "We always point the finger at fast food when we talk about the overweight problem in this country, but it has more to do with our increasingly inactive lifestyles," says Dr. Rippe. "Something as simple as walking can help prevent the weight gain we associate with middle age."

Don't think that walking can burn enough calories to whittle your waistline? Consider this: Brisk walking—about 4½ miles an hour—actually burns more calories than running at the same pace, according to a study from Washington University in St. Louis.

A younger heart. Probably the best benefit of regular walking is a stronger, healthier heart. The Centers for Disease Control and Prevention in Atlanta reports that walking just 3 hours a week at an easy pace can cut your risk for heart attack and stroke by almost one-third. The same 3 hours, when you walk a little faster, can cut these risks in half.

"It doesn't matter how old you are, walking can improve your cardiovascular fitness, control blood pressure, lower cholesterol, and improve the tone of your arteries," says Dr. Rippe. "All of those things not only help you live longer but also help you look and feel healthier and younger."

Healthy blood sugar. A regular walking program is one of the best strategies for easing symptoms of diabetes as well as preventing it in the first place, says Dr. Rippe. In a study of more than 1,400 men and women, researchers at the University of South Carolina in Columbia found that taking a daily walk significantly improved how well the body used insulin to regulate blood sugar.

Sound sleep. When we are young and without worry, we generally sleep straight through the night (and sometimes well into the morning!) without much trouble. As we get older, the responsibilities that come with age can rob us of this restful luxury. Regular walking can give it back, says Dr. Yetter. Researchers at the University of Arizona have found that regular walking lowers the risk for all kinds of sleep problems, including fitful and interrupted sleep.

Fewer aches and pains. At least 80 percent of people in this country will get waylaid by back pain at some point. And let's face it, the more years we live, the better the chances that our backs will let us down. But instead of resting on your behind and waiting for your back to feel better, going for walks, in most cases, will strengthen your back, shed some of those

Eight Ways Walking Makes You Young

1. Reduces excess weight
2. Lowers blood pressure
3. Cuts cholesterol
4. Boosts energy
5. Takes you outdoors
6. Reduces stress
7. Improves sleep
8. Relieves aches and pains

back-straining pounds, and generally make you feel better, says Dr. Yetter. (Don't forget to stretch before going for a walk—stretching adds flexibility to your back.)

Walking Younger, Walking Stronger

You took your first steps somewhere around your first year of life and have been striding around ever since. That's the beauty of walking. You don't need to learn a thing. You can just step out your door and go. The other great thing about walking is that you can always pick up new tips and techniques to make this simple exercise even better, says Bonnie Stein, a walking coach in Redington Shores, Florida.

"Any kind of walking can be good for you," she says. "But if you want to really lose weight and feel fitter and younger, you have to adjust your technique and pick up the pace a little bit."

Rock on your feet. You'll burn more calories if you put your whole body into your stride. "Concentrate on pushing off. Think about rolling from your heel, through the outside of your foot, to the ball of your foot, and then pushing off from the toes," says Stein. Your front stride will be short and quick rather than long and leisurely.

Swing your arms. Normal walking is great for strengthening your legs. But if you want to give your upper body more youthful tone, you have to get your arms involved. "Swinging your arms can improve the effectiveness of your walking 100 percent. You'll go faster and get some firming and toning of the upper arms," says Stein.

Start by bending your arms at about a 90-degree angle. Hold your arms in close enough to your body so that your thumbs brush just under your waistband as your arms move forward and back. Close your fists loosely and bring them up just about to the level of your sternum on the upswing. Swing them slightly behind the side seams of your shorts on the downswing. "Concentrate on streamlining your body like a rocket by keeping your elbows pulled in and your arms swinging smoothly and rhythmically," Stein says.

Stand tall. An upright posture makes your walking more efficient by opening up your chest, which allows your lungs to expand fully. Imagine that there's a string attached to the top of your head and that it's pulling you slightly skyward with every stride. Also, tighten your belly and tuck in your rear by slightly squeezing your gluteal muscles, Stein says. Keep your eyes up and focused 12 to 20 feet ahead of you. This will keep your neck aligned properly.

Take the "talk test." Walking is supposed to be invigorating and fun. You shouldn't be gasping for air, but your body shouldn't be bored, either. "On a scale of 1 to 10, with 1 being lying in bed and 10 being all-out exertion, I tell people to aim for about a 7," Stein says.

One way to determine if you're hitting the right stride is to do the talk test, she advises. "When you're walking at a 7, you should be breathing harder than normal, but you should still be able to carry on a simple conversation."

Walk every day. In order to get the best results from walking, you really should try to do it every day, says Stein. "If you aim to do it every day, you'll probably get 5 or 6 days in every week. If you shoot for fewer, you'll walk fewer."

Take a 10-minute walking break. Obviously, the longer you walk, the more fit you'll get. But in a busy world, it's not always possible to break away for ½ hour at a time. Don't sweat it. Just take a 10-minute walk around the block, says fitness researcher Marie H. Murphy, Ph.D., an exercise physiologist at the University of Ulster at Jordanstown, Northern Ireland. British researchers have found that short bouts of brisk walking—say, three 10-minute walks—yield fat-burning benefits similar to walking the same amount all at once.

"We've found that taking 10-minute walks might even be better in the long run," says study coauthor Dr. Murphy. "If you're set on the idea of walking 30 minutes a day and then you miss a session, you've missed a full

Living Proof
PANEL

An Energizing Walk

Instead of taking a coffee break, I'll take a walk break in the middle of the afternoon. I actually write it in my daily schedule.

It makes a big difference in my productivity because it's that time of day when I'm stiff from sitting behind a desk, my energy is flagging, and I need to do something. A brisk 15-minute walk completely rejuvenates me.

Delma L. Gorden

Walking is my time to work out the stress of the day. I go to the walking track, I put some great music on my Walkman, and I really get moving. I feel much calmer and more energized when I'm finished. Sure, sometimes it's hard to take those first steps out the door, but it's always worth it.

Pat Mast

My walks have helped me lose a lot of weight. I had started by doing power walks in the evenings. Then I decided to pick up the intensity a little. I'm now running for a while, then walking for a stretch, and I keep alternating. By walking, I can work out longer than if I just tried to jog the whole time. And throwing in a little jogging has let me vary my routine and burn a few more calories.

Anna Reese

30 minutes that week. If you miss one 10-minute session, you've missed much less."

Make It Fun!

Once you have started walking regularly, there are literally dozens of ways to keep it fresh and maximally effective. Here are some ideas to get you started.

Take a hike. Hiking can be described as adventurous walking where the sidewalk ends. It's a wonderful way to enjoy the benefits of walking to the fullest and explore the great outdoors, says personal trainer Michelle Edwards of the Cooper Institute. "There are hiking clubs in almost every community. You can join them on dayhikes along the most beautiful trails in your area," she says. Hiking also burns tons of calories: about 400 per hour for a 150-pound person going at a leisurely pace. To get a list of hiking clubs in your area, you can go to the Web site www.americanhiking.org.

Go to the mall. Not a big fan of the outdoors? Many shopping malls open their doors (but not their stores) early in the mornings so that people can come in and walk, says Edwards. "That way, you can lighten your waistline without lightening your wallet."

Try pole walking. A fun way to add some zip to your step and burn almost one-quarter more calories is to walk with trekking poles, says Edwards. These are rubber-tipped ski poles designed for walking. Studies have found that the effort it takes to swing the poles while you walk burns more calories and increases your heart rate by about 15 percent.

Tune in to tunes. It's not the best idea to wear headphones when you're walking outdoors because it's too hard to hear what's going on around you. But inside, when you're mall walking or walking on a treadmill, music can make the time fly. "People work out longer and at a higher intensity while listening to music, even when they don't mean to," Edwards says.

Make walking feel like play. When you were a kid, you didn't go out and play in order to think about your homework. You did it to stretch your body, air out your mind, and have some fun. Treat walking the same way, says Dr. Yetter. "Treat it as a break from the daily grind. Make it as fun as possible by exploring new neighborhoods and parks. Admire the way different people decorate their yards. Watch birds. Clear your mind and relax."

No More Dieting

FACT: LOTS OF AMERICANS SAY THEY ARE DIETING. SURVEYS SHOW THAT AT ANY ONE TIME, ABOUT 30 PERCENT OF MEN AND 40 PERCENT OF WOMEN ARE ATTEMPTING TO LOSE WEIGHT.

Fact: More Americans than ever are overweight. About one in five people are now considered obese (which means they have a body mass index greater than 30). The percentage of Americans who are overweight increased by one-third between 1991 and 1998, from 12 percent to 17.9 percent—a figure that is considered to be a low estimate. Some researchers are calling our widening bottoms and expanding bellies a national epidemic.

How do we make sense of these two contradictory, uncontested facts? Whatever those "dieters" are doing—or not doing—just isn't working. If it were, the U.S. population would be slimming down, not getting heavier, right?

One large national study of almost 108,000 men and women sheds some light on the matter. The truth is that people who say they are dieting are not really doing what it takes to lose weight, according to the study, which is part of the Behavioral Risk Factor Surveillance System at the Centers for Disease Control and Prevention.

Some are eating less fat, but they aren't cutting calories in the process. In fact, people are eating an average of 200 calories more a day now than 10 years ago, says John P. Foreyt, Ph.D., director of the Behavioral Medicine Research Center at Baylor College of Medicine in Houston and coauthor of *Living without Dieting*. "Keep it up, and you'll gain 20 pounds in a year."

Most aren't gaining that much that fast. But many gain a pound or two a year between ages 20 and 60, and in a few years, that starts to add up. One reason for the overeating, Dr. Foreyt believes: "Portion sizes have gotten so big that people no longer have any concept of the amount of food that actually makes up a normal portion."

People also aren't getting enough exercise. Although two-thirds of the people trying to lose weight report using physical activity, only 42.3 percent of men and 36.8 percent of women report doing enough to make an impact on weight—30 minutes at least five times a week. "Just this exercise alone would be enough to counter the weight gain most adults experience over the years," says weight-loss expert Dr. Ross Andersen of Johns Hopkins University School of Medicine.

Today's mostly sedentary desk jobs and home conveniences make exercise a necessity—we don't chop wood or scrub floors anymore. Heck, we don't even get up to change TV channels.

So if most "dieters" are not exercising sufficiently and only a few are actually cutting calories, what the heck are they doing?

Many are stuck in a cycle of start-stop, try-fail. "They had a rough weekend, they overdid it, and they start a diet on Monday," says Dr. Andersen. "By Tuesday night, however, when the gang goes out for happy hour after work, they're so hungry that one beer leads to a plate of chicken wings and then a hamburger. And by the time they get home that night, they decide they've blown it—it's called the what-the-hell effect—and they might as well forget about this attempt to go on a diet. They start again the following Monday and do the same thing."

Some of the people caught in this cycle are looking for the traditional version of a diet—a quick fix that will take the pounds off and then allow them to get back to eating-as-normal.

"They will eat nothing but cabbage soup for days if they think that will work," says Dr. Foreyt. "They go way too low on calories. Unfortunately, very restricted diets such as these leave people feeling seriously deprived. And before long, it grinds people down, and they abandon the diet. There has never been a study that showed that dieting in the traditional sense works."

Even if people lose weight by cutting calories, they tend not to be able to keep the weight off if they don't develop regular exercise habits. Experts also cite other obstacles to weight loss.

Snacking too much. For some, it turns into nonstop nibbling, says Madelyn H. Fernstrom, Ph.D., director of the Weight Management Center at the Uni-

Living Proof
PANEL

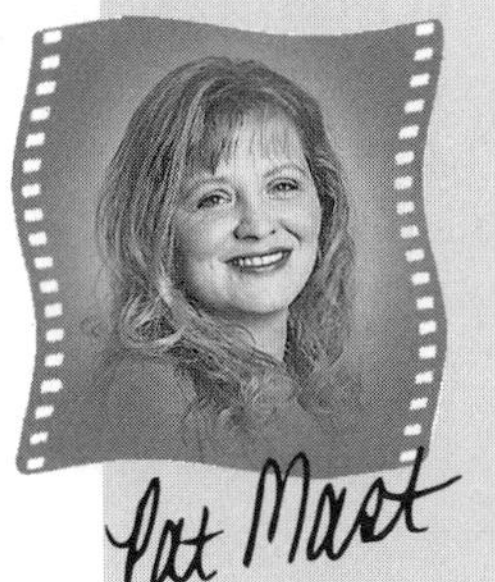

Diets Don't Work—I Know Because I Tried Them

Like lots of people, I've spent time watching what I eat. And for me, that has meant trying to eat lots of fruits and vegetables and not much junk. That strategy worked pretty well until I stopped smoking. Then, I put on 40 pounds in 2½ years.

I tried the cabbage soup diet and actually liked it, because I like cabbage soup and fruits and vegetables. And that's what the diet was. I lost 7 pounds in 7 days but managed to keep it off for only a few weeks.

Then I tried Weight Watchers. Again, I had early success—6 pounds in the first 2 weeks. But I stalled for the next 16 weeks and finally gave up.

Most of the other diets I tried involved simply making healthier food choices. I knew what to do from going to Weight Watchers. My biggest downfall was premenstrual bingeing on sweets and other high-calorie foods. So I would start out at the beginning of my cycle with good intentions, only to find it all falling apart during the last week.

What's different this time? For me, probably the biggest thing is the fiber. I just never paid much attention to it before as part of my eating plan. I fill up on high-fiber cereal for breakfast. And for snacks, fruits and vegetables. Without realizing it, I have munched and crunched my way through five or more servings of fruits and veggies by the end of the day. Am I totally stuffed? Yes. There's not much room for more.

versity of Pittsburgh Medical Center. "If you snack, it's important to plan your snacks as carefully as you do your meals."

Have no more than about 200 calories during a snack, and eat about every 4 hours, says Dr. Fernstrom. Some people find that they have better control of their food intake if they don't snack at all, especially on tasty high-fat, sugary foods, which we all find hard to put limits on.

Eating too many high-fat foods. High-fat foods pack a lot of calories in a small amount of food. So they are an easy way to eat more calories than you ever intended to eat. You need to know where the fat is, even when it's not obvious.

Unfortunately, the list is long and includes some foods that may surprise you: bran muffins, Chinese food, creamy coffee drinks, so-called lean ground beef. Even salads get fat fast when you add fatty dressing or too much cheese or croutons.

Overeating at mealtimes. It's a natural instinct to want to clean our plates, empty the bag, lick our fingers. "But in doing so, we tend to eat beyond the point where our hunger is satisfied. In fact, some of us don't perceive a signal to stop until we are stuffed—we can't eat another bite," says Dr. Fernstrom.

That's why it's important to have only a reasonable amount of food available when you sit down to eat. Use a smaller plate if you need to. And take your time eating. At restaurants, divide large portions in half before you dig in. Stow half the portion in a doggie bag even before you begin eating.

Eating for emotional reasons. People eat for all sorts of reasons besides being hungry. Some turn to food when they're feeling angry, lonely, or frustrated. You'll need to tune in to the emotions that are driving you to food, and then find ways to express your emotions appropriately or make yourself feel better without food.

What's the Alternative?

Many weight-loss specialists are abandoning the word *diet* altogether. They're also leaving behind the diet mentality—the drastic short-term changes that fail to produce long-term results. Instead, they are focusing on subtle, healthy lifestyle changes that people can incorporate slowly—and painlessly—into their daily lives to produce permanent changes.

"We have people make changes that they hardly notice, even when they are losing weight," Dr. Foreyt says.

Here is what experts suggest you focus on.

Make small changes. You don't need to eat cabbage soup to lose weight. In fact, you don't need to go on any bizarre, restrictive, one-food-only diet.

"You just have to cut portion size a little bit to reduce calories," Dr. Foreyt says. "We take what the person is eating now and simply cut 100 calories from it in the form of fat, meaning a little less butter or margarine, or a little more fat off the meat."

You do have to get moving. Dr. Foreyt asks his patients to expend at least 100 calories a day in exercise by walking or doing some other physical activity for 20 minutes. Even if you never get beyond this level, combined with a small reduction in calories, you'll be reversing the weight-gain trend, he says. Plus, you'll be improving your health and longevity in countless ways.

Rearrange your environment to support your good intentions. In today's world, we are surrounded by enticements to eat, eat, eat. It's easier to sidestep those enticements when you have to go out of your way to indulge, Dr. Andersen says.

You don't need to eat cabbage soup to lose weight.

"In the beginning, especially, it can be important to remove the cues that lead to overeating," he says. That may mean not keeping goodies in the house. If TV commercials have you screaming for ice cream, you'll have to go out for it. If you do, buy just one serving.

Or it may mean not stopping at fast-food places if you can't make do with a broiled chicken breast and diet soda. It may mean taking the foods you want to eat to work with you—not ordering out, where a dazzling array of selections could lead you into temptation.

Examine your attitude before you start. "If you are someone who has abandoned a program five times in the past 5 months, you need to reflect and say, 'What is going on? What am I going to do differently this time?'" Dr. Andersen says.

Such reflection can lead you to a more serious attempt at weight loss. "If you are not ready and willing to get serious about getting your weight down, you would be better off moving into a maintenance phase for a period of time," he says. "You can start the weight-loss phase when you feel ready to do the work that is involved."

Go for the Goals: The Get Thin, Get Young Eating Plan

THE APPROACH OF THE GET THIN, GET YOUNG EATING PLAN IS SIMPLE AND STRAIGHTFORWARD: EAT SMALLER MEALS MORE OFTEN. CONTROL THE PORTIONS YOU EAT. AND CONCENTRATE ON THE FLAVORFUL, ENJOYABLE FOODS YOU SHOULD EAT INSTEAD OF TRYING TO DEPRIVE YOURSELF OF FATTENING FOODS THAT YOU SUPPOSEDLY SHOULDN'T EAT.

You'll learn how to cut back on calories through portion control (vital for weight loss) as well as how to create a moderate-fat diet that includes the foods you enjoy (vital for weight maintenance). You'll also get the nutrients, such as vitamins, minerals, and phytochemicals, that you need to live longer and feel younger.

Best of all, this sensible approach is geared to the long run. It will help you break bad habits and establish a new way of eating, a way that will help you not only take off pounds but also keep them off. Here's why.

The Get Thin, Get Young Eating Plan

Here is a summary of the goals for the Get Thin, Get Young Eating Plan. Details on the scientific evidence that shows how each daily goal helps you get thinner and younger, complete with simple, practical tips on how to achieve the goal, are found in the chapters indicated.

Use this as a quick daily reminder. Photocopy it and place it on your refrigerator door. And incorporate the goals into your food diary as a simple checklist that you can mark off each day.

EACH DAY

- Master portion control (page 120)
- Get 30 grams of fiber (page 153)
- Eat four servings of fruit (page 189)
- Have five servings of vegetables (page 189)
- Include six servings of whole grain products (page 227)
- Eat two to three servings of lean protein (page 252)
- Factor in fun (page 259)
- Have one to three servings of healthy fat (page 296)
- Eat five or six mini-meals or three meals with two snacks (page 318)
- Drink eight glasses of water (page 349)

EACH WEEK

- Eat fish twice
- Have beans three times
- Try one new fruit or vegetable

"Weight loss and weight maintenance are different metabolic states," says Barbara Rolls, Ph.D., professor of nutrition at Pennsylvania State University in University Park and author of *Volumetrics*. In other words, what you do to lose weight won't necessarily help you keep it off.

That's why so many fad diets fail. When it comes to weight loss, there are no magic foods. It doesn't matter whether you eat fewer carbohydrates or less protein or fat when you're trying to lose weight. All that matters is that somehow you take in fewer calories than your body's burning. That way, your body has to burn your fat stores for energy.

Fiber fills you up fast, so you eat less. Plus, you feel full longer.

What you're eating does make a difference for weight maintenance, however. That's because keeping your weight steady is both physical and psychological. "Let's face it. The scale is a lot more motivating when your weight is going down than when it's steady," Dr. Rolls says. "Just fighting the regain is tough."

People often breathe a sigh of relief and go back to their old eating habits once they have reached their goal weights. Or, they give up on their diets before they reach their goals because the dietary changes were too tough to stick with.

That's the beauty of this real-life approach: The small changes you make over the next 12 weeks can become part of your everyday lifestyle.

Here are some of the key concepts behind the plan.

Choose foods with flavor. "People will not stick with a weight-loss plan they do not enjoy," says weight-loss expert Dr. Ross Andersen of Johns Hopkins University School of Medicine.

If you want to lose weight, don't waste calories on food that doesn't taste good. Look for lower-calorie, nutrient-packed foods you love, like strawberry-banana yogurt smoothies, grilled sea bass, or fresh tomatoes, onions, and basil tossed with olive oil and balsamic vinegar.

Fill up on fiber. Vegetables, fruits, and whole grains are loaded with fiber. And fiber is absolutely crucial for successful weight loss.

"Increasing the fiber content of meals makes a huge difference in weight loss. Most people don't realize this," Dr. Rolls says. Fiber fills you up fast, so you eat less, and it digests slowly, so you feel full longer.

Go on a culinary adventure. Yes, you do have to eat your vegetables. But you're an adult now, so you don't have to eat Brussels sprouts if you don't like them. There are dozens of other vegetables to choose from. Look around your produce aisle, or better yet, go to a farmers' market or health food store. Odds are that there are numerous vegetables or fruits there that you've never tried before. Talk to the grocer and find out the best way to prepare the one you select. Then, next week, try a new whole grain.

Don't deprive yourself. Research at Pennsylvania State University shows that the more you restrict a food, the more kids want it. "Adults aren't much different," says Dr. Rolls. There's no need to deny yourself the pleasure of higher-calorie foods, as long as you practice portion control and modify your meal accordingly.

For instance, if you're going out and you want dessert, order it. Just balance it with a light entrée, like a broth-based soup and a leafy green salad.

Choose a plan you can live with. Weight-loss winners—those who lose weight and keep it off—have one thing in common: They eat the same way at their goal weight as they did when they were losing weight. Many people make the mistake of reverting to their old habits once they achieve their desired weight loss. So it's important while losing weight to develop a meal plan full of foods you enjoy.

Stay with it. Realize that you are going to have setbacks. You are going to lose control one day and eat an entire bag of chocolate kisses instead of just one or two pieces.

No, that won't help you lose weight. But neither will giving up on your new eating plan.

"People have to get out of that mindset of giving up on their weight-loss plan when they make one dietary mistake or when they regain a few pounds," says Dr. Rolls.

Go for a walk or run. Exercise helps control appetite. At your next meal, get right back on track with reasonable portions of lean protein, fresh vegetables, and whole grains.

Master Portion Control

DESPITE WHAT SOME FAST-FOOD CHAINS MIGHT WANT YOU TO THINK, WE AREN'T BORN TO SUPER-SIZE. A STUDY OF 32 PRESCHOOL CHILDREN IN UNIVERSITY PARK, PENNSYLVANIA, FOUND THAT THE EATING HABITS OF THOSE UNDER 5 YEARS OLD WERE NOT INFLUENCED BY LARGER PORTION SIZES. THEY ATE ONLY AS MUCH AS THEY WANTED.

But the study also showed that children over age 5 ate more food than they craved when they were presented with larger portions. Researchers theorize from this that children *learn* to overeat—and unfortunately, that's a lesson that can lead to a lifetime of weight problems.

"Portion control is one of the biggest reasons people can't lose weight," says Karen Miller-Kovach, R.D., a registered dietitian and chief scientist for Weight Watchers International in Woodbury, New York. "They tend to focus more on what they eat rather than how much."

Here's an example: When you eat out, you order the heart-smart option, spaghetti with marinara sauce. Confident that you've chosen a healthful, low-fat meal, you down the entire plate.

The only problem is, that plate of spaghetti holds 4 cups, or *8 servings,* of pasta. That's more than your entire daily requirement for grains (6 servings) in one meal, and all that pasta is not even high in fiber. It's like eating 15 slices of white bread (about 800 calories). And that's not taking into account the sauce, the salad, and the bread you dipped in olive oil. They're all healthful choices, but you just ate more than 1,400 calories in one sitting.

Those extra calories not only will add pounds but also may subtract years from your life, research suggests.

In order for you to lose weight, you're going to have to master portions. That means learning what an official serving size from each of the food groups looks like and how many portions you can eat and still lose weight.

GET THIN

We tend to overestimate our consumption of low-calorie foods such as fruits and vegetables and underestimate our intake of higher-calorie foods such as steak, olive oil, peanut butter, and even bagels, according to Miller-Kovach.

It's not necessarily our fault. "Everything is super-size, from your sirloin to your cereal bowl," she says.

And it's not like we're scooping out the casserole with a measuring spoon. We live in a hurry-up-and-get-it-done society, and that applies to meals, too. So we eat too fast, reaching for seconds before our stomachs can send signals to our brains that we're full.

We're also intent on getting value for our money. And in a restaurant, that means an overflowing, oversize plate. For instance, in 1955, an order of McDonald's french fries weighed a little more than 2 ounces. Today, it is three times that size.

Cutting back on portion sizes would help us lose pounds overall, but that's not all. Given the results of one study on monkeys, conducted at Wake Forest University in Winston-Salem, North Carolina, chances are that we would lose those pounds in our stomachs. That's the most dangerous place to carry extra body fat, putting us at significantly higher risk for heart disease, diabetes, and colon cancer than if it landed on our hips and butts.

Super Serving Sizes

Nearly everything is super-size these days. Most restaurants dish out at least twice the official government serving size. In some cases, it can be four times as big, says Jerome Agrusa, Ph.D., associate professor of hospitality management at the University of Louisiana in Lafayette.

FOOD	USDA SERVING	TYPICAL RESTAURANT SERVING
Bagel	1 oz	4–5 oz
Chips	1 oz	3+ oz
French fries	1¾ oz	6–8 oz
Pasta	½ cup	4 cups
Pasta sauce	½ cup	2 cups
Popcorn	2 cups	8–12 cups
Meat	2–3 oz	6–16 oz
Muffin	1 oz	4–6 oz
Soda	8 oz	16+ oz

Get Young

Want to live longer? Eat less. Restricting calories is the only method known to slow aging in mammals.

In hundreds of animal studies, eating less food not only enabled animals to live longer but also kept them healthier throughout their lives. They had significantly reduced rates of serious conditions such as heart disease, diabetes, various cancers, kidney diseases, and autoimmune diseases—all leading killers of human beings, according to Richard Weindruch, Ph.D., a researcher in the department of medicine at the University of Wisconsin Medical School and Wisconsin Regional Primate Research Center, both in Madison.

The reason that limiting calories works? Our bodies begin aging on the inside long before we see gray hair, age spots, and wrinkles. Researchers think that aging is connected to metabolism's vandalistic by-products, free radicals. Desperate to replace particles they lack, free radicals roam our bodies snatching pieces of other molecules, damaging them, and creating more free radicals in the process, says Dr. Weindruch.

Some of these damaged molecules make up our DNA, the blueprints for every cell in our bodies. It's tough building healthy new cells with only part of the architectural plan.

Limiting calories prevents this damage, one University of Wisconsin study suggests. It found that feeding mice low-calorie diets prevented 70 percent of the changes in genetic activity associated with aging and kept mice alive 50 percent longer. Although this study used rodents, experts believe overeating accelerates aging in humans, too.

Controlled human studies have not yet begun, however, says Dr. Weindruch.

In the meantime, a preliminary study conducted in Biosphere 2, a man-made ecosystem with eight men and women sealed inside, showed that restricting calories lowers levels of cholesterol, glucose, and insulin—risk factors for age-related diseases such as heart disease, stroke, and diabetes.

And it's not as though those were the results of starvation. In Biosphere 2, the inhabitants ate 20 percent fewer total calories but were still able to sustain 60- to 70-hour work weeks and do hard physical labor (manual farming) 3 hours a day, 6 days a week. If you eat 2,000 calories a day, reducing your calories by 20 percent is equivalent to giving up your morning bagel with cream cheese.

It's critical that in all these studies, including those involving animals, calories, not nutrients, were restricted. In Biosphere 2, for example, inhabitants ate top-of-the-line-healthy foods such as papayas, whole wheat porridge, and goat's milk. Nary a Twinkie nor a Coke gained entrance.

Go for the Goal

It's increasingly difficult in our super-size society to intuitively understand what an appropriate portion of food is. A serving is not how much you eat in one sitting or how much fits in your bowl. One serving of cold cereal, for instance, is typically about 1 cup, according to most cereal manufacturers.

Yet, we are more likely eating about 2 cups of cereal each morning, Miller-Kovach says.

It's not a problem as long as we recognize that we've just eaten more than two times our grain allowance for the day. Here are some quick and easy ways to avoid the overeating trap, according to Miller-Kovach.

Take a measure. Used to a heaping bowl of pasta? Measure out ½ cup and put it in your bowl. That's probably not going to be enough for dinner, so measure out another ½ cup. Then mark how high the pasta comes up in the bowl with a permanent magic marker and use that bowl every time you eat pasta.

You can do the same with cereal, rice, vegetables—anything that fits in a bowl. Don't want to scar your dishes? Get a good mental picture. Or take a Polaroid and stick it on your refrigerator. Be sure to retest your portion intelligence monthly since our eyes tend to inflate portions over time.

Get a grip on portions. The Get Thin, Get Young Eating Plan sets targets for how much of each type of food you should eat. The idea is simple: Concentrate on eating pleasurable, flavorful versions of the foods you're most likely skimping on now, and you won't have to fret about *not* eating foods that will make it difficult to lose weight and keep it off.

The daily targets are: four servings of fruit, five servings of vegetables, two to three servings of lean protein, six servings of whole grains, and one to three servings of healthy fat.

When there's a range, start with the lowest number of servings (for example, two servings of lean protein). If you find that you're still hungry, add another portion of fruits or vegetables first before you move on to grains, proteins, or fats. And make sure that you are adding single portions, not second helpings.

But how do you know what a serving size is? Are you condemned to carry measuring cups and spoons around with you for the rest of your life?

Not hardly. You already have all the information you need at hand. Literally. Your palm and fingers contain the approximate serving sizes for all the major food groups.

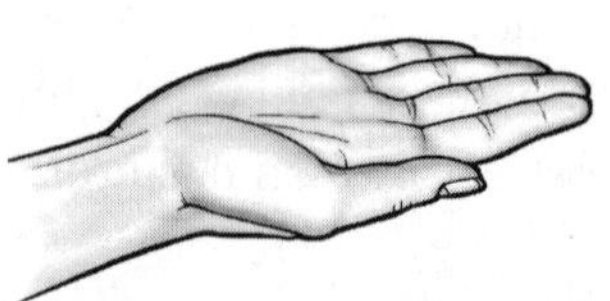

Palm of hand = one serving (3 ounces) of meat, fish, or poultry

Tip of thumb to first joint = 1 tablespoon of oil (a serving of salad dressing equals 2 tablespoons)

Tip of finger to first joint = 1 teaspoon, one serving of oil

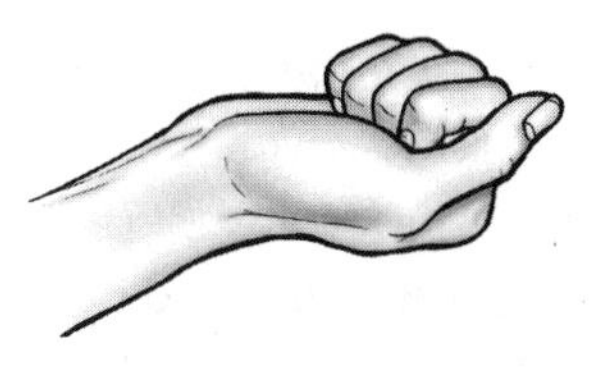

Clenched fist = two servings (1 cup) of potatoes, rice, or pasta

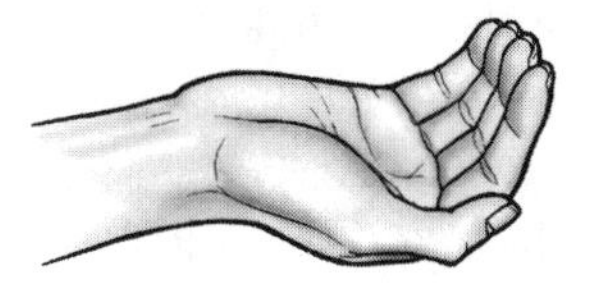

Cupped hand = one serving (½ cup) of pasta, chopped fruit, or cooked vegetables

Of course, this doesn't mean a petite 5-foot woman can use the hand of her 6-foot-5 linebacker husband to portion out her meal. This rule of thumb is built proportionately. You have to use your own hand.

Cut your meat. Three ounces is considered a serving of meat, but good luck trying to find 3-ounce servings at the supermarket or a restaurant.

Here's a quick tip: Figure that beef shrinks about 25 percent when it's cooked. So that 16-ounce steak you bought will be about 12 ounces when it arrives on your table. Cut it into quarters before you cook it, freeze in individual bags, and you'll never have to guess at a serving size again.

Eating out? Ask the waiter to bag half of your meal in the kitchen so that you're not even tempted. Going for the chicken? It doesn't take much to meet your daily protein requirement—an average boneless chicken breast will do the trick.

Stack a sandwich in your favor. Ever order a sandwich so big that you couldn't open your mouth wide enough to take a bite? Restaurants typically layer 4 ounces of meat on sandwiches.

You can easily cut that in half: When ordering, ask your waiter to wrap half to go, or ask that the sandwich be prepared with only 2 ounces of meat. Restaurants keep close tabs on their portions, so you can figure the odds are good that they have a scale back in the kitchen to weigh your cold cuts.

Divide and conquer portions. If you're at a dinner party and can't remember what appropriate servings of each food group are, visually divide your plate: reserve half for vegetables, one-quarter for whole grains, and one-quarter for beef, fish, poultry, or beans.

Bring your own. Stock a snack drawer at work so that you always have healthy, low-fat options on hand. Avoid the economy size, however. Instead, buy single-serving packs of pretzels, raisins, fruit cups, or fig cookies. Or divide that super-size pretzel bag into single ½-cup servings at home and take them to work. If your snack stash is portion-controlled, you're less likely to overeat.

Make your weakness a strength. Most of us have foods that make us lose all self-control. Chocolate-covered graham crackers, pumpkin cheesecake, Buffalo wings, fresh-baked baguettes. So limit how much is easily available. Put two graham crackers into a plastic bag and freeze the rest. Buy individual slices of cheesecake from the bakery instead of a whole one. Cut that baguette into 10 pieces and freeze 8 of them.

Week Two

On the Road

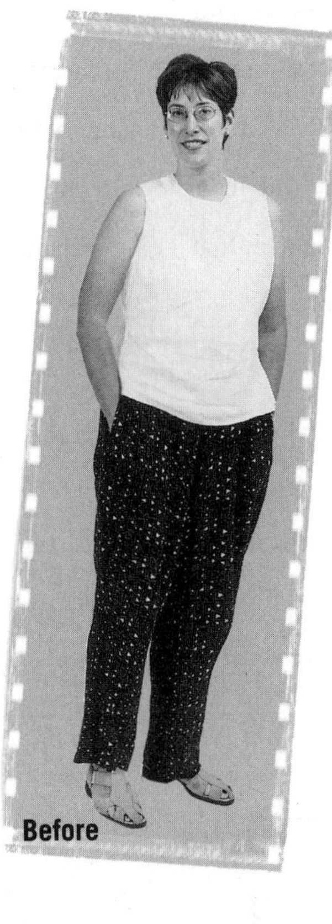

Before

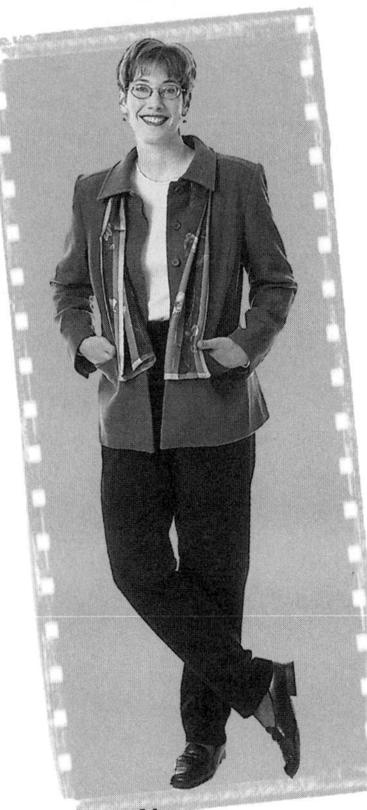

After

WHEN MY HUSBAND RUNS HIS HANDS OVER MY BODY, HE COMMENTS ON HOW MUCH FIRMER AND TIGHTER IT FEELS!

—Deb Gordon

Week Two

It's Week 2 of The *Prevention* Get Thin, Get Young Plan, and you're on the road to a slimmer you! Perhaps you've never made it this far before when trying to lose weight. Then again, maybe you have. Whether your program derailed after the first week or the first month, this time it will be different. You're making gradual lifestyle changes that you can easily adopt as healthy, lifelong habits.

This week, you'll learn a few more simple adjustments that will reap a wealth of benefits. For instance, if you add a little strength training to your fitness regimen, you will sculpt a younger-looking, shapelier body—faster. And boosting your intake of heart-healthy, high-fiber foods will encourage the pounds to slide off you more quickly. Plus, you can create the illusion of a slimmer you right now by choosing clothes that complement your personal body type.

Changing the Way You See Yourself

WHICH WOULD YOU RATHER HAVE?

A. A THINNER BODY

B. AN EXTRA 3 TO 5 YEARS ON YOUR LIFE

PSYCHOLOGY TODAY FOUND THAT OF THE 4,000 PEOPLE THEY SURVEYED, ABOUT ONE-QUARTER OF THE WOMEN SAID THAT THEY WOULD HAPPILY LOP 3 YEARS OFF THEIR LIVES FOR SLEEKER BODIES.

That same survey also found that about two-thirds of the women and more than half of the men were unhappy with their weight, and a whopping 89 percent of the women said that they wanted to lose weight.

The numbers add up to an overwhelming conclusion: We're not exactly big fans of our bodies. And it doesn't seem to matter what shape or size they are. "A person who is 20 pounds overweight may be more dissatisfied than a person who is 100 pounds overweight," says David B. Sarwer, Ph.D., assistant professor of psychology at the Center for Human Appearance at the University of Pennsylvania in Philadelphia.

So if you scowl at yourself in a mirror day after day, prodding and pinching those not-so-firm areas, know that you are not alone.

You'd think this dissatisfaction with our status quo would motivate us into a weight-loss frenzy. Interestingly enough, it does the exact opposite. All those hours scrutinizing our bodies saps the youthful energy right out of us, with one study from the University of Pennsylvania School of Medicine in Philadelphia showing that the more dissatisfied a woman is with her body, the more likely she is to report symptoms of depression and lower self-esteem.

Your weight does not determine your value or worth.

Not exactly the mindset to get you excited about walking a mile or preparing a healthy meal.

But if you feel good about your body—even if you think that you could lose a few pounds—you're more likely to be successful at losing that weight. A Stanford University study found that people who were happiest with their bodies at the start of a weight-loss program were more than twice as likely to lose weight as those who were least satisfied with their bodies.

Why? Because with high self-esteem, you feel as if you could conquer the world—and that includes losing weight.

Although it sounds as though you're going in two opposite directions—acknowledging that you'd like to lose weight yet accepting yourself as you are—it can be done, says Clara Gerhardt, Ph.D., a clinical psychologist and associate professor of human development and family studies at Samford University in Birmingham, Alabama.

You just need to view weight loss as an investment in a valuable item—yourself.

Silence Your Harshest Critic

It's often said that we are our own harshest critics. And when it comes to our bodies, that couldn't be more true, says Steve Sultanoff, Ph.D., adjunct professor of psychology at Pepperdine University in Malibu, California, and president of the American Association for Therapeutic Humor. Who hasn't spotted a fault that others probably couldn't find under a microscope?

This self-criticism may seem harmless, but it's not. It can negatively affect your self-image. "When you give yourself these negative messages, you actually create a psychological impact of which you may not be aware," says Dr. Sultanoff.

Just as those negative thoughts take a toll on your psyche, so can positive thoughts and actions chip away at poor self-esteem to build a truer and happier sense of self, he says. To do that, try the following advice.

Watch your language. You'd never tell a friend that she looks fat and old, so why do you tell yourself that? "Stop picking on yourself and putting yourself down," says Judy Rosenberg, Ph.D., a clinical psychologist in Beverly Hills, California. Not only does it bring you down, making it hard to get and stay motivated, but it reinforces the idea that you can't lose weight. "If you have negative 'fat' thoughts, then the outcome is fat," she says.

Pat yourself on the back. Announce to the world what you enjoy and cherish about yourself: your talents, your parenting skills, your ability to forgive, your collection of Elvis wine glasses. And forget about the notion that you shouldn't toot your own horn. "There is pressure not to brag or boast," Dr. Sultanoff says. It's a ridiculous idea.

If you're not comfortable drawing attention to your best traits in public, write them down in a list and read it over when you feel the I'm-a-terrible-person-because-I'm-overweight thoughts invading. Tell yourself, "While I may want to change my weight, my weight does not determine my value and worth. I am the same person, having the same value, no matter what my weight. Whether I gain or lose 20 pounds does not affect who I am as a human being."

Or, Dr. Sultanoff recommends, ask yourself, "How does my losing or gaining weight make me a better or worse person?" Of course, it does neither. Your weight does not determine your value or worth, he asserts.

Splurge on yourself. People who dislike their bodies tend to withhold nice things from themselves as a form of punishment. That just makes you feel worse, says Elena Ramirez, Ph.D., a clinical psychologist and weight-management researcher at the University of Vermont in Burlington. Treat yourself to massages, take a bubble bath, buy that outfit you've always wanted. These small rewards will not only lift your spirits but also make you feel better about your body.

Challenge your own ideas. "I am a bad person because I can't lose weight." Dr. Ramirez suggests you think about that common refrain for a minute. Murderers are bad people. Child abusers are bad people. But caring, contributing members of society like you are not, even if you do weigh a few pounds more than you would like.

"A woman will say, 'No one will ever love me.' It's an irrational thought," says Dr. Ramirez. When you find yourself equating your body with dread and doom, argue with yourself. If you think you're a bad person, list all the good things you do. If you think no one will ever love you, then what is your husband, your children, your mother, or your dog doing?

Ask the same questions about yourself when you judge your body. Is your stomach really the size of a watermelon? By understanding just how inaccurate these thoughts are, you can begin silencing them, Dr. Ramirez says.

Balance likes with dislikes. A study of 79 overweight women at the University of Pennsylvania found that more than half of those surveyed hated their waists or abdomens. But what about the percentage of people who think they have great legs, beautiful eyes, or nice hair? Instead of focusing on what you don't like about your body, focus on what you *do* like.

"When you look at yourself, you could be saying, 'While my stomach is not as flat as I would like it to be, I think my eyes are pretty,'" says Dr. Sarwer. Before long, you'll start to think more about what is right about your body instead of what is less than perfect.

Give up control. Face it: You have your mother's crooked nose, your grandmother's short and stocky legs, your aunt's round face. There are some parts of your body and appearance that you just can't control or change. Accept them as traits that make you an individual.

What about the Rest of the World?

How you see yourself also is affected by what you *think* others are thinking of you, Dr. Sultanoff says. The truth is, they probably don't spend much time analyzing how you look or how much you weigh. In fact, they're probably better than you at seeing your beauty. So stop worrying about what others think and start enjoying your own life.

Wear what you fear. In body-image therapy, clients often are instructed to wear the one thing they feel most uncomfortable in: a pair of shorts, a bathing suit, a fitted top. Then they go out in public wearing it. Most soon realize that the world doesn't stop to stare. In fact, says Dr. Sarwer, hardly anyone notices.

Don't call attention to yourself. You don't want anyone to see your thighs, so you wear ankle-length sweatpants to the beach. Hate to break it to you, but you are the only person wearing ankle-length sweatpants on the beach—and everyone is staring at you. "People who cover up and make an issue of hiding weight often bring more attention on themselves," Dr. Sarwer says. If you wore the bathing suit, you'd look just like everyone else.

Living Proof
PANEL

Her Body, Her Friend

Delma A. Garda

For all my body's flaws, it is mine. It has carried and nursed three children, and for that I think it deserves some battle marks!

So when I started the program, it wasn't because I hated my body. I joined for many reasons: It motivated me to exercise; it was a good way to meet people since I had just moved to a new area; and, yes, it would be nice to go down a dress size and just feel a little less than my age.

What I am finding, though, is how much more pleased I am with my body. Parts no longer jiggle. When I wear bicycle shorts, I don't feel I have to wear a T-shirt that reaches my knees. And when my husband runs his hands over my body, he comments on how much firmer and tighter it feels!

Stop comparing. You compare yourself with the woman in the office with the tightest butt or the mom across the street who has washboard abs after having two kids. Notice that you never compare yourself with the woman in the office with tree-trunk legs or the mom whose waistline broadcasts to the world that she's had three kids.

"We often compare ourselves with the thinnest or most beautiful person and then only those features we dislike the most," Dr. Sarwer says. But everyone is different, so the comparison doesn't mean much. "While comparing ourselves to others is often automatic, it is a dangerous practice that leads us to being upset. Many times, it is better to realize that this game is one we can't win. Therefore, we should try not to play. Once we are aware that we are comparing, we are better able to curb this tendency."

Disregard numbers. Guess the weight of the person next to you. Chances are, you can't. "We forget that people don't know how much we weigh by looking at us," says Dr. Sarwer.

Even though Dr. Sarwer works with overweight patients all the time, he still can't calculate people's weights just by looking at them. "The exact numbers on the scale aren't always what's important," he says. "A 3- to 5-pound difference is probably not going to make a significant difference to your health and body image."

So while you sit there convinced that people are mentally chiding you for being over your ideal weight, they probably don't have a clue.

Get indignant. Your husband calls you, "My little fatty." Or your mother-in-law slyly notes that you don't *really* need that piece of cake, do you? Don't smile politely. Get mad. Real mad.

"Say, 'How dare you! Get out of my face,'" Dr. Rosenberg says. "You have to have boundaries. Develop a feeling of indignation, and don't let anyone cross that line."

These little insults and put-downs—even those supposedly said in jest—erode your self-esteem, she says. By refusing to accept them, you say to yourself and others that you don't deserve to be treated that way.

The Joy of Strength Training

MOST PEOPLE DON'T KNOW THAT MARILYN MONROE LIFTED WEIGHTS. THAT'S RIGHT. THAT AMERICAN ICON OF FEMININITY, BEAUTY, AND GLAMOUR HOISTED DUMBBELLS REGULARLY. OBVIOUSLY, SHE DIDN'T WANT BIGGER MUSCLES OR TO LOOK MORE MASCULINE. SHE JUST KNEW WHAT MILLIONS OF WOMEN ARE DISCOVERING TODAY—THAT BUILDING MUSCLE IS AMONG THE BEST WAYS TO KEEP A YOUNG, TRIM FIGURE.

Forget everything you've heard about muscle and bulk. Muscle tissue is what keeps you thin. Each pound of lean muscle tissue in your body burns about 50 calories a day, even when you're doing nothing more than sitting around. On the other hand, each pound of fat tissue burns only 2 calories.

This is one of the reasons that you could eat more when you were younger and not gain weight. Pound for pound, you naturally had more calorie-burning muscle tissue. The problem is, when women reach their forties, they start losing small amounts of muscle and replacing it with fat. After age 40, you naturally lose about ½ pound of muscle a year. Some women lose up to 1 pound a year after they hit menopause. At that rate, by age 55, you could be down 15 pounds of muscle and burning 600 fewer calories a day.

Luckily, it doesn't have to be that way.

"So many women in their late thirties and forties come to see me saying, 'I've never had a weight problem in my life, and now I do, even though I'm not doing anything different,'" says certified fitness instructor Kelly Bridgman, wellness director for the Peggy and Philip B. Crosby Wellness Center at the YMCA in Winter Park, Florida. "Well, they may not be doing anything different, but their bodies are. The metabolism is slowing down. And the only way to really rev it back up is with strength training."

Muscle Makes You Trim and Shapely

Not only will strength training give you your old body back, it will give you a better body back. Aerobic activity can burn calories and fat, but only strength training will tone you and give you a great shape.

"Exercise physiologists used to emphasize aerobics as the best way to get in shape. But we're finding that strength training is at least as effective for total health and fitness," says exercise physiologist Robert Brosmer, vice president of health and wellness at the Central Florida YMCA in Orlando and coauthor of *Health and High Performance*. "Only strength training and sensible nutritional habits really change the way you look."

Though men have been taking advantage of the toning effects of weight lifting for years, women are just starting to discover that it's just what they're looking for to fight the effects of age and gravity, especially in their curves.

"Women are very specific about the body parts that they want to make better," says Majid Ali, a certified fitness instructor in Los Angeles. "They want to firm their butts and lift their breasts and stop places from jiggling. Though aerobic exercise can certainly help you lose weight all over, the best way to hit these spots is to build those muscles."

Muscle Makes You Young

Building muscle does more than give you a younger-looking body. It also gives you a younger-feeling body.

"People can't believe how much physical improvement they notice once they start resistance training," says Laura Senft, a registered physical thera-

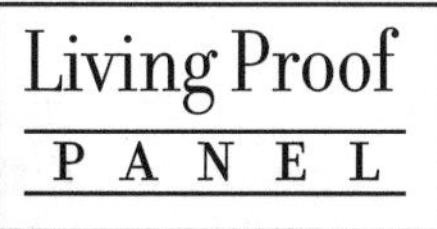

It's Fun and Easy!

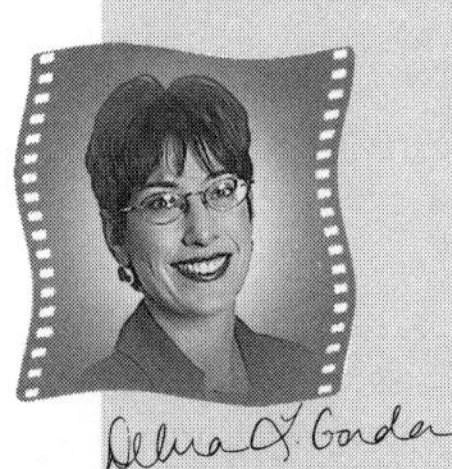

The exercises are easy. They take only 15 minutes. You can do them anywhere. And my 3-year-old likes to play with the extra balls while I do them.

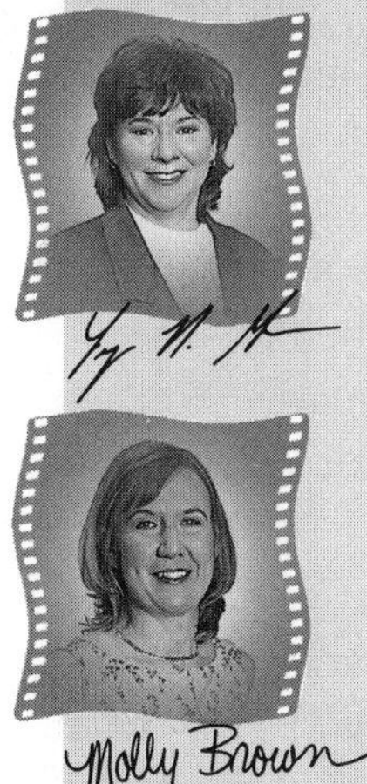

The exercises seemed so simple, I wasn't sure they'd work. But after just a few times, I felt stronger and my back didn't hurt at the end of the day like it normally did.

The combination of walking and weight training has made me feel really great. I found the medicine balls so effective that I even took them on vacation when I went to Maine.

pist at the Kessler Institute for Rehabilitation in West Orange, New Jersey. "They can do everything better, from climbing stairs to playing with their kids. They have more energy. And because they're reducing body fat, building bone, and increasing muscle, they're a whole lot healthier."

Here are some ways that weight lifting helps make your body young.

Revs your metabolism. As you've read, strength training gives you more lean muscle tissue, which burns tons of calories every day. But it also gives your metabolism an extra calorie-burning boost for about 30 minutes after you're done working out. In fact, your body continues to burn more calories after ½ hour of strength training than it does after ½ hour of jogging.

"By building muscle and burning fat, you can get to a point—even in your forties and fifties—where you aren't losing lean body tissue and you aren't gaining fat body tissue," says Brosmer. "So your body looks and feels younger."

Builds younger bones. All women are at risk for osteoporosis. As bones age, they lose calcium and other minerals. This makes them more porous and likely to break. It's also what causes some women to "shrink" as they age, a result of vertebrae compressing.

Of course, it's important to get enough calcium. And walking can help increase bone density. But strength training is the best strategy for keeping your bones strong. "Working out with some weights twice a week is all it takes to lay down bone in your arms and legs, where women are most likely to get weak," says Senft.

Improves self-confidence. "Resistance training is great for building self-esteem," says John Yetter, M.D., medical director at SSM Rehab Sports Medicine in St. Louis. "You can see yourself getting stronger, not just when it comes to lifting weights, but in everyday life. You can climb stairs more easily. You can open jars and pick up heavy household objects. It gives you little morale boosts all day long."

Promotes better balance. When we're young and running around all the time, balance isn't much of a problem. As we get a little older and more sedentary, however, our brain-to-muscle connections can get weak from disuse. Strength training can prevent that from happening. In a study of men and women in their late seventies, researchers found that those who strength-trained three times a week for 16 weeks were able to improve their balance by almost 70 percent.

Strengthens joints. When it comes to aches, pains, and injuries, your body's weakest links are its joints. Strength training—you guessed it!—helps keep joints strong and pain-free. "It's important to strengthen your muscles, ligaments, and tendons because they're what you rely on to move through this life," says Dr. Yetter. "You won't walk, play, or work very well if your joints or muscles are weak."

Have a Ball!

Most people are convinced that the only way to get the benefits of strength training is to spend hours at the gym. Nothing could be further from the truth. Sure, free weights and Nautilus machines are perfectly fine ways to build muscle and burn fat. But you can get all the same benefits—with minimal gear—right at home. It's quick. It's easy. And best of all, it's fun.

That's right, fun. You don't need barbells anymore (although a lot of people still enjoy using them). Many women are now exercising with small (4- or 6-pound), brightly colored medicine balls. They are easy to carry and fun to use. Using them feels a whole lot more like playing than like working out.

"If I could have only one thing to train with for the rest of my life, medicine balls would be it," says Michael Romatowski, director of personal training at Athletic Express Health Club in Gaithersburg, Maryland, and author of *Secrets of Medicine Ball Training*. "The motions and the ways you use your hands when using them are much more like the things you do in real life."

10 Easy Exercises

The key to making your body its youngest and shapeliest is to exercise and tone all the major muscle groups, in both your upper and lower body. Women's risk of osteoporosis—and the hunched-over posture it can cause—makes building muscle in the upper body important. And lower-body exercises can help trim and tone the stomach, hips, and thighs—the trouble spots where most women have a tendency to add pounds.

Think you don't have time for such a complete workout? Think again. Only professional bodybuilders need to spend hours in the gym, says Senft. With the 10 simple exercises shown on the following pages, done two or three times a week, you can hit all of your muscle groups. Plan on doing one set of 10 to 15 repetitions for each exercise. (Each time you lift a weight, it's one repetition.) It will take you 20 minutes tops, then you're done.

Incidentally, even though the following exercises specify using medicine balls, you can easily substitute 5- or 10-pound dumbbells. The weight you use should be heavy enough so that the last four repetitions are fairly hard.

So, let's get started!

Half Squats

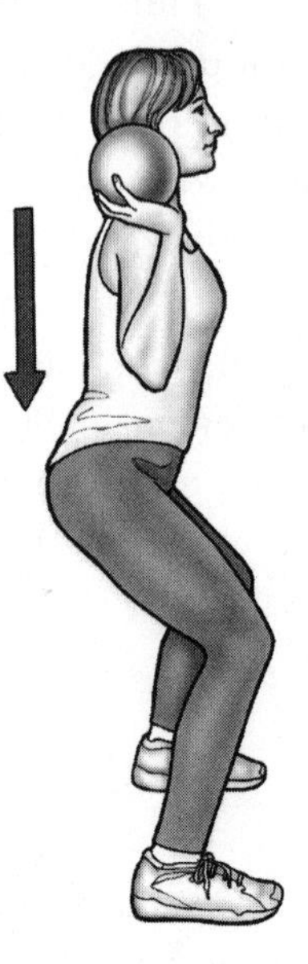

Stand with your back facing a chair (without armrests). Keep your feet flat on the floor and positioned slightly more than shoulder-width apart. Hold the medicine balls up at your shoulders with your palms facing up. Keep your head in line with your upper body, facing forward.

Keeping your back straight, slowly bend at the knees and hips, as though you were sitting down. Don't let your knees extend beyond your toes. Stop just shy of sitting on the chair. Hold for a second, then return to the starting position. Repeat.

Muscles worked: Hip muscles, quadriceps (front of thighs), hamstrings (back of thighs), gluteals (buttocks), and lower-back muscles

Chest Presses

Lie on your back, with your knees bent and your feet flat on the floor and about hip-width apart. Hold the balls up over your chest with your arms extended and your palms facing the ceiling. Your thumbs should face each other.

Bend your elbows and slowly lower the balls. Stop when the balls are about even with your shoulders. (If you're lying on the floor, your arms will be resting on the floor.) Slowly return to start. Repeat.

Muscles worked: Chest and shoulder muscles and triceps (back of upper arms)

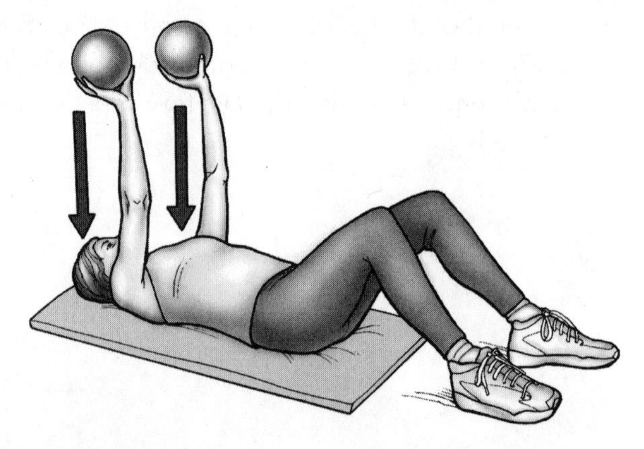

Bent-Over Rows

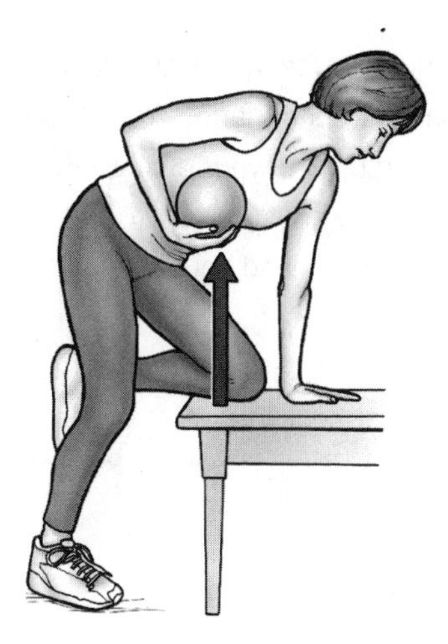

Hold a ball in your right hand, with your palm facing up, your thumb facing out, and your elbow pointed back. Rest your left knee and left hand on a chair or bench for support. Place your right foot on the floor, with your knee slightly bent. Keep your back straight. Your head should be down and in a straight line with your back. Let the arm holding the ball hang down toward the floor.

Slowly pull the ball up to your chest. Your right elbow will point toward the ceiling as you lift. Hold for a second, then lower to the starting position. Complete a full set, then switch sides and repeat with the other arm.

Muscles worked: Back and neck muscles

Biceps Curls

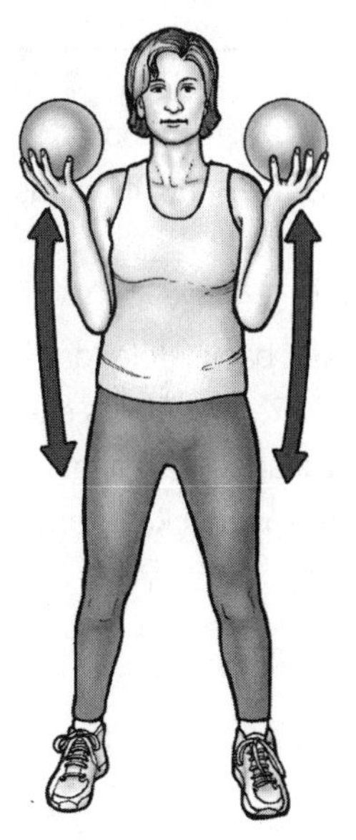

Stand with your knees slightly bent and your feet about shoulder-width apart. Hold the balls down at your sides, with your palms facing up and your thumbs facing out. Keep your body erect and your head up and facing forward.

Keeping your elbows at your sides, slowly lift the balls upward toward your collarbone. Don't arch your back. Hold for a second, then slowly lower to the starting position. Repeat.

Muscles worked: Biceps (front of upper arms)

Overhead Triceps Extensions

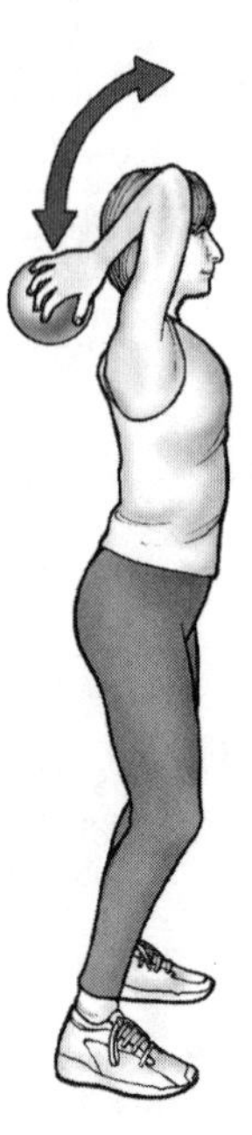

Stand with your knees slightly bent and your feet about shoulder-width apart. Hold one ball over your head with both hands. Your arms should be extended, with your palms facing up and your elbows slightly bent and close to your head.

Keeping your arms close to your head, slowly bend your elbows and lower the ball behind your head as far as it will go. Hold for a second, then return to start. Repeat.

Muscles worked: Triceps (back of upper arms)

Shoulder Presses

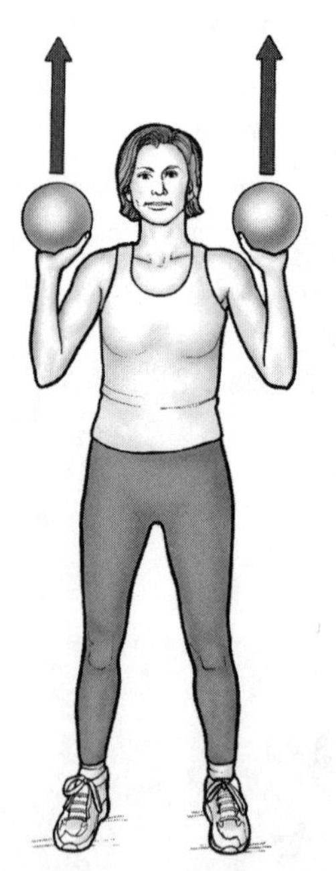

Stand with your knees slightly bent and your feet about shoulder-width apart. Hold the balls at shoulder height, palms facing up and thumbs facing each other.

Slowly press the balls up until your arms are fully extended. Don't lock your elbows or arch your back. Hold for a second, then lower to the starting position. Repeat. If this exercise is difficult, you may try it seated instead of standing.

Muscles worked: Shoulder muscles, triceps (back of upper arms), and upper-back and neck muscles

Downward Chops

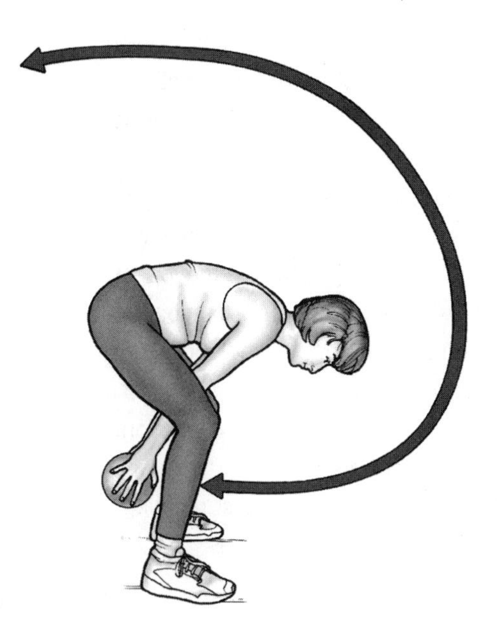

Stand with your knees slightly bent and your feet about shoulder-width apart. With both hands, hold one ball over and behind your head, with your elbows bent about 45 degrees.

Moving with control, bend at the waist and swing the ball down between your legs, as though you were chopping wood. Then swing it back up behind your head. Repeat. The speed should be slow to moderate for beginners. At the bottom of the movement, the position is similar to hiking a football backward through your legs.

Muscles worked: Abdominals (including obliques), back and shoulder muscles, gluteals (buttocks), and hamstrings (back of thighs)

Diagonal Chops

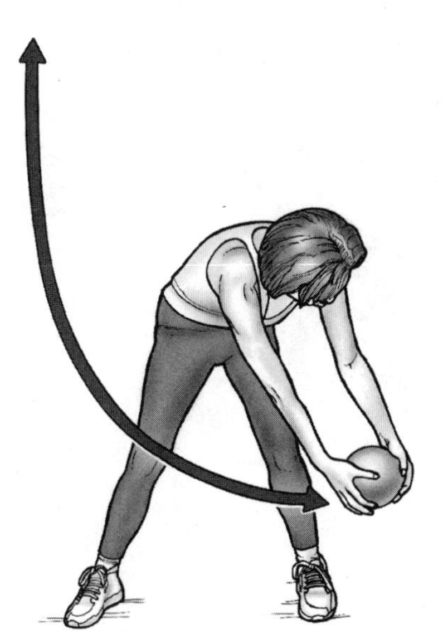

Stand with your knees slightly bent and your feet about shoulder-width apart. Hold one ball high above your right shoulder with both hands. Your elbows should be slightly bent.

With control, swing downward along a diagonal path until the ball is outside your left knee. Let your head and eyes follow the path of the ball as you swing it down, then back up above your right shoulder. Perform equal repetitions on both sides.

Muscles worked: Core muscles in your abdomen, back, and shoulders and supporting muscles in your buttocks and thighs

Chops and Twists

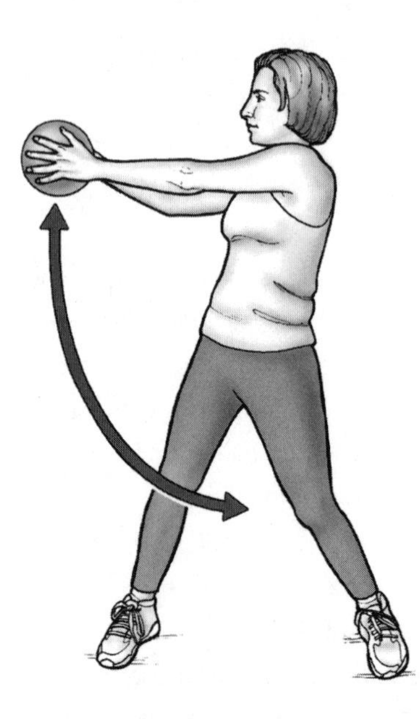

Stand with your knees slightly bent and your feet about shoulder-width apart. With both hands, hold one ball over and behind your head, with your elbows bent about 45 degrees.

With control, swing the ball down between your legs (see downward chop illustration on page 143). As you swing it back to the top, twist to the right, as though you were going to toss the ball backward over your right shoulder. Swing back down through your legs, then swing up and twist to the left. Continue in a smooth motion.

Muscles worked: Core muscles in your abdomen, back, and shoulders and supporting muscles in your buttocks and thighs

Classic Crunches

Lie on your back on a mat or carpeted floor, with your knees bent and your feet flat on the floor, about hip-width apart. Clasp your hands loosely behind your head, with your elbows facing out. Tilt your pelvis slightly to flatten your back against the floor. Slowly curl your shoulders about 30 degrees off the floor. Don't pull up on your neck. Hold for a second, then slowly lower. Repeat.

Muscles worked: Upper abs

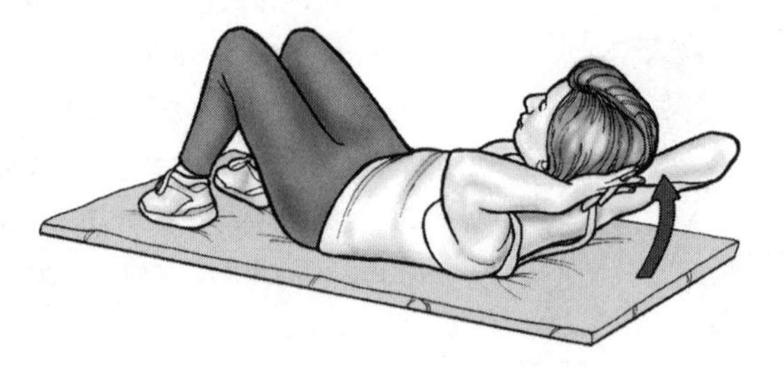

Bad Foods and Other Myths

CONSIDER, IF YOU WILL, THE JEKYLL-AND-HYDE SAGA OF THE EGG. A PERFECT SOURCE OF PROTEIN. EASY TO PREPARE. AND CHEAP. BUT THE EGG DEVELOPED A REAL IMAGE PROBLEM AT ABOUT THE SAME TIME DOCTORS STARTED RECOMMENDING THAT WE CONSUME ONLY 300 MILLIGRAMS OF CHOLESTEROL PER DAY IN ORDER TO REDUCE THE RISK FOR HEART DISEASE.

Our own brand of scientific deduction went something like this, says Susan Adams, R.D., a registered dietitian in Seattle and spokesperson for the American Dietetic Association. Cholesterol is bad. Eggs have cholesterol (213 milligrams per egg). Therefore, eggs are bad. The flaw in this type of one-dimensional nutritional policing is that foods, eggs included, also contain healthy nutrients, she says. Besides cholesterol, each egg contains protein, iron, unsaturated fats, essential amino acids, and folate and other B vitamins.

"Actually, eggs are a very good food," she says.

So don't believe everything you hear about other so-called bad foods like white bread, red meat, and chocolate. They also can fit into a healthy eating plan.

"There are no junk foods. There are only junk diets," says Frances Berg, a licensed nutritionist in Hettinger, North Dakota; author of *Women Afraid to Eat*; and editor of *Healthy Weight Journal*.

More than ever, we're realizing that what we eat does make a difference in the way we look and feel. But we're also confused. Foods touted as healthy one week may be branded downright unsafe next month. This black cloud of conflicting information can drown out the fun in food if you let it.

The quick-fix approach to weight control has a 95 percent failure rate.

"Food is beautiful, and eating is fun," says John La Puma, M.D., a Chicago physician who is the founder and medical director of the CHEF (Cooking, Healthy Eating, and Fitness) Clinic, which uses a cutting-edge approach to weight loss based on putting flavor first. "No food by itself is bad. How you eat it and how often is what gets you into trouble."

The notion that some foods are inherently bad or good remains one of the biggest myths about nutrition. It's a misconception held by 77 percent of Americans, according to the American Dietetic Association's 2000 trends survey.

Misguided or not, the black-and-white approach to a healthy diet is actually a logical product of the confusion generated by the steady stream of headline-making health studies in our sound-bite culture.

"We generally have a couple of reactions to the nutrition news that makes the headlines," says Adams. "We tend to avoid things because we think they're bad, or eat more of something because we think it's good."

So as you start making lifestyle changes to lose weight and feel better, it helps to know nutritional fact from fiction. Here's a quick primer on some of the most common mistakes that people make.

Myth: Dieting Is the Only Way to Lose Weight

If you subscribed to a daily newspaper, and it only made it to your doorstep 20 days out of the entire year, you would cancel it, right? Well, diets deliver even less often than that. Restrictive dieting—the quick-fix, short-term, "on-again, off-again" approach to weight control—has a 95 percent failure rate.

The good news is that the message may be sinking in. Fewer Americans are dieting, according to a survey by the Calorie Control Council. In 1986, 37 percent of adult Americans were on diets. That number dropped to 27 percent in 1998, while another 39 percent said that they were making serious efforts to control their weight without dieting.

Why do we fail at weight loss? We're not exercising enough. We're eating too much fat. And we're eating too much, period. Our calorie intakes keep going up, currently more than 2,000 calories a day compared to about 1,800 in the 1970s.

For the best chance of weight-loss success, give up dieting and normalize your eating patterns for life, says Berg. The goal is to tune in to internal signals of hunger and satiety, eating when hungry and stopping when satisfied.

"One of the benefits of normal eating is that you think less about food," she says.

Myth: Eating Healthy Is Boring

With the right blend of skills and planning, healthy fare is delicious and fun to prepare, Dr. La Puma says. He discovered that when he took some time off and went to cooking school.

There, he learned how to make healthy food taste delicious. When he lost 30 pounds while enjoying the process, he knew he was on to something.

"People need to learn the skills to change their habits," says Dr. La Puma.

He developed a pleasure-packed approach to weight loss that trains people in everything from planning to shopping to cooking. When he tested his innovative program on a group of overweight people, they dropped an average of 24 pounds in 22 weeks without counting a calorie, banning a single food, or dodging a single restaurant. The best part? They had fun doing it.

Myth: I Can Eat as Much as I Want as Long as It's Low-Fat

This might be true if we were filling up on naturally low-fat foods such as strawberries. At 136 calories per pound, you could eat them by the bucket and still lose weight.

But in the real world of processed food, 93 percent of us are eating re-

How Myths Originate

Like the dreaded *Rocky* sequel, some version of the high-protein diet reemerges every 5 years as the new "breakthrough" formula for weight loss, says Dr. Carol Boushey of Purdue University, who tracks the origin of popular myths about nutrition.

But there's nothing new about it. Nor will it work for permanent weight loss, she says. Yet, eager for a solution to get rid of those stubborn pounds, people try it. They do lose weight. But it's mostly water and lean tissue, not fat. And even though they will probably regain the weight shortly after the diet ends, the myth remains intact.

Confusion about the significance of new research helps breed new myths and perpetuate old ones. These days, the media informs us about every new study, particularly those concerning the health effects of diet and lifestyle. Eventually, we get the message that if only we can change our habits to keep up with the latest research, we'll stay well. The problem is, in the world of science, one study is just a tiny piece of a big puzzle.

duced-fat or fat-free versions of typically high-fat foods. "The issue isn't just fat, it's total calories," says Carol Boushey, R.D., Ph.D., assistant professor of food and nutrition at Purdue University in West Lafayette, Indiana. Low-fat often doesn't equal low-calorie. Smear 2 tablespoons of reduced-fat peanut butter on a slice of bread, and you'll end up with the same calorie count as the full-fat version.

But it doesn't stop there. When our eyes see low-fat, our brains say, "Eat more." To test how low-fat and high-fat labels affected eating, Barbara Rolls, Ph.D., professor of nutrition at Pennsylvania State University in University Park, and her colleagues at the university gave 48 women three indistinguishable raspberry-flavored yogurts.

When the women ate the yogurts labeled "low-fat," they consumed significantly more calories during the subsequent lunch and dinner than they did after eating the yogurt labeled "high-fat." When the yogurts weren't labeled for fat content, these differences didn't occur.

Low-fat foods can help promote weight loss, but only if they are also low

"Like a soap opera, you can forget to watch for a few weeks and never miss a thing. The same is true of scientific research," Dr. Boushey says.

So how do we make ourselves myth-proof? The short answer is to be more skeptical. To look at research with the reserve of the scientist, follow these tips.

Be cautious. Inconsistency is common in scientific research, particularly epidemiological research (the kind that tracks patterns in a population) about diet and lifestyle. Remember that the papers in medical journals are often works in progress for other scientists and aren't intended to be the final word for the public.

Wait for the sequel. As soon as a study is published, news of its conclusions (though virtually none of its qualifying details) hits the airwaves. Within hours, millions of people consider eating more oat bran to fend off disease. Don't change your lifestyle habits based on the results of one study.

"In time, all the studies will come together and a consensus will be reached," says Dr. Boushey. Usually, it will come in the form of a recommendation from a government agency or a nonprofit health organization such as the American Heart Association.

in calories, you eat them in normal portions, and you don't consider them a license to overeat later, says Dr. Boushey.

Myth: Eating a Certain Type of Food Will Help You Burn Fat

This is the hook that promoters of the grapefruit diet used to reel in a hopeful public.

"While it's true that you do burn calories digesting your food, the amount is just a small percentage of the calories you've eaten, so it won't affect your weight," says James O. Hill, Ph.D., associate director of the University of Colorado Health Sciences Center in Boulder. The grapefruit diet, the cabbage soup diet, the rice diet, the fruit diet, and the high-protein diet all have one thing in common: "They go against healthy balance," says Adams. "They don't make sense for lifelong change in habits to develop new eating patterns."

Myth: Eating at Night Will Make It Harder to Lose Weight

Even some experts believe this common diet myth, but research doesn't confirm it. It's the total number of calories that you eat every day and the total number you expend in activity that count—not when you eat.

Not convinced? In a study of 7,000 people, those who ate 64 percent or more of their calories after 5:00 P.M. were no more likely to gain weight over a 10-year period than those who ate only 25 percent of their calories after 5:00 P.M. Our national average, by the way, is 46 percent of calories eaten after 5:00 P.M.

If your schedule means that you have to eat a late dinner, don't worry, says Dr. Boushey. Calories consumed at night will simply be burned when needed. And by the way, you do burn calories while you sleep—about 50 per hour, depending on your weight and other factors.

Myth: Cravings Are the Body's Natural Response to Nutritional Deficiencies

If this were true, then what nutritional void does chocolate candy, the most frequently craved food, fill?

"Everyone likes the idea of the wisdom of the body," says Marcia Pelchat, Ph.D., a sensory psychologist at Monell Chemical Senses Center in Philadelphia. But researchers are still hard-pressed for a scientific explanation as to why cravings arise and what purpose they serve. And the missing-nutrient theory doesn't seem to hold up under scientific scrutiny.

In one study, Dr. Pelchat asked people to consume nothing but a nutritionally complete, sweet vanilla beverage and water for 5 days. The participants reported craving foods such as pizza and steak—foods with a different aroma and texture—over sweet foods like ice cream or cookies. These cravings arose in the absence of nutritional need.

But there is hope: Cravings become less frequent and easier to deal with as we age, Dr. Pelchat says.

Myth: All Fat Is Bad

According to one survey, fat and how to eat less of it seems to be our number one nutrition concern. All we have to do is cut the fat, and our weight-loss woes will be over—or so we think. But the function of fat goes way beyond making food taste good. Our bodies need fat—for a healthy heart, stronger bones, better vision. Fat coats every nerve and is the major part of every cell membrane. It can even help us lose weight.

"One of the reasons you tend to overeat on low-fat diets is that you're hungry all the time. Adding essential fats into your diet actually encourages weight loss by promoting a feeling of fullness and satiety," says Ann Louise Gittleman, C.N.S., a clinical nurse specialist, a nutritionist, and author of *Eat Fat, Lose Weight*. "You are satisfied for longer periods of time—up to 4 hours."

The key is to replace unhealthy saturated and trans fats found in red meat, dairy, margarine, and baked goods with healthy fats such as those found in olive and flaxseed oils, salmon, almonds, and dark green, leafy vegetables.

Overweight people who avoid fats might eat more and gain weight. Researchers at the Children's Hospital and Tufts University, both in Boston, fed 12 obese teenagers test meals and then let them eat whenever they felt hungry over the next 5 hours. Those who had been given a high-starch meal took in 81 percent more calories during this period than those who initially ate a meal that was higher in fat. The finding may help explain why so few French people are overweight despite their high-fat diets.

Myth: Vitamins Give You Energy

Feeling tired and run-down? A friend is sure to advise you to take vitamins to boost your energy. Though essential for health, vitamins lack the crucial ingredient necessary to produce energy: calories.

"Calories come from fat, carbohydrates, and protein," says Patricia Hart, R.D., a nutritional consultant and chef in San Francisco. In other words, food. Vitamins are just the supporting cast in the metabolic process. As you digest your meal, they assist the enzymes that release the energy from food.

No vitamin will undo the excesses of a lousy diet—high fat, extra calories, or too much sodium.

Myth: Eating a Healthy Diet Costs More

Four out of 10 people think that fruits, vegetables, fish, and other foods that fit into a healthful diet cost more than what they're currently tossing into their grocery carts. That's not necessarily true, says Adams.

When researchers from Pennsylvania State University and the Mary Imogene Bassett Research Institute in Cooperstown, New York, gave 300 people with high cholesterol instructions on cutting fat from their diets, those whose cholesterol dropped the most lopped an average of $1.10 per day from their food bills. For a family of four, that comes to a yearly savings of $1,600.

Myth: Fresh Vegetables Are More Nutritious Than Canned or Frozen

Fact: Nine out of 10 people buy into the belief that fresh is better than frozen or canned. That's not necessarily true when it comes to nutritional value, says Adams. Many fresh vegetables that end up in the produce aisle are harvested before they're ripe, trucked thousands of miles, and stored for long periods. All these factors diminish nutrient values, particularly vitamin C levels.

When well-handled by the processor, canned and frozen produce retains most of its vitamins and minerals.

"It's a direct trip from field to processing plant. Nutrients are more or less locked in," says Adams. "Canned beans, pumpkin, corn, pineapple, tomatoes, spinach, and beets, to name just a few, are actually quite nutritious."

Fill Up on Fat-Fighting Fiber

"A MILD, SMOKY FLAVOR WITH AN OVERALL BEGUILING QUALITY." IN A SOUTHWEST VERSION OF THE PEPSI CHALLENGE, THAT'S HOW SANTA FE CHEFS DESCRIBED THE FLOR DE MAYO, ONE OF THE TOP CONTENDERS IN A BLINDFOLD TASTE TEST.

And what exactly was this exotic-sounding, tasty dish? Here's a hint: People eat the tin-can version of its plainer cousin around the campfire.

Yes—the bean. Who would have thought that nature's quintessential fiber food could go gourmet?

Chances are that the idea of eating fiber-rich food brings a different picture to mind. Perhaps bathroom regularity and excessive intestinal gas. Euell Gibbons jokes aside, if the thought of filling up on fiber sounds as appetizing as gnawing the bark off a tree, read on and maybe you'll change your mind.

Instead of thinking of fiber as the digestive equivalent of the Roto-Rooter man, think fat-fighting power. That's right. Fiber may be your best weapon in the battle of the bulge. And you're probably not getting enough of it. The average American consumes less than half of the Daily Value of 25 grams that experts and the American Dietetic Association recommend.

"People have heard about fiber—remember the oat-bran mania of the

Give Yourself a Quick Fiber Checkup

Use this easy counter to see if you're getting 30 grams of fiber each day. Fill in the number of servings of each particular food you eat each day and multiply it by the number of grams of fiber to get each answer. Then add up all your amounts for your total daily fiber intake.

1.5 g fiber	×	_____	servings of fruit	=	_____	g
1.5 g fiber	×	_____	servings of vegetables	=	_____	g
2.5 g fiber	×	_____	servings of whole grains	=	_____	g
(whole wheat bread and pasta, brown rice)						
1 g fiber	×	_____	servings of refined grains	=	_____	g
(white bread and pasta, white rice)						
5 g fiber	×	_____	servings of dried beans	=	_____	g
Fiber in a serving of your breakfast cereal				=	_____	g
YOUR DAILY FIBER TOTAL				=	_____	**g**

1980s? Yet, they don't quite understand what fiber is," says Gayle Reichler, R.D., a registered dietitian and consultant in New York City and author of *Active Wellness*.

So what, exactly, is fiber? Once known as roughage, fiber is found only in plant foods: fruits, vegetables, whole grains, legumes (beans, peas, and lentils), nuts, and seeds. It's the part of the plant that we can't digest, which is why people once assumed it had no nutritional value. But as you'll see, fiber has a bulk of benefits in helping you get thinner and younger.

Get Thin

A typical person who doubled his fiber intake could lose 9 to 10 pounds over the course of a year without reducing his calorie intake. Fiber cuts calories by blocking the digestion of some of the fat and protein consumed with it.

Think of fiber as many fine threads. As they travel through the intestinal tract, the threads wrap around each other like a piece of twine, tying up calories in the process. For best results, aim for 30 grams of fiber daily, spread out over the day.

Fiber cuts calories in more straightforward ways as well. Most high-fiber foods are low in calories and fat, so if you eat more of them, you'll eat fewer calories and less fat. And because of their bulk, high-fiber foods tend to satisfy hunger quickly, before you have a chance to overeat.

Get Young

Want to keep your heart healthy? Eat a bowl of high-fiber cereal or oatmeal at least five times a week, says Regina Ragone, R.D., a registered dietitian and food editor for *Prevention* magazine. Harvard researchers who studied the fiber intake of 68,782 women in the Nurses' Health Study found that those who ate the highest amount of fiber from cereal had a 34 percent reduced risk for developing heart disease.

Fiber can help keep your body young in other ways, too, by reducing your risk for age-related conditions such as stroke, cancer, and diabetes, says Andrew Weil, M.D., director of the program in integrative medicine at the University of Arizona in Tucson.

When you're talking health benefits, there are two kinds of fiber: soluble and insoluble. "Breaking fiber into categories is tricky, however, since many foods contain both kinds," explains Dr. Weil.

Insoluble fiber—found in prunes and apple skins, carrots, cabbage, and whole grain products—keeps your body's digestive tract humming. Soluble fiber—the kind found in oatmeal, oat bran, beans, peas, citrus fruits, and strawberries—binds with cholesterol in the intestines, preventing its absorption into the blood.

Go for the Goal

You can easily—and tastefully—get at least 25 grams of fiber a day with an array of delectable fruits, vegetables, beans, and nuts. Whole grain foods

The Fiber Hall of Fame

The following cereals rank among your best choices for a high-fiber start to your day.

CEREAL	CALORIES	FIBER (g)
General Mills Fiber One (½ cup)	65	14
Kellogg's All-Bran Bran Buds (⅓ cup)	80	13
Kellogg's All-Bran (½ cup)	80	10
Kellogg's Raisin Bran (1 cup)	200	8
Post 100% Bran (⅓ cup)	80	8
Post Raisin Bran (1 cup)	190	8
Post Shredded Wheat 'n Bran (1¼ cups)	200	8
General Mills Multi-Bran Chex (1 cup)	200	7
Quaker Shredded Wheat (3 biscuits)	220	7
Quaker Oat Bran (1¼ cups)	210	6

such as whole wheat bread, high-fiber cereals, and whole wheat pasta also are excellent sources.

"Aim to boost your fiber intake by taking a look at where high-fiber foods can replace lower-fiber choices," says Ragone. "It's not that important to know what kind of fiber you're getting. The best rule of thumb is to aim for a wide variety of high-fiber foods."

Top your cereal with prunes, blackberries, strawberries, apple slices (including skins), or chopped pears; add chickpeas to your salad; or top your baked potato with chopped broccoli. And try these creative fiber boosters.

Eat the breakfast of champions. The quickest, absolutely easiest way to get a jump on your fiber intake for the day is to start with a bowl of high-fiber cereal, says Ragone. Many people who never touch whole wheat pasta or brown rice think nothing of eating a whole grain cereal such as shredded wheat.

Look for a whole grain cereal that has at least 5 grams of fiber per serving. Top it with a handful of raspberries, which have more than 6 grams of fiber per cup, and you're more than a third of the way to your goal.

"Watch out though," cautions Ragone. "It's really easy to eat too much cereal and add extra calories." Read the label to check serving size and use a measuring cup to get the right amount in the bowl. If you use the same bowl every morning, you'll know how far to fill it.

Mix it up. Are you a kid at heart when it comes to breakfast cereal? Do you long for the sweet taste and primary colors of your youth? Then try the art of cereal blending, says Ragone. By mixing one of your sweet favorites with a sensible high-fiber cereal, you'll come up with a great-tasting hybrid that has 5 or more grams of fiber per serving. Here are three suggestions to get you started.

■ Shredded Crunch: ¼ cup Cap'n Crunch, ⅚ cup Shredded Wheat 'n Bran (5.6 grams of fiber, 170 calories)

■ Fiber Charms: ⅓ cup All-Bran Extra Fiber, ⅓ cup Lucky Charms (8.9 grams of fiber, 73 calories)

Living Proof
PANEL

My Partner in Weight Loss

When I learned that fiber could help me lose weight, I reevaluated the choices I made in food.

The first change I made was at breakfast. Cheerios had always been my cereal of choice, but it had only 3 grams of fiber in a cup. Now I eat more than a cup of high-fiber cereal (a mix of Fiber One, Raisin Bran, and Basic Four for optimal fiber and taste), and I get 12 grams under my belt before I even leave for work in the morning. That's almost half of my daily goal of 30 grams.

Then I tackle the rest of the day. Instead of crackers, I have a couple of pieces of fruit during the day. I eat a healthy lunch with a green salad and have a nutritious dinner, such as low-fat tacos with refried beans. With these changes, I make my fiber goal by the end of the day.

Now I look at the dietary fiber content of everything I buy, and I try to get the most fiber I can from my food. My friends and coworkers comment on how much I eat—and I still lost weight.

- Count Fibrula: ⅜ cup Fiber One, ¼ cup Count Chocula (9.8 grams of fiber, 75 calories)

Veg out. "One thing I really try to promote is eating your fruits and vegetables," says Ragone. "That's going to be your ticket."

An average serving of fruits or vegetables contains about 1.5 grams of fiber. Double up on fruits and vegetables—that's about 9 daily servings—and you'll easily make your daily fiber quota.

Some of the best high-fiber choices are pears, apples, oranges, berries, baked potatoes (with skin), peas, and Brussels sprouts.

Read the whole label. Replace half or more of your refined carbohydrates with whole grain carbohydrates, says Ragone. There are hundreds of whole grain products on the shelves—bread, pasta, cereal, rice, and snacks.

Start by reading the ingredient list. The first ingredient should include the word *whole.* If it doesn't, the product has mostly refined flour. Words such as *unbleached, enriched, stone-ground,* or *wheat* may sound good, but they don't mean "whole grain."

Can it. Now is a good time to use the fiber-filled contents of those cans of beans that are gathering dust on your pantry shelves, says Ragone. Add color, texture, and flavor to your meals by mixing beans into salads, sauces, and rice dishes.

Make a quick burrito with fat-free, vegetarian refried beans. Check gourmet shops for high-quality dried beans like the Flor de Mayo grown by New Mexico bean expert Elizabeth Berry.

Sprinkle it on. Sprinkle a couple of tablespoons of freshly ground flaxseed on your cereal, soup, or salad, says Reichler. It has a nutty taste, similar to sesame seed, and a mere ¼ cup will give you 6 grams of fiber.

Besides containing heart-healthy and brain-boosting omega-3 fatty acids and beneficial phytoestrogens, flaxseed is a good source of fiber, offering more than 3 grams per tablespoon. Also try pumpkin seeds, wheat germ, pistachios, or almonds for a fiber bonus. But watch out for the extra calories, especially from the nuts.

Drink plenty of water. If you don't drink enough water, fiber can actually promote constipation, says Ragone. So make sure that you get your eight 8-ounce glasses a day.

Take it slow. "The main complaint I get from people about eating fiber is that it is gas-producing. It's no secret that fiber can result in flatulence," says Dr. Weil.

When bacteria in the gut attack and digest the complex carbohydrate molecules in fibrous foods, methane gas is released. Tolerance to fiber can

Choose to Boost Your Fiber

You can significantly boost the amount of fiber in your daily diet by making small, simple substitutions. For example, make the following smart choices in the course of a single day, and you increase your fiber intake by a whopping 21.8 grams.

EAT THIS . . .	INSTEAD OF THIS . . .	FIBER BOOST (g)
Bagel, oat bran (2 oz)	Bagel, plain (2 oz)	6.2
Bread, whole wheat (1 slice)	Bread, white (1 slice)	2.0
Crackers, Triscuit (7)	Crackers, Ritz (10)	2.4
Pasta, whole wheat (1 cup)	Pasta, white (1 cup)	4.3
Popcorn, air-popped (3½ cups)	Potato chips (10)	3.3
Potato with skin	Potato without skin	2.5
Rice, brown (1 cup)	Rice, white (1 cup)	1.1

vary greatly from person to person. The best way to manage it is to build up fiber intake slowly.

If you're accustomed to eating a low-fiber cereal like Kellogg's Special K (only 1 gram of fiber), Reichler suggests making the shift in steps. Instead of grabbing a box of Fiber One off the shelf, try something with a medium amount of fiber like Cheerios or Whole Grain Total instead.

Satisfy your sweet tooth. Yes, you can get a good dose of fiber even when you indulge. And for each gram of fiber substituted for simple carbohydrates, you can block the absorption of 7 calories, says David J. Baer, Ph.D., a research physiologist at the U.S. Department of Agriculture Human Nutrition Research Center in Beltsville, Maryland, who studied the effects of fiber on 17 people. That's because fiber "crosses out" calories by speeding them through your digestive system before they can be absorbed and stored as fat, he explains.

Try these fiber-rich treats: one slice of blackberry pie (401 calories, 4.5 grams of fiber), a 1.7-ounce Almond Joy (227 calories, 4.3 grams of fiber), or a Weight Watchers brownie (190 calories, 4 grams of fiber).

Fashion Secrets: Clothes That Slim, Clothes That Add Pounds

IMAGINE GETTING DRESSED IN THE LATE 19TH CENTURY. YOU WRAP WHALEBONE AROUND YOUR WAIST, SUCK IN YOUR STOMACH, AND HANG ONTO THE BEDPOSTS WHILE YOUR MAID TIGHTENS YOUR CORSET UNTIL YOU GET THE FASHIONABLE 14-INCH WAIST.

Luckily, we don't need bones and strings to look thinner in today's world. Nor do we have to wait until we actually lose as much weight as we want to enjoy the benefits of looking thinner.

A certain color, a particular cut, or a specific fabric is all it takes to minimize our hips and thighs, shrink our waists, and give us more height. It's simply a matter of knowing how to create the illusion.

Start with Your Mirror

Stand at least a body length away from a full-length mirror in a well-lit area—totally naked.

"It's like being in a museum," says Laurie Krauz, an image consultant in New York City. "You get to see the entire artwork."

Are you tall or short? Broad or narrow? Is the line from your shoulder to your hip straight or curvy? "Instead of trying to fix your body," she says, "you need to learn about your body. Understand the line of your body so you can select clothing that agrees with that line."

To do that, you need to determine your body shape. There are four body shapes: pear, hourglass, apple, and rectangle. To narrow your choices, check out your waist.

"I call them waist or waist-nots," says Catherine Schuller, a fashion retail editor of *Mode* magazine and author of the *Ultimate Plus-Size Modeling Guide*. "Either you have an indentation above your hips or you're straight up and down."

If you have an indentation, you're classified as a pear or an hourglass. If you don't, you're an apple or a rectangle. Here's how to tell where you fit.

The Pear

- You have an indentation above your hips.
- Your waist is 10 to 12 inches smaller than your hips.
- Most of your weight is distributed below your waist.

The Hourglass

- You have an indentation above your hips.
- Your weight is evenly distributed between your bust and hips.

The Apple

- You don't have an indentation above your hips.
- Your waistline is the widest part of your body.
- You have thin arms and legs.

The Rectangle

- You don't have an indentation above your hips.
- Your hips, bust, and waist are in proportion to each other.

Once you've figured out your shape, accept it, says Jan Larkey, author of *Flatter Your Figure*. No matter how much weight you gain and lose, your basic structure won't change.

Shop Till You Drop

Now comes the fun part: choosing the clothes that most flatter *your* body type.

Frame your face. "One of the kindest things we can do for ourselves is to wear a collar," says Judith Rasband, an image consultant in Orem, Utah, and author of *Fabulous Fit* and *Wardrobe Strategies for Women.* It lifts people's attention to our faces instead of our bodies.

Choose a V-neck collar because the vertical line is very slimming to everyone, says Claudia Kaneb, wardrobe head at NBC's *Today* show. Or wear a chain with a small pendant or a knotted scarf draped down like a necklace over a shirt with a high collar for the same effect.

Waist not, want not. Your body type will determine the clothes you choose to minimize your waistline. Follow these guidelines.

Pear. Keep patterns and textures above your waistline and solid colors below. "Anything loud or bulky below the waist adds dimension," Schuller says. Wear skirts and pants without pleats.

Hourglass. You're evenly proportioned, says Schuller. You can wear the same clothes as a pear-shaped woman, and you can wear patterns below your waistline.

If you have a flat stomach, try a fluted trumpet skirt. Its long, straight style, flaring out from midcalf to ankle, is very slimming, says Princess Jenkins, an image consultant at Majestic Images International in New York City.

Apple. Look for clothes with an overall downward taper ending at the end of the garment—whether it is at the bottom hem of a blouse, skirt, or even a sleeve, says Schuller. You are as wide as your widest line, wherever that falls. Avoid horizontal stripes—they add dimension there and make you look wider.

Rectangle. Schuller suggests choosing column dresses—those that go straight up and down and don't taper—made of fabrics like velveteen, matte jerseys, and heavy silks that move as your body moves, creating fluidity.

Get hip. Avoid horizontal lines at the hips, such as tops with patch pockets and sideways stripes, Jenkins says, because they add weight to every shape. Clothes that slim your hips include A-line skirts, long jackets that cover the hips, loose-fitting tunic tops, and slightly padded shoulders.

To minimize thighs, Jenkins suggests choosing pants with a semi-full leg, staying away from those that taper at the bottom.

Scale the fashion heights. If you're short, don't wear long shirts over long skirts, Larkey says. Your waist gets lost, and you'll look even shorter. Accentuate your waist instead with an A-line blazer or a belt and wear skirts that show an extra inch or two above the ankles.

Or try pantsuits, says Kaneb. Unless you're under 5 feet 4 inches tall, pantsuits with longer jackets that cover your hips and thighs will make you look taller and slimmer.

Find the right fabrics. Anyone carrying extra weight should avoid fabrics such as fleece, tweeds, leather, metallics, and nubby knits, which add visual pounds, Jenkins says, as well as busy patterns such as large floral prints, checks, and polka dots. Here are some of her general guidelines for specific body types.

No matter what your figure type, don't wear clothes that cling.

Pear and hourglass. Choose softer fabrics, such as thin wools, cotton jerseys, and lightweight silks.

Apple and rectangle. Choose stiffer, thicker fabrics, such as crisp cottons, stiff silks, and lightweight linens.

Make It Fit

The right fit helps those fabulous clothes hang well on your body and do what they were meant to do—create an illusion of thinness. "If you wear things too tight, you look large," says Schuller. "If you wear things too big, you look large."

It won't be easy. Designers cut clothes for the proportional woman, someone who is eight heads tall (her head is exactly one-eighth of the length of her body) with shoulders and hips of the same width. So finding clothes that fit *your* body, not Cindy Crawford's, can be a real challenge—especially since the same size from different manufacturers may fit differently.

But don't give up. "Women go shopping and put something on. And if it doesn't fit, they blame their bodies," Krauz says. "Instead, women should realize that it's the fault of the manufacturer."

Here are some ways to get the right fit every time.

Give yourself enough room. No matter what your figure type, don't wear clothes that cling. A loose fit won't outline the bulges that our figures acquire as we age, Rasband says.

Shop for separates. "It's ridiculous to design clothing for women where the top and the bottom are the same size," Krauz says. "The only people it works for are the symmetrical body types."

Search different departments. Don't be afraid to go between the juniors', misses', and women's departments for the clothes you need. For instance, blouses in the larger, "women's" sizes tend to have bigger armholes. So if you're an apple, you may need to buy your tops in the women's department and your skirts in the misses' department, says Larkey. If you're a pear, you may do just the opposite.

Give it the fit test. Once you've found clothes that seem to fit well, put them to the test, says Jenkins. Roll your shoulders forward and make sure that the fabric doesn't pull. Raise your arms and make sure you have a comfortable reach. Check that the buttons and zippers are not pulling at the chest or hips.

Get it tailored. You might have to take measures beyond the department store for a good fit. While men can get a suit altered anywhere, women usually have to search for a seamstress and pay extra.

But it's a worthwhile expense, Jenkins says, because fit is so important. Once you own a piece of clothing that fits perfectly, you'll never want to wear another ill-fitting garment again.

Be careful with jackets and blazers, however. Make sure that they at least fit in the shoulders, even if you're going to have them altered, because shoulders are difficult to alter. Also, look at how the front of the blazer falls against your chest. You don't want the seamstress to have to restyle the jacket.

It's All in the Details

They're why we love to shop: color, style, and that special something that makes an outfit truly ours. Those same details can help camouflage many an imperfection.

Choose the right color. Color makes a statement. Color has energy. And color can be slimming. "Everybody thinks black is the only color that's slimming," says Mari Lyn Henry, professional member of the Association of Image Consultants International. "That's nonsense. If you wear a solid color—dark green, wine red, navy blue, royal purple, teal—it molds to your body and gives you a shadow effect." Vibrant colors can add youthfulness, while light, washed-out colors tend to age you.

Be color consistent. Wear the same or similar color top and bottom to look thinner, Jenkins suggests. Splitting your body in half with dark pants and light-colored shirts makes you look wider.

Buy the best. Higher-quality fabrics hang better on your body, flowing where they should and hugging your curves just right. "The designer spent time creating a pattern and sewing it in a way that's going to make you look good," Jenkins says.

Get Rid of the "Fat Dress"

It might be a pair of jeans, a roomy sweatshirt, or even a dress—your "fat dress." We all have one. Something we wore at our biggest. You hang it in the back of your closet and feel comforted that it's there in case of emergency (like a cookie-eating binge).

"I have clients who have three different types of clothes in their closets: current clothes, thin clothes, and fat clothes," says Jan Larkey, author of *Flatter Your Figure.*

But times are changing. You've made a commitment to lose weight, and it's time to put your fat clothes to rest. Permanently.

Here are some creative—and liberating—ways to do it.

- Burn them in a quiet ceremony with the comfort of friends.
- Drive your car over them half a dozen times.
- Donate them to an organization that provides career clothes to poor women.
- Cut them up, turn them into a collage, frame it, and hang it on the wall or refrigerator as a constant reminder of why you're changing your lifestyle.
- Make them into a quilt or a throw pillow.
- Cut them up into rags, then burn calories by cleaning your house or waxing your car with them.

They are expensive, however, and it can be hard for many of us to buy just one blazer when we know we could get a whole suit, including an extra blouse and a pair of shoes, for the same money.

"I have a hard time doing it," Kaneb admits, "But if it's a good blazer or a good coat, something I'll wear for years and years, I just have to spend the money." You can also pick up bargains at end-of-season sales or in resale shops.

Judge the quality of a garment with the wrinkle test. Ball it up in your hand. If it wrinkles too much, you don't want it. Heavy rayon and brushed silks are good fabrics because their wrinkles disappear as you wear them, says Kaneb.

Week Three

Turning Back the Clock

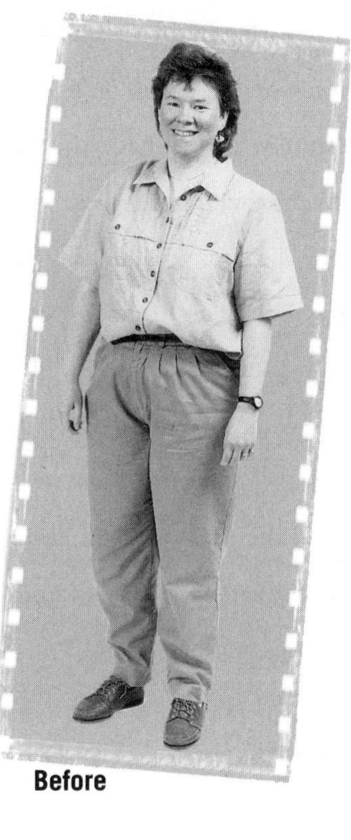

Before

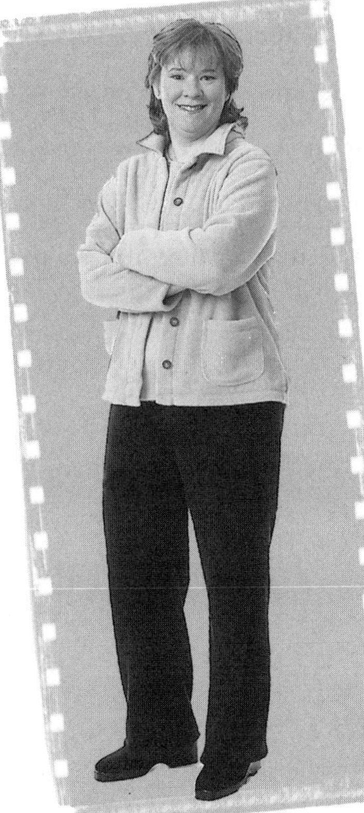

After

NOW I'M THINNER, HEALTHIER, AND HAPPIER, AND I HAVE MORE TIME DURING THE WEEK.

—Lynn Gano

Week Three

Appearing thinner is an important factor in looking younger, but it's not the only one. You can do many things in addition to exercising and eating healthfully to turn back the clock. This week focuses on some of those youth-enhancing strategies.

For starters, you'll learn that having a positive attitude can give you a more youthful appearance. And you'll discover the three basics to keeping radiant, youthful skin—as well as tips for applying makeup to look thinner. If you would like to go beyond walking and add some variety to your aerobic workout, you can narrow your choices by reading the overview of some of the most popular aerobic activities. Plus, you'll find a strategy to help you plan your meals each week so that you'll never have to scramble for a quick and healthy meal.

A Youthful Mind, A Youthful Body

WHEN A DOCTOR TOLD SUPREME COURT JUSTICE AND AVID TENNIS PLAYER HUGO BLACK THAT THE SPORT WAS ILL-ADVISED FOR SOMEONE IN HIS FORTIES, THE JUSTICE QUIPPED, "IN THAT CASE, I CAN'T WAIT TO TURN 50 SO I CAN PLAY AGAIN."

The late judge wasn't about to let his age—or someone else's misconceptions about his age—keep him from doing what he loved, and neither should you.

Now more than ever, your age merely chronicles the number of years you've been on this planet. It doesn't tell you how you feel, how you look, or how you think.

And if you want to lead a healthier, more active lifestyle—the kind that results in not only losing pounds but also keeping them off for good—you need to think younger. If you do, in a very real sense, you'll *be* younger.

"If you get up and you say, 'I am old and I can't do these things,' then you can't. I can see two older people who are basically the same age and even at the same physical level, and one's attitude is 'I can do it.' And the other's attitude is 'I can't.' And guess what? The one will, and the other won't," says Dana G. Cable, Ph.D., professor of psychology at Hood College in Frederick, Maryland. "I see those who are 60 who feel they can't do anything, and I see those in their nineties who aren't about to give up on anything."

Science is finding more and more that our thoughts really do affect our health. One study found that HIV-positive men stay healthier longer if they are optimistic. Another study discovered that heart patients who improve their attitudes and control their hostility lower their blood pressures.

"Part of it is that we physically do respond better when the attitude is right," Dr. Cable says.

You're surrounded by real-life examples of this fact. Chances are that you've gasped when you learned the age of someone who you thought was much younger. And you've probably had an experience where you pegged someone to be much older than their years. It's not just their physical appearance that throws you off, it's the way they act, the vibes they give off.

That's because the mind emits a physical aura that skews how old you appear, Dr. Cable says.

"I Think, Therefore I Can"

Remember the children's tale *The Little Engine That Could*? While the bigger engines refused to head up the steep mountain and said, "I cannot," the little blue engine took on the challenge, repeating his mantra: "I think I can, I think I can . . ." That positive thinking got him over the mountain, which he celebrated by saying, "I thought I could . . ."

That same youthful spirit and determination fuels your weight-loss success. "I believe that the attitude you go in with—even for something like losing weight or changing habits—if you really have that strong belief that you can do it, you will," Dr. Cable says.

We all know the mathematics for getting thinner. Cut back on calories and increase exercise. Yet it doesn't come that easy for most people. Why? For some, it's their attitudes. If you go into a weight-loss effort thinking it can't be done, then it can't.

If you think it will be torture, then it will be. "How many times aren't people successful, and suddenly they try and they are. Why is it different? There's a different mental state," Dr. Cable says.

It's not the attitude itself that takes pounds off. But having a positive, youthful outlook makes doing the things you need to do easier.

"If you believe that becoming physically active will help you be successful, then you'll stick with it. You'll say, 'I can do this,'" says Ross An-

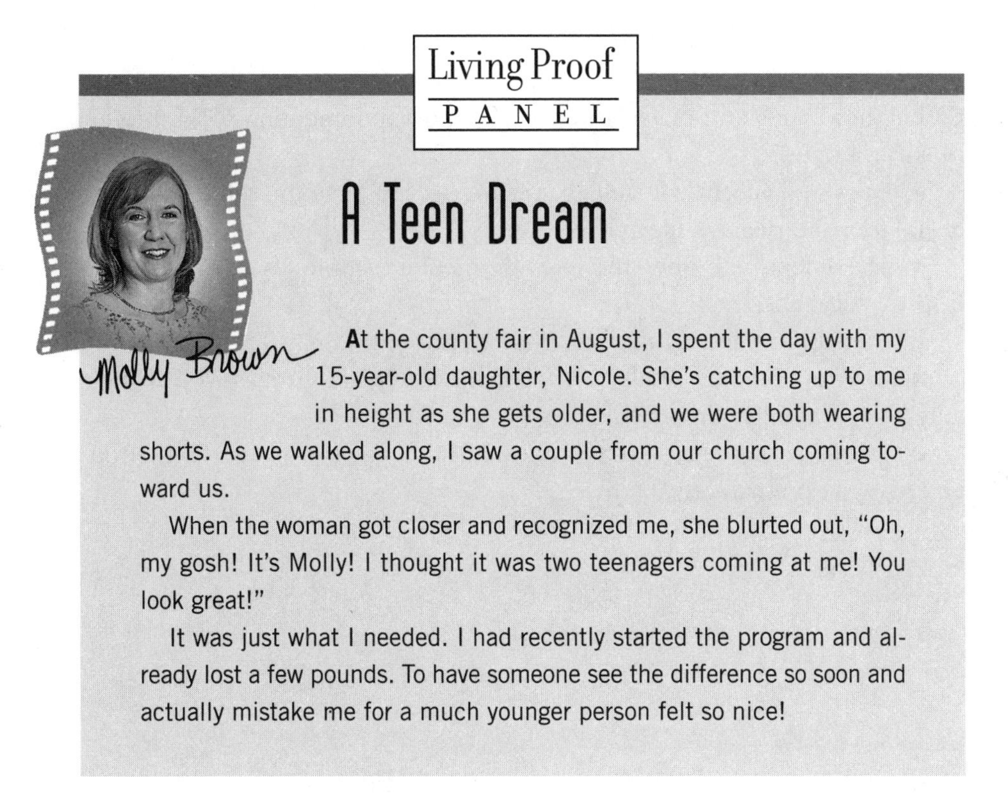

Living Proof PANEL

A Teen Dream

Molly Brown

At the county fair in August, I spent the day with my 15-year-old daughter, Nicole. She's catching up to me in height as she gets older, and we were both wearing shorts. As we walked along, I saw a couple from our church coming toward us.

When the woman got closer and recognized me, she blurted out, "Oh, my gosh! It's Molly! I thought it was two teenagers coming at me! You look great!"

It was just what I needed. I had recently started the program and already lost a few pounds. To have someone see the difference so soon and actually mistake me for a much younger person felt so nice!

dersen, Ph.D., assistant professor of medicine at Johns Hopkins University School of Medicine in Baltimore and one of the nation's leading researchers on lifestyle activity and weight loss.

Once that attitude takes over, the pounds start to fall away, and the younger you comes shining through, he adds.

A New Attitude

Working the muscles between your ears as well as the muscles all over your body is what will make this weight-loss effort different from all the rest.

"In general, people look at losing weight as exercising or lowering calories. They often don't think about how they view the process and how their attitudes will be so important to their success," says Steve Sultanoff, Ph.D., adjunct professor of psychology at Pepperdine University in Malibu, California, and president of the American Association for Therapeutic Humor.

Here's just a sample of how your mind can help you find the thinner, younger you, says Dr. Sultanoff.

- Open yourself up to all types of adventures, such as trying new foods, finding new ways and places to exercise, and experimenting with different looks and styles.
- Enjoy and accept yourself as you are, so you have the self-esteem and desire to make positive lifestyle changes.
- Experiment with new and exciting mental techniques such as visualization, yoga, and meditation.
- Find support and motivation from friends and family.
- Strive to meet new goals that will keep you fit and firm as well as mentally and physically stimulated.
- Manage your stress so that it doesn't sabotage your weight-loss efforts and age you prematurely.

The Joy of Aerobic Exercise

THE HUMAN BODY MAY BE THE ONLY MACHINE THAT LASTS LONGER THE MORE YOU USE IT. BY MOVING YOUR BODY EVERY WAY YOU CAN, AS OFTEN AS YOU CAN, YOU BECOME TRIMMER AND LIGHTER INSTEAD OF HEAVIER AND SLOWER. YOUR ARTERIES REMAIN SUPPLE AND CLEAR INSTEAD OF HARDENING AND BLOCKING. YOUR BONES GET STRONGER INSTEAD OF WEAKER. YOU HAVE MORE ENERGY INSTEAD OF LESS. AND YOU CONTINUE FUNCTIONING LIKE A YOUNG, HEALTHY, WELL-OILED MACHINE.

The catch is that in today's world, it's not easy to use our bodies as often as we used to," says exercise physiologist Robert Brosmer, vice president of health and wellness at the Central Florida YMCA in Orlando and coauthor of *Health and High Performance*. "In just one generation, we've managed to computerize life to the point where the only thing many of us use all day is our fingertips."

Increasing daily activity by taking stairs instead of elevators, for example, or by parking farther away from stores to get some extra walking in is definitely one of the antidotes to this modern sedentary life. But for those who want even better results, the answer is regular aerobic exercise. That means getting out a few days a week to raise your heart rate and get your blood pumping more vigorously throughout your body.

Aerobic exercise is truly a health tonic, says John D. McPhail, senior health educator at the Michigan Public Health Institute in Okemos. "Even small daily doses done regularly throughout the week can do wonders for your health. But for even better results, like increased weight loss, it helps to increase the dose."

The Calorie Equation

Why is aerobic exercise so helpful for getting thinner and healthier and feeling younger? Because it burns calories, says McPhail. "Research has found that the more calories you burn, the less likely you are to get some cancers, lung disease, stroke, and diabetes. Even suicide rates are lower for people who burn more calories."

Plus, the more calories you burn, the more likely you are to keep zipping up those favorite jeans without a problem. Burn enough, and you'll need a smaller size. Consider this: Someone weighing 150 pounds who starts taking a brisk 1½-mile walk (20 to 30 minutes) each day will lose about 12 pounds in a year—even if she doesn't eat a crumb less. "If you can't carve out a 30-minute stretch, take two 15-minute walks or three 10-minute walks," McPhail adds. "All that matters is that you do it on a regular basis."

And remember, if you want the best calorie burn for your time and effort, keep the pace a little faster. When you walk at a moderate pace of 3 miles an hour, you burn 238 calories an hour (assuming you weigh 150 pounds). Pick it up a notch, so that you're striding strong at 4½ miles an hour, and you'll burn more than 300 calories an hour. Pump your arms and power down the block like a racewalker, and you'll burn an impressive 400 (or more) calories an hour.

Can't tell how fast you're going? Judge your efforts by your exertion. Rate them on a scale from 1 to 10, with 1 being very little effort and 10 being the hardest you can go. To burn the most calories without burning yourself out, try to stay around a 6 or 7. "Your breathing should just be slightly harder than it was at a slower pace," says Michelle Edwards, a certified personal trainer and a health educator for the Cooper Institute for Aerobics Research in Dallas. "If you're panting and heaving, you're going too hard."

Exercise Smart, Exercise Healthy

Sometimes people get so excited about starting an exercise program that they plunge into it with everything they have. "It's great to be enthusiastic, but you need to treat your body right," says personal trainer Michelle Edwards of the Cooper Institute. And remember, check with your doctor first if you are new to exercise. Here's what she recommends.

Warm up. This can't be stressed enough. Start your activity slowly to give your muscles time to warm up and stretch out.

Talk, and keep talking. During your workout, periodically do the "talk test," Edwards suggests. "When jogging or walking briskly, you should be able to keep up a conversation comfortably. If you're too breathless to talk, you're exercising too hard."

Beat the heat. When the mercury rises, exercise in the morning or evening, when temperatures are cooler. Drink more than the usual eight glasses of water a day. Wear light, cool clothing. And if you feel dizzy, weak, or light-headed, slow down or stop for a while. These could be signs of heatstroke.

Layer up. When temperatures dip, put on several layers of clothing. This keeps you warm and allows you to remove a layer once you get moving and warm up. Wear gloves to protect your hands and a hat to keep body heat from escaping.

Give yourself time to digest. You should wait at least 2 hours after a meal before exercising vigorously.

Spring for quality shoes. "Good shoes can be the difference between enjoying exercise and quitting," says Edwards. "Buy quality shoes to fit your activity—and remember the four basic rules of good footwear: cushioning, stability, wearability, and fit."

Stop for pain. "Exercise should never hurt," she says. If you feel pain in your muscles or joints, stop. If you feel chest pain or pain in your left shoulder or arm or in the left side of your neck, stop and consult a doctor immediately. These symptoms could be a sign of a heart attack.

Living Proof
PANEL

Molly Brown

It's Fun to Be Active Again

For a while, I just fell away from being active, and I was carrying around unwanted extra weight as a result. Starting to engage in regular exercise again has made all the difference in my weight.

I started out by walking with my daughter, and I felt better almost immediately. When we wanted to do something besides walking, we'd get some aerobics videotapes and do those together. I even got my husband into the act—we started taking swing dance classes. It's fun to be active again.

And it has really paid off. I lost all the weight I wanted to lose without major or unpleasant changes to my diet or lifestyle. My family and I haven't given up our favorite treats like ice cream and my mother's homemade pies. You don't have to worry as much about occasional indulgences when you're exercising regularly. Plus, you don't really feel like eating as much junk food when you're exercising.

Getting more aerobically active is definitely good for the whole family.

Feel Younger Fast

The research is overwhelming. If you want a magic bullet to make your body thinner and younger, aerobic exercise is it. "If all the benefits of exercise were available in a pill, I wouldn't be able to write prescriptions fast enough," says James Rippe, M.D., associate professor of medicine at Tufts University School of Medicine in Boston; director of the Center for Clinical and Lifestyle Research in Shrewsbury, Massachusetts; and author of *Fit over Forty*. "People only have to take that first step to start realizing their goals."

What can regular aerobic exercise do for you?

Trim your figure. Ask most people how to lose weight, and the first word out of their mouths will likely be "diet." What they really should be saying is "exercise." "The increase in obesity in this country during the past 20 years has more to do with our inactive lifestyles than our eating habits," says Dr. Rippe. "Certainly, eating a healthful diet will speed up weight loss, but more than anything, you have to move."

Canadian researchers, for example, found that when overweight men and women walked about 40 minutes every day for a year, they lost an average of 10 pounds—even though most of them actually ate more during the study than they did before.

Keep your heart young. Your heart is the motor that keeps your body running. The stronger and more efficiently it works, the healthier and more energetic you are. Consider how an active person's heart works compared to the heart of someone who's inactive. In 1 minute, a sedentary person's heart beats 70 to 75 times. An active person's heart, on the other hand, is so strong that it can pump the same amount of blood in only 45 to 50 beats. That's 36,000 fewer beats every day—13 million fewer a year. The easier it is for your heart to do its work, the longer it'll keep on beating, and the better you'll feel.

What's more, active people have significantly lower blood pressures, lower cholesterol levels, and less risk for stroke and heart disease than their inactive counterparts. And the benefits of aerobic exercise happen superfast. When researchers at the University of Pittsburgh started 12 overweight women walking or stationary cycling for an hour a day, the women's blood pressures fell 4 points in just 1 week.

Give you a youthful attitude. Anyone who exercises regularly will tell you that there's nothing like it for shedding stress, boosting your mood, and just plain feeling good about yourself. Regular exercise is so effective, in fact, that psychologists have begun prescribing it to treat mild to moderate depression as well as anxiety disorders and alcohol abuse.

"Even more than the obvious physical changes, the inner changes in women who exercise are remarkable," says Michael Bourque, certified personal trainer and personal training coordinator for the Center for Health and Wellness of the Central Florida YMCA in Oviedo. "They're happier with their bodies. They walk confidently. And they just exude self-confidence."

Sharpen your memory. Your brain is not a muscle, but regular aerobic exercise can keep it strong like one. When researchers at Case Western Reserve University in Cleveland compared the lifestyles of people who had Alzheimer's disease with those who didn't, they found that the healthy individuals were significantly more physically active than those who had the disease. Regularly participating in activities like jogging, biking, golfing, weight training, ice-skating, swimming, and playing racquetball or tennis all appeared to have a protective effect.

Help you kick old habits. Cigarette smoking may be a habit that people pick up when they're young and "invincible," but it's one that soon saps the youth right out of them. Research has shown that people who start aerobic exercise find it easier to quit smoking without gaining a lot of weight—one thing that discourages many women from quitting.

In one study, researchers at Brown University in Providence, Rhode Island, divided smokers into two groups. Women in one group attended a 12-week behavioral stop-smoking program and started exercising. Those in another group did the behavioral program and attended health lectures. At the end of the study, the exercisers were about twice as likely to have stayed smoke-free as the nonexercisers. Plus, they gained only half as much weight.

Start It Up

There's no doubt about it: The toughest part of starting an aerobics program is . . . getting started. You can make it easier by following just a few steps.

Pick your days. To shed weight most quickly, you should try to do your favorite aerobic activity for 20 to 60 minutes, 3 to 5 days a week. You'll have a much easier time making that happen if you pick your workout days right at the beginning. "If you just say, 'I'm going to try to exercise 3 days this week,' it'll never happen," says Brosmer. "But if you plan ahead and mark your calendar, you'll do it."

Be sure to plan your days off, too, he says. "It's nice to look at your calendar and say, 'Okay, Wednesday I'm taking a break.' "

Ease into it, ease out of it. No matter if you're walking, swimming, or playing racquetball, you have to give yourself a chance to warm up and cool down. "Too many people go out and try to walk or play as hard as they can as soon as their shoes are tied," says McPhail. "After 2 minutes, they feel awful. They chalk it up to being in terrible shape, and they quit. All they really needed to do was warm up."

Start out slowly for the first 5 to 10 minutes. Walk slowly. Take a couple of easy strokes. Volley back and forth lightly. Then turn up your efforts as you feel your body warming up and becoming more limber. Wind down the same way at the end of your activity. Stopping abruptly can cause dizziness.

Pack your shoes. Life is unpredictable, but your exercise routine doesn't have to suffer because of it. "Simply take your walking shoes with you wherever you go," says Dr. Rippe. "Whether you're on business or on vacation, you're going to have some downtime when you can get out for an invigorating walk. If you have your shoes with you, you can fit exercise into even the most hectic schedule."

Make it a family affair. With advances in technology, it's easy to take young children along, whether you're biking, hiking, or walking. "You can buy baby joggers, baby backpacks, off-road strollers, bike seats, and bike attachments that let your child sit in the back and pedal, too," says McPhail. "When you include your kids, you're not only getting great exercise but also teaching your children a healthy way of life."

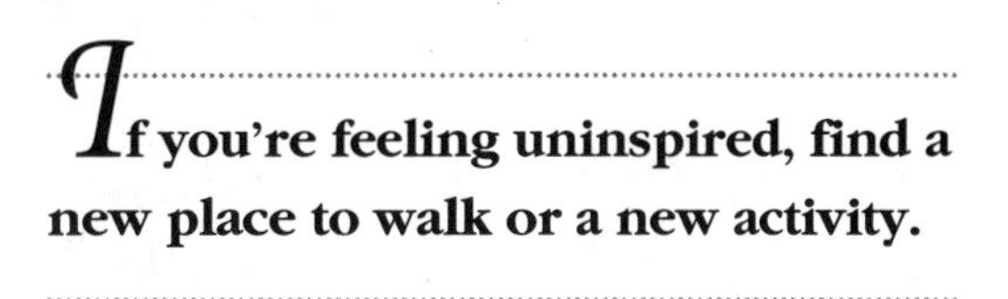
If you're feeling uninspired, find a new place to walk or a new activity.

Move to music. If aerobic exercise feels tiring and tedious—and it often does when you're on a treadmill or exercise bike—simply add music. "Research shows that when people listen to music while exercising, they don't feel as if they're working as hard," says Brosmer. "And they exercise longer."

Mix it up. You may love pizza, but if you eat it every night, you'll soon get sick of it. The same is true for aerobic exercise, says certified personal trainer Jana Angelakis, founder of PEx Personalized Exercise in New York City. "The same walking routine that you couldn't get enough of when you started can feel stale after a few months," she says. "If you're feeling uninspired, don't immediately blame the exercise. Blame boredom. Find a new place to walk, or try a whole new activity. It will invigorate you immediately."

Aerobics for Everyone

In order to stick with aerobic exercise, the single most important factor is finding something that you really like to do. "Don't do something you hate just because it's good for you," says Angelakis. "You'll just get frustrated and discouraged. When you do something you like, you always make time for it, and you feel great doing it."

Not sure what it is you like to do? You're not alone. "Picking an activity can be confusing when you're just starting out," she says. "Your best bet is to find a few activities that interest you and try them on for size."

Here are some of the most popular aerobic activities. (Note: The calorie figures given below are based on someone who weighs 150 pounds.)

Walking. This is by far the easiest exercise—just put one foot in front of the other, says Brosmer. "It's easy on your joints. And you can do it absolutely anywhere."

Living Proof
PANEL

Moving to the Music

I have always liked to exercise. But it's not as if I could just dash out the door and go exercise. I have a child to care for, after all.

So it has been a matter of getting my husband, John, to take care of our son, Sam, for an hour or two so that I can get the exercise I need. John, I must say, has been really supportive in that way.

We got a treadmill, which has really helped me keep exercising during the winter months. It's nice because I can put Sam up for his nap, then go work out on the treadmill for an hour. I know some people get bored working out on a treadmill, but I've kept it interesting by frequently changing the music I listen to while I'm on it. Depend ing on my mood, different music is motivating for me on different days. But usually it's upbeat, happy stuff that just makes me want to move.

Some days it has been harder than others to get myself motivated to do it. There have been times when I've gotten Sam down for his nap that I've just wanted to go to sleep myself. But I know that after doing my workout, I will have a lot more energy and will get a lot more accomplished during the rest of the day.

What you need: A good pair of walking shoes.

Calories burned: 200 to 400 an hour, depending on your pace.

The price tag: About $70 for the shoes.

Special benefits: Walking is extremely social, says McPhail. "It's easy to find buddies. And almost every community has walking clubs. Check at your local mall, community education office, or park office."

Jogging. The advantage of jogging is that it lets you burn more calories in a shorter amount of time than walking, says Brosmer. It's harder on your joints than walking, however, so skip the pavement and stick to dirt trails and gravel tracks.

What you need: Running shoes.

Calories burned: 500 to 600 an hour at a moderate pace.

The price tag: About $70 for the shoes.

Special benefits: Runner's high. "The psychological benefits of pushing yourself a little bit are real," says Deborah Saint-Phard, M.D., an exercise physiatrist for the Women's Sports Medicine Center at the Hospital for Special Surgery in New York City. "All those feel-good hormones (called endorphins) kick in, and you feel great."

Swimming. Exercising in water uses all your major muscles and is a great aerobic-conditioning exercise, says Brosmer. One thing to keep in mind, however, is that swimming generally doesn't heat your body as much as exercising on land does (because the water is cool). As a result, swimming doesn't burn as much fat as other exercises. It's best to combine it with another activity.

What you need: A bathing suit and a place to swim.

Calories burned: 400 to 550 an hour swimming freestyle laps at a slow to moderate pace.

The price tag: Pool memberships vary in price, but you can swim year-round at your local YMCA for about $25 a month.

Special benefits: Swimming is easy on your joints, and the water is supportive, so even people who are very overweight find that they feel comfortable doing it.

Bicycling. Invigorating and scenic, bicycling is easy on your joints, and it makes you feel like a kid again.

What you need: A bike and a helmet.

Calories burned: 400 to 550 an hour at a moderate pace.

The price tag: Approximately $200 and up for a bike, and $30 and up for a helmet.

Special benefits: You can get the same benefits by riding a stationary bike if you don't want to ride outside. Or, better, join an indoor Spinning class.

Dancing. Aside from the great music and it being tons of fun, dancing is a super workout.

What you need: A little space and some music.

Calories burned: About 375 an hour if you're doing ballroom, disco, folk, or square dancing, and about 200 if you opt for the slow, romantic variety.

The price tag: Free at home. Private lessons start at about $25 an hour.

Special benefits: "Dancing isn't just good for your body, it's good for your soul," says Dr. Rippe. "It's one of the most positive mind-body exercises you can do."

Playing tennis. Volleying with a friend is a great way to enjoy an afternoon and burn some extra weight. "You don't even have to keep score," says Dr. Saint-Phard. "Just enjoy hitting the ball back and forth."

What you need: A tennis racquet, balls, and a court to play on.

Calories burned: About 500 an hour playing singles.

The price tag: About $70 for a racquet and $3 for a can of balls. Community courts are free. Sometimes the U.S. Tennis Association offers free lessons in some areas.

Special benefits: Great for your lower body—tennis is a fantastic workout for your butt and legs.

Hiking. It can be nothing more than walking on a trail, but of course, you also get to see beautiful landscapes and enjoy the outdoors.

What you need: Boots and drinking water.

Calories burned: 400 to 500 an hour at a moderate pace.

The price tag: $75 for boots. No need for a special pack for short day-hikes. Just use a fanny pack for snacks and water.

Special benefits: Super toning for your legs and butt.

Inline skating. An updated version of a favorite childhood pastime—roller-skating—inline skating is fast, fun, and easy on the joints. And it can burn as many calories as jogging.

What you need: Skates, helmet, and pads.

Calories burned: 400 to 600 an hour, depending on your pace.

The price tag: Skates and safety equipment can cost about $250. Some sporting goods stores offer free lessons and let you rent skates for the day, so you can try them out before you buy.

Special benefits: Your kids will love it, too.

Doing aerobics. Forget what you remember about bouncy twentysomethings in Lycra thongs. Aerobics classes have come a long way. "Most exercise facilities offer a wide variety of classes for people of all levels," says Bourque. And there's more to choose from, such as salsa dancing or sports-inspired classes like kickboxing.

What you need: Aerobics or cross-training shoes.

Calories burned: About 450 an hour doing a high-impact workout.

The price tag: About $70 for the shoes. Classes at the YMCA are about $25 a month.

Special benefits: It's supervised exercise, so you'll know you're doing it right. And you can meet new people and have a great time.

Planning for Mealtime Success

It's 6:00 P.M. Do you know where your healthy dinner is? You check the cupboard and find pasta but no sauce. You go to the fridge and find lettuce but no tomatoes, carrots, peppers, or salad dressing. Odds are that you're probably not setting your table for weight-loss success.

And you're not alone: 25 percent of Americans lack the ingredients to throw together even one home-cooked meal, according to a survey by the Grocery Manufacturers of America in Washington, D.C.

With all the quick but unhealthy options available—a fast-food restaurant on every corner, pizza delivery at your fingertips, and hot dogs at gas stations—having a healthy eating plan is a great way to keep you from packing on pounds, says John La Puma, M.D., a Chicago physician who is the founder and medical director of the CHEF (Cooking, Healthy Eating, and Fitness) Clinic, which uses a cutting-edge approach to weight loss based on putting flavor first.

"A successful plan becomes like the wallet in a man's back pocket. It's just part of what he carries around with him without giving it a second thought until he needs it," Dr. La Puma says.

Your Tools for Success

Michelangelo couldn't have painted the Sistine Chapel without the proper paint and brushes. And you can't become an artist in the kitchen without the right tools, even if you have the right foods on hand. Here are 10 tips from culinary experts to help you whip up a masterpiece every time.

Cut to the chase. Optimize your slicing and dicing time by using the right 8- or 10-inch chef's knife. Before you buy a knife, pick it up and do a slicing motion. It should feel comfortable and balanced in your grip, says Pierre LeBlanc, associate professor at the Culinary Institute of America in Hyde Park, New York. When you find a fit that works, go with it.

Stick with nonstick. You won't need to add butter when you have nonstick pans. Keep a small and a medium saucepan on hand, along with a frying pan and a big pot for cooking soup and chili, says Jyl Steinback, author of *The Fat-Free Living Cookbook* series. Pamper your pans by using wooden and plastic spoons instead of metal ones.

Go for a wok. Use a 3,000-year-old healthy cooking method—the wok. Its shape keeps the heat on the bottom and lets you quickly cook meat and vegetables with little or no oil. Try adding fat-free broth, water, or wine as a great substitute for oil.

Master micro-dinners. Cut your cooking time by defrosting meat, heating vegeta-

But where do you begin, especially if your idea of planning ahead is to set aside enough time to microwave frozen burritos for dinner? Start early, so you can think at your own leisure about what you'd like to eat, instead of digging through the cupboards when the stove's already hot and your stomach's rumbling.

Here are some ways to make sure that you always have healthy, slimming foods on hand.

Take some time. You plan meetings, doctor's appointments, and parties—so why not what you're going to eat? That's what senior nutritionist Linda Antinoro, R.D., tells her clients at the nutrition consultation service at Brigham and Women's Hospital in Boston when they tell her they don't know how to plan meals.

bles, cooking rice, and warming up leftovers in your microwave oven. But don't use it to cook meat, fish, and eggs, LeBlanc says, because the food won't cook evenly.

Make it steamy. Cooking delicious vegetables in a steamer on your stove preserves nutrients and avoids added fat. The steamer holds the vegetables above the water so that the vitamins aren't lost in boiling.

Shake things up. Use a blender to whip up fresh fruit smoothies, homemade salad dressings, sauces, and soups.

Perfect your slice. Use a food processor for more complicated chopping ventures, such as slicing cabbage for coleslaw or cutting fresh herbs. Or buy shredded cabbage and precut vegetables. The time you save is worth the few extra pennies you spend.

Go slow. Add vegetables and broth to a slow cooker to make soup, or use beans and sauce for chili, and then go for a walk, see a movie, or visit some friends. When you come home, a healthy meal will be waiting.

Be a gourmet griller. Whether you're on the patio or at your stovetop, grill vegetables, potatoes, and lean burgers for delicious, healthy meals.

Pop in some fun. Make a guilt-free version of movie popcorn. Pop some corn in an air popper, add a little butter-flavor cooking spray, sprinkle with salt, Butter Buds, fat-free grated Parmesan cheese, or spices, and you have a fun, low-calorie snack, Steinback says.

Want to get in touch with your inner child? Throw each piece in the air and catch it in your mouth.

Set aside 15 to 30 minutes on the weekend to plan what you're going to eat for the next week.

And don't forget your pencil and paper. "Writing things down makes it more of a commitment," says Melanie Polk, R.D., director of nutrition education at the American Institute for Cancer Research in Washington, D.C.

Keep your daybook handy, too, as a reference. It will help you plan for emergencies. If you have a busy day on Wednesday, plan to prepare leftovers, Antinoro suggests. If you're going to be in your car at lunchtime, take a cooler with a sandwich and fruit.

Be specific. Start with Monday and list what you're going to eat for breakfast, lunch, and dinner, Antinoro says. And be as specific as you can. Instead of writing "yogurt" for breakfast, write "½ cup of fat-free plain yogurt with fresh strawberries."

Since you're not in a hurry as you plan, take the time to come up with some creative variations for your meals, and plug them into the rest of the days of the week. When you have different kinds of meals planned for each day, you're less likely to fall into a nutritional rut.

Make your list. Once you have a detailed menu for the week, use it to make your grocery list. Write down all those items that are on your plan but absent from your kitchen, and make sure that you buy them before Monday.

Creating a list from your plan will also keep you on track while you're shopping. With a detailed list, you'll get in and out of the store faster, and you'll be less likely to fall prey to impulse buying, such as those ever-tempting chocolate chip cookies that are on sale, Antinoro says.

Leverage your leftovers. Will you have steak left over from Monday's dinner? Then plan beef stew for Tuesday. Do you have a leftover chicken breast? Toss it with grilled peppers and onions for chicken fajitas. Then, says Antinoro, you won't have to summon up every meal from scratch if you use leftovers wisely.

Save money and calories. Instead of turning to the Sunday circular before you make your grocery list, wait until after you've written it, says Antinoro. That way, you'll only search for the food you've already planned. Bypass the frozen pizza and go right to the frozen broccoli that you need for dinner on Thursday.

Use a varied palette for your palate. Strive for a vivid combination of colors and textures in each meal.

"Whitefish, mashed potatoes, and cauliflower is a balanced meal, but it doesn't look very exciting," Antinoro says. "Try steamed broccoli, squash, rice, and chicken. Anything that helps make it look more exciting and more enticing will help with the enjoyment."

Toss yourself healthy. You don't have to chop and wash lettuce every night if you want salad with dinner. Make a big salad on Sunday and keep it in the fridge for later in the week. Once you've washed and thoroughly drained the lettuce, it will stay fresh in the fridge for up to 5 days.

Add carrots, beets, radishes, and celery to the salad right away. They stay fresh in the fridge for about 5 days. Antinoro suggests waiting to add tomatoes until just before dinner for freshness.

Wrap it up. You could save even more time by doubling a recipe, then

Living Proof
PANEL

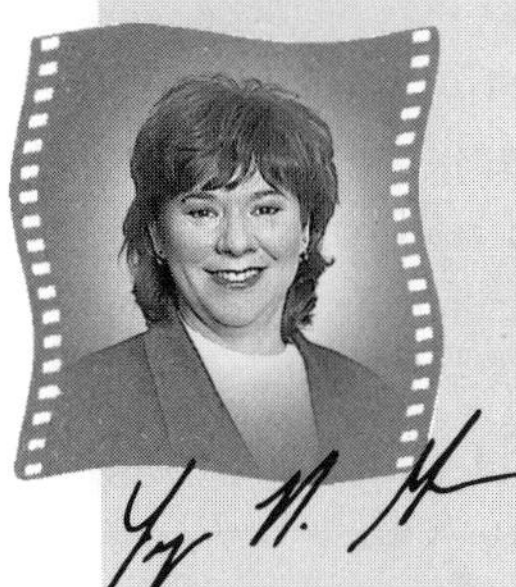

Sunday Planning Saves Time All Week

My old eating habits kept me from losing weight, and they gave me hunger pangs. With no breakfast and a small lunch, I used to come home from work ravenous. I'd end up eating a big meal late at night and munching on potato chips.

I needed to start planning my meals ahead of time, so I began taking a few hours on Sunday to plan and cook for the week. It made all the difference.

Now on Sundays I pull a few recipes—such as stir-fried vegetables and rice, and roasted chicken and sweet potatoes—and I use them as a guide for my grocery list. I also tack on cereal and milk and a dozen pieces of fruit for snacks and dessert. Because I buy healthy lunches at work, I don't have to worry about planning for them on Sunday.

When I get home, I cook the meals and separate them into the correct portions. Once they're sealed in containers in the fridge, I don't have to think about dinner again until I'm ready to eat—and then all I have to do is warm it in the microwave oven. Now I'm thinner, healthier, and happier, and I have more time during the week. It sure beats eating Pop-Tarts.

wrapping the extra food and keeping it in the freezer for up to 10 days, says Jyl Steinback, a personal trainer in Scottsdale, Arizona, and author of *The Fat-Free Living Cookbook* series. To ward off freezer burn, she wraps leftovers in foil before putting them in plastic bags, then labels them with masking tape, sometimes even adding how long they should be microwaved.

If you do this on the weekends, preparing dinner during the week is a snap. Just defrost your meal in the refrigerator or microwave oven and then warm it on the stove or in the oven.

Store soup for later. Freeze homemade soup in 2- to 4-cup containers, and for up to 3 months, you'll have a delicious meal waiting to be eaten.

When you're ready to eat it, either let the soup defrost in the fridge for 2 days or run the frozen container under warm water, empty the soup into a saucepan with ½ inch of water, and reheat on high to boiling. Watch it carefully. Immediately reduce the heat to low and simmer for 5 to 10 minutes.

Most soup ingredients will keep their texture and flavor for up to 3 months, says Steinback, except for potatoes, pasta, green beans, and lima beans, which can get mushy after freezing.

Don't forget dessert. As you plan, keep your eating habits in mind. If you can serve yourself one scoop of frozen yogurt, eat it slowly, and be satisfied, then it's safe to keep ½ gallon in the freezer, Polk says. If that puts too great a strain on your willpower, schedule a stop at the corner store during the week and buy one ice cream sandwich or an individual serving of your favorite dessert so you won't overeat.

Plan for your life. Whatever you do, create a plan that's reasonable and allows for variance. Some days, you'll eat more calories than others, Polk says, and a plan that allows for a little give-and-take will last a lifetime.

Double Up on Fruits and Vegetables

ONE CHOCOLATE CHIP COOKIE OR A PINT OF FRESH STRAWBERRIES? LET'S SEE: THE STRAWBERRIES WOULD FILL YOU UP MORE. KEEP YOUR MOUTH BUSY LONGER. MAKE YOU FEEL SATISFIED AND NOURISHED. HMM, TOUGH CHOICE. AT A MEASLY 107 CALORIES PER PINT, YOU CAN EAT YOUR FILL OF SWEET, RIPE STRAWBERRIES AND STILL NOT COME CLOSE TO THE CALORIE COUNT IN ONE COOKIE. PLUS, YOU GET A HEALTHY DOSE OF FIBER, POTASSIUM, AND VITAMIN C.

Okay, maybe that one's a no-brainer, but you get the idea. Even the least nutritious fruit beats a low-fat cupcake hands down.

When you opt for fruits and vegetables, you can simply eat more food and still lose weight, says James J. Kenney, R.D., Ph.D., a nutrition research specialist at the Pritikin Longevity Center in Santa Monica, California. Your focus immediately shifts from what you can't eat to how much you can eat.

And when it comes to fruits and vegetables, you can eat as much as you want. Maybe you've heard this before: According to those who have successfully lost weight, it's probably the single most practical food strategy to manage your weight and your appetite.

A group of 21 people who lost 25 percent of their body weights and kept it off for at least 4½ years was asked, "What really, really works?" Two strategies made the difference between previous attempts that didn't work and their final attempts that did—exercising and eating a lot more fruits and vegetables than before.

"Get into the habit of asking yourself, 'How am I going to get my fruits and veggies today?'" says Evelyn Tribole, R.D., a nutritionist in Irvine, California, and author of *Healthy Homestyle Cooking*. This healthy habit works better than counting calories, reducing fat, or cutting down on portions.

Your goal is to aim for 9 servings of fruits and vegetables every day, says nutritionist Melanie Polk of the American Institute for Cancer Research. Generally, a serving equals ½ cup of fresh or cooked vegetables, 1 cup of raw leafy vegetables, a medium-size piece of fruit, or ½ cup of canned or fresh fruit.

Get Thin

When you fill up on fruits and vegetables, the amount of fat and calories in your diet will automatically decrease, says Polk. Why? Because with their high fiber and water content, fruits and vegetables fill you up better and longer than refined foods like chips, crackers, candy, and cookies.

Evidence shows that there's a direct relationship between how many vegetables you eat every day and how thin you are. Researchers at Tufts University in Boston studied the food choices of 71 healthy adults and compared them with their body mass indexes (BMIs, as the folks in the white lab coats call them).

People who ate a wide variety of vegetables were more likely to be thin, while those who ate a wide variety of sweets, snacks, entrées, and carbohydrates were more likely to be overweight.

Get Young

Increase the amount of fruits and vegetables that you eat, and you can add 10 years to your life, says Paul Lachance, Ph.D., executive director of the Nutraceuticals Institute at Rutgers University in New Brunswick, New Jersey.

Playing the Farmers' Market

Picking which fruits and vegetables to eat is a lot like saving for retirement. You want to have a diversified portfolio. But, instead of healthy mutual funds, you want to choose a wide range of phytochemicals and nutrients that will protect you from nose to toes.

For the broadest health benefits, Dr. Paul Lachance of the Nutraceuticals Institute at Rutgers University has developed a food-centered approach to cash in on eight key nutraceuticals that increase your chances of feeling better and living longer: antioxidants, fiber, allylic sulfur compounds, isothiocyanates, terpenes, flavonoids, phytoestrogens, and saponins.

Each day, eat at least one serving from each of the following groups.

Garlic, onions, leeks, and chives. These pungent foods contain allylic sulfurs, natural compounds that help lower cholesterol.

Citrus fruits and berries. These are loaded with antioxidant vitamin C and folate, which have been shown to lower the incidence of several types of cancer and reduce the risk of heart disease. Good choices include oranges, red grapefruit, kiwifruit, mangoes, and strawberries.

Deep orange and dark green fruits and vegetables. Beta-carotene and the other carotenoids that give these foods their deep color fight cancer and macular degeneration, an age-related disease that can lead to blindness. The best sources are cantaloupe, pumpkin, carrots, spinach, Swiss chard, beet greens, turnip greens, and dandelion greens.

Cruciferous vegetables. Foods like broccoli, cabbage, kale, and cauliflower provide the cancer-fighting power of isothiocyanates, indoles, and flavonoids.

Legumes. These foods from the bean and pea family supply fiber and protein. Eating a handful of nuts such as peanuts (which are also legumes) three times a week can reduce your risk of having a heart attack by 40 percent.

The reason is that fruits and vegetables are loaded with an array of disease-fighting compounds that help your body stay young and energized.

Studies—literally hundreds of them—repeatedly show that people who consume diets loaded with fresh fruits and vegetables are the healthiest. Many

The Most Nutritious Fruits

Any fruit is a good fruit. But if you're looking for the most nutritious, check out this list compiled by the Center for Science in the Public Interest in Washington, D.C. They have ranked 47 items based on levels of carotenoids, vitamin C, folate, potassium, and fiber.

THE BEST

1. Guavas
2. Watermelon
3. Grapefruit, pink or red
4. Kiwifruits
5. Papayas
6. Cantaloupe
7. Apricots, dried
8. Oranges
9. Strawberries
10. Apricots, fresh
11. Peaches, dried
12. Blackberries
13. Grapefruit, white
14. Raspberries
15. Tangerines
16. Persimmons
17. Mangoes
18. Honeydew melon
19. Star fruit

STILL PRETTY GOOD

20. Apricots, canned
21. Lemons
22. Blueberries
23. Plums
24. Bananas
25. Cherries
26. Limes
27. Peaches, fresh
28. Grapes
29. Rhubarb
30. Avocado
31. Pears
32. Pineapple, fresh
33. Apples
34. Figs, fresh

BEATS A CUPCAKE

35. Figs, dried
36. Nectarines
37. Pomegranates
38. Currants, dried
39. Pineapple, canned
40. Prunes
41. Peaches, canned
42. Dates, dried
43. Raisins
44. Fruit cocktail, canned
45. Pears, canned
46. Cranberry sauce, sweetened
47. Applesauce, unsweetened

fruits and vegetables supply ample amounts of calcium, iron, magnesium, and vitamins that prevent age-related chronic diseases. Packed into every spinach leaf, every spear of broccoli, and every slice of tomato are thousands of other health-giving, disease-fighting compounds called phytochemicals.

"No other food is so closely linked to vitality," says Elizabeth Somer, R.D., a registered dietitian and author of *Age-Proof Your Body*.

And it's never too late to enjoy the benefits of their nutrient riches. "Improvements in health risks are noted within weeks of adding more fruits and vegetables to the diet," says Somer.

Why can't you just take a supplement? "You can't get the nutrients and protective phytochemicals you need from pills. We don't even know what all these substances are, how they work, or whether they work best together. The best thing you can do is eat a variety of foods," says Polk.

Go for the Goal

If the word *vegetable* conjures up images of some kind of flaccid green matter relegated to a small corner on your dinner plate, think again.

"We're in a new age of vegetables—not just what Mom used to make but new varieties (not cooked until they're mushy) and new flavors," says Polk. "We're using herbs and spices to add flavor, not drowning them in butter."

Fruits and vegetables can be the most flavorful, exciting part of your diet. Here's how.

Plan ahead. Include at least two fruits or vegetables at every meal and two more for snacks. This is one of the easiest and most effective ways to get produce into your daily diet, says Somer.

Pick the freshest. If you're a tomato lover, you know the bliss of sinking your teeth into the first real tomato of the summer. Vine-ripened or not, those hothouse versions pale in comparison. To satisfy your tastebuds, select the freshest produce available, says Dr. Lachance.

"When you buy anything fresh, it's alive. When you take a bite out of an apple, it ought to say, 'Ouch,'" he adds.

There are two different degrees of fresh: garden fresh and market fresh. Garden fresh is definitely more nutritious than market fresh, says Dr. Lachance. You'll notice it right away because it just tastes better. That corn on the cob from Florida or the grapes that came from Chile may still be breathing, but they've paid a price to get to you. Out of season, it's better to eat market-fresh produce than to not eat fruits and vegetables at all.

For the most vitamin-packed fruits and vegetables, a good place to start is your local farmers' market. Look for produce that feels heavy for its size, smells fragrant, and is not wilted, shriveled, brown, or bruised.

Tune in to living color. When it comes to the vitamin content of fruits and vegetables, the more vibrant the color, the better. Extra color is a sign of extra nutrients and phytochemicals, says Katherine Tucker, Ph.D., associate professor of nutrition at Tufts University. These protective chemicals take the form of pigments in the vegetables, so the deeper the color, the more benefit you'll get.

Choose red grapes instead of green. Romaine or watercress instead of iceberg lettuce. Red cabbage instead of green. Dark orange carrots over pale ones.

Count the colors on your plate. You don't need a calculator to keep track of the nutrients you're getting at each meal. Just think in terms of color.

"Sometimes people don't do real well when they have to classify things such as eating cruciferous vegetables like broccoli, cabbage, or Brussels sprouts," says Polk. If that happens to you, try counting the colors on your plate, in your stir-fry, or in your salad. Go for a range of greens, reds, purples, yellows, and oranges.

If you have three or more colors, you're probably eating a healthy balance of nutrients.

Expand your tastebuds. Every time you go to the grocery store, buy a vegetable or fruit that you have never tasted before, says Dr. John La Puma of the CHEF (Cooking, Healthy Eating, and Fitness) Clinic.

His vegetable picks are broccoli sprouts, fennel, Hubbard squash, jicama, kale, sweet potatoes, Swiss chard (a big hit with his patients), and tomatillos.

Side with protein. When someone asks what's for dinner, our first answer is typically the meat: meat loaf, pork chops, hamburgers, or chicken. Protein usually has the starring role during a meal. To make the shift toward incorporating more vegetables and fruits into your diet, think of meat as a condiment.

"It is really a question of looking at food in a different way," says Polk. Take a somewhat Mediterranean approach to meal planning and build your entrée around produce first. Try this: The next time you make a stir-fry, call it a vegetable stir-fry with chicken instead of a chicken stir-fry with vegetables.

Be a sneak. A few years back in Pennsylvania, some clever folks (no doubt with an overabundance of squash in their gardens) came up with the idea of celebrating Sneak Some Zucchini onto Your Neighbor's Porch Night in August. Here's a better idea: Sneak some zucchini or other vegetables into your diet.

Living Proof PANEL

Double the Pleasure

Before I went on the Get Thin, Get Young Plan, I probably ate two or three servings of fruits and vegetables daily. But once I got started, I became much more aware of how many fruits and vegetables I ate.

So now, on a good day, I eat five or six servings. I usually take fruit with me to work so that I'll be less tempted to indulge in the cookies, candies, and other sweets that invariably show up in the workplace. Snacking on fruit makes it easier for me to stay on track and reminds me to eat a good lunch rather than simply opting for fast food. At home, instead of opening the refrigerator and just grabbing anything within reach, I'll go for a carrot or a piece of celery.

I still have an occasional piece of chocolate, but I don't keep ice cream or other sweets around the house. I would rather go out and work in the yard or run around the block than eat those things.

I try to vary what I eat so I don't get bored. So, for instance, if I've had my fill of carrots, I'll switch over to celery or strawberries. When I do find that no single fruit or vegetable appeals to me, I'll throw some yogurt, fruit juice, and a few frozen fruits together in the blender and make a smoothie. That takes care of five or six servings in one shot.

If you're like many people, potatoes account for about half of the vegetables you eat. Expand your horizons by sneaking some more green (and orange) matter into your diet, Tribole advises.

Here are some of her favorite ways to incorporate three of nature's nutrient powerhouses into your diet inconspicuously.

■ Spinach: Snip it like basil and add it to soups and tomato sauces.

■ Cauliflower: Mix cooked cauliflower with baked potato. Stuff the mixture back into the potato skin, sprinkle it with a little cheese, and bake it again.

■ Carrot: Carrot juice is a terrific spiking agent. Use it when you make gelatin or smoothies.

Wake up. If you don't start with breakfast, you don't have a chance of making it to 9 to 10 servings a day, says Dr. Lachance. The easiest way is to toss a handful of berries or a sliced banana onto your cereal in the morning.

Another way is to try some vegetables for breakfast. Prepare an omelette with thin slices of antioxidant-rich sweet red and yellow peppers, cut-up broccoli, or chopped tomatoes.

Hold the mayo. Spread a tablespoon of mashed avocado on your sandwich instead of light mayonnaise. At less than 23 calories a tablespoon, avocado will save about 22 light-mayo calories and provide about 1 gram of fiber and a healthy dose of monounsaturated fat, says Polk.

The Secrets to Radiant, Youthful Skin

JUST *ONE* DAY.

JUST ONE UNPROTECTED DAY IN THE SUN IRREVERSIBLY DAMAGES SKIN CELLS AND DNA—THE SAME DAMAGE THAT CREATES WRINKLES AND AGE SPOTS AND THAT MAY LEAD TO SKIN CANCER. THAT'S WHAT A STUDY AT THE DERMATOLOGY CLINICAL RESEARCH CENTER AT BOSTON UNIVERSITY MEDICAL CENTER FOUND.

JUST ONE DAY.

It goes to show that while we search for baby-smooth skin in a bottle, something as simple as sun protection truly sustains the promise of youthful skin. Even those who can afford expensive face-lifts and chemical injections won't look any younger if they don't heed basic everyday precautions.

"Do you know what a woman with aging skin who gets a face-lift but doesn't follow the basics looks like? She looks like a woman with aging skin and a face-lift. The basics go a long, long way," says Barney J. Kenet, M.D., a dermatologic surgeon at New York–Presbyterian Hospital/Weill Cornell Medical Center in New York City and author of *How to Wash Your Face*.

Those basics are sunscreen, sun protection, and a good daily skin-care regimen. That's what will keep your skin youthful and glowing. Then, with the aid of makeup, you can further turn back the clock and even appear to have shed a few pounds.

There Goes the Sun

Sun worshipers can forget about becoming patients of Leslie Baumann, M.D., assistant professor of clinical dermatology and director of cosmetic dermatology at the University of Miami. "If you don't intend to practice sun avoidance, then don't even bother coming in to have wrinkles looked at. It's a waste of your money."

Sun damage contributes about 90 percent to the aged appearance of skin. While genetics and aging do play a part in how old you appear, they account for only a small percentage. Most wrinkles, age spots, crow's-feet, sallow skin, blotches, and broken blood vessels come from the sun's rays, not the aging process itself.

"I have 80-year-old patients who have beautiful, young skin, all because they stayed out of the sun," says Roger I. Ceilley, M.D., clinical professor of dermatology at the University of Iowa in Iowa City and past president of the American Academy of Dermatology.

But don't fear if you've spent a good deal of your life running to the sun instead of ducking for cover. Even after years of sunbathing, if you start wearing sunscreen today and every day hereafter, you'll see a marked improvement in the quality of your skin.

"I've seen some remarkable turnaround with just sunscreen. The skin can repair itself to a degree. And because of that, it is never too late to start," Dr. Ceilley says.

You may wonder what the point is of having beautiful skin if you can't bask in the sunshine. You want to be on the beach, on the tennis court, or out in the yard with the kids. Or perhaps you have a job that requires you to spend time in the midday sun. Well, no one is asking you to stay locked up in a dark cellar while the rest of the world romps in the warm sun. You can still enjoy the daylight while protecting your youthful looks.

But you must protect yourself with the best antiaging product on the market: sunscreen. The study at Boston University also found that using sunscreen every day made the patients' skin react as if it hadn't been exposed to the sun at all.

Sunscreen: What to Buy

Forget the days when baby oil was the only "sunscreen" you took to the beach. Now you need a product that offers maximum protection from the sun's rays. The problem isn't where to find it. Just about every drugstore and cosmetic counter is lined with sunscreens and sunblocks in every form imaginable.

What you want is the right sunscreen that covers all your youthful-skin needs. Use the following criteria, and you'll enjoy the sun's rays in peace, knowing you're protected.

Purchase broad-spectrum sunscreens or sunblocks. The sun comes at your skin with two types of ultraviolet (UV) rays: UVA and UVB. The UVB rays burn or tan your skin, producing free radicals, which are molecules that damage skin cells and elastic tissue.

UVA rays won't make you burn. Instead, they penetrate deep within the skin, resulting in wrinkles and other signs of premature aging. Although both rays do their part in adding years to your skin, the UVB type is the most harmful during the summer, and UVAs bombard your skin year-round.

To fight both UVA and UVB damage, sunscreen should include ingredients such as avobenzone, zinc oxide, or titanium dioxide. But don't worry about remembering highly scientific monikers when perusing rows of sunscreens. Simply look for the words *broad-spectrum,* Dr. Ceilley says. That means the product blocks both UVA and UVB.

Go for SPF 15 or higher. SPF stands for "sun protection factor." To calculate how it works, multiply how long it would normally take you to burn by the SPF number. For instance, if you burn in 10 minutes, an SPF of 15 would allow you 150 minutes in the sun.

If you put on a thick layer and don't wash or rub it off, an SPF of 15 is as low as you should ever go, Dr. Ceilley says. If you have fair skin or you spend a lot of time out in the sun, wear a product with an SPF of 30. (Only if you have very fair skin or a history of skin cancer should you use something with a higher SPF. You won't have to apply quite as heavy a layer, either.)

Moisturize with sunscreen. If you're thinking, "Oh, great. Another skin product I have to stuff in the medicine cabinet"—think again. Many products now combine a sunscreen with a daily moisturizer. Use one to moisturize and protect your skin at the same time, Dr. Ceilley suggests.

Grab some sunscreen lip balm. Your lips need protection from the sun as well. But sunscreen lip balm with an SPF of 15 serves another novel yet practical purpose: Apply the lip balm around your eyes. It won't run or burn when you sweat, and it's easier to apply than lotion or gel.

Sunscreen: Wear It Well

Choosing the right sunscreen is only half the battle. If you don't use it correctly, your skin still catches those age-inducing rays. One study found that most people use only 50 percent of the recommended amount of sunscreen—meaning, they are only receiving half of the SPF. While their bottles of sunscreen may last longer, they're wasting their youthful looks.

Follow a few simple guidelines, and you'll get the maximum from your sunscreen. Your skin will thank you every time you look in the mirror and don't see a new wrinkle.

Apply 20 minutes before you go out. Using sunscreen doesn't mean that you have immediate protection. It takes at least 20 minutes for the active ingredients to soak into your skin. Slather on sunscreen first thing in the morning to ensure that it has enough time, Dr. Ceilley says.

Don't be stingy. If your bottle of sunscreen lasts a year or so, you're not using enough. For full-body protection, use 1 ounce, or one shot glass full of sunscreen, Dr. Ceilley says. When applying to just your face, use a marble-size amount, he adds.

If you put on an SPF 15 but don't use enough, it's the same as if you used a sunscreen with an SPF of 8—about half as much. A study at Dryburn Hospital in Durham, England, found that people who didn't put on the recommended amount of sunscreen only received between 20 and 50 percent of the SPF protection on the label.

Reapply. A study at the Queensland Institute of Medical Research in Herston, Australia, found that reapplying sunscreen every few hours offered 2½ times better protection from UV rays than using a single application. If you're working out, sweating, swimming, or doing anything strenuous, reapply every 2 hours. Even waterproof sunscreens eventually wear off, Dr. Ceilley says.

Wear it all days and all seasons. Clouds do not protect you from UV rays. Cold, blustery winter days do not protect you from UV rays. As long as the sun is in the sky—even if you can't see it—those rays will break through and into your skin. Make sunscreen a daily and yearlong habit, Dr. Ceilley says.

More Than Just Sunscreen

Sunscreen is powerful, but it's just one part of a sun-protection program. The rest is up to you. "There is much more that you can do to protect yourself," Dr. Ceilley says. Here's how.

Stay out of the midday sun. Don't shun the sun like a vampire during the day, but be conscious of how much time you're out between the hours of 10:00 A.M. and 4:00 P.M., when the sun's rays are the strongest. Take a break in the shade, or go inside every hour or so, Dr. Ceilley says.

Wear a hat. A fashionable hat not only will make you look younger but also will keep those age-ravaging rays away from your face and neck altogether. Sport a hat with at least a 4-inch brim that goes all around your head. It should completely shade your ears and the back of your neck, Dr. Ceilley says.

Don your glasses. The sun's rays have been shown to promote cataracts, another sign of aging. But on top of that, squinting exacerbates crow's-feet and other lines around the eyes, Dr. Ceilley says. Put on shades with UV protection when in the sun.

Cover up with clothes. When possible, wear long-sleeved shirts and long pants, Dr. Ceilley says.

The Fountains of Youth

If Ponce de León were around today, he wouldn't have to travel halfway around the world in search of the mythical fountain of youth. A quick hop to the local mall would be as far as he would have to go to hear tales of magic potions and waters that reverse the marks of time.

But even today, finding a true fountain of youth could prove just as elusive as de León's ancient quest, even though countless ads clamor about products that claim to have the true youth serum. Yet, Dr. Baumann says, only two products have been scientifically shown to bring back a youthful look and glow to aging skin. These two antiaging products can help erase some of the signs of time, such as wrinkles, lines, and age spots. Here's how they work and how to use them.

Alpha hydroxy acids. As far as over-the-counter antiaging ingredients go, alpha hydroxy acids (AHA) reign supreme. These natural acids—the most popular of which is glycolic acid—make you look younger in several ways.

They increase exfoliation of the skin, accelerating the removal of the

Save Your Money on Topical Vitamin C

Back in the good old days, you found vitamin C in your orange juice or morning multivitamin. Now it's in everything from your moisturizer to your makeup.

The question is: Is it doing anything?

The answer is no, according to Dr. Leslie Baumann of the University of Miami.

"Vitamin C is my pet peeve. Most of the products do not get absorbed. It becomes inactive very rapidly," she says.

The theory behind vitamin C in beauty products makes sense. Vitamin C is an antioxidant, so theoretically, it should help eliminate the free radicals that damage your skin, causing wrinkles and age spots.

The problem is that like many other things in life, what works in theory doesn't always pan out in reality. Many vitamin C formulations lose their effectiveness when the bottle is opened and the product is exposed to air.

"I haven't been able to find one that is stable and absorbed," she says. Until a better product is made—or better research confirms that topical vitamin C has any effect—she recommends saving your money. "Use it to purchase sunscreen," she adds.

outer layer of skin and revealing smoother, softer skin. They moisturize, helping to diminish the appearance of fine lines, and soften dry, sun-damaged skin. And in higher concentrations, they increase the thickness of the skin's second layer, called the dermis, which gives skin its youthful, glowing, healthy look.

But not all AHA products are created equal. Depending on the product, the amount of AHA varies and will have different results. For instance, one study compared a product with 5 percent glycolic acid to one containing 12 percent. While the 5 percent product did improve the skin's surface, the 12 percent concentration had more dramatic results, as it altered two layers of the skin.

Research has suggested that you need at least a 10 percent AHA concentration to stimulate the formation of collagen, which could help restore a youthful appearance. While you may see a difference in skin smoothness, an over-the-counter product with less than 10 percent won't help to erase lines or wrinkles.

There are a few over-the-counter AHA products—Alpha-Hydrox and Aqua Glycolic are two—that do have concentrations of 10 percent glycolic acid. But most contain less than 10 percent.

What should you do? Start with one of these over-the-counter 10 percent products. Keep in mind that you may need to use it for a few weeks to a couple of months to see results. If it doesn't work or you have had a lot of sun exposure, talk to your dermatologist, who can prescribe treatments with a much higher concentration, Dr. Kenet says.

Retin-A and Renova. You have to make a trip to your dermatologist's office if you want to get one of these, but it may be well worth the visit. Retin-A and Renova are prescription drugs that contain tretinoin, a derivative of vitamin A.

In various studies, Retin-A reversed sun damage, increased collagen formation, improved fine and coarse wrinkling, erased age spots, and evened out skin discoloration.

Retin-A was—and still is—an acne treatment. After dermatologists noticed its youth-promoting effects, they prescribed it for aging skin. Retin-A's sister product Renova was created solely for the purpose of treating wrinkles and aging skin. Follow the directions carefully and check with your dermatologist to see how these treatments may interact with other skin products you use.

You can find over-the-counter products containing retinol, another byproduct of vitamin A. But no evidence shows that it works as well as its prescription siblings, Dr. Kenet says.

If you want to start with an over-the-counter brand first, give it a try, Dr. Baumann says. If you don't see any improvement, ask your doctor for a prescription for Retin-A or Renova.

The Getting Younger Skin-Care Program

Dr. Kenet's message when it comes to daily skin care is to keep it simple. Instead of convincing patients that they need an arsenal of skin-care products, he says that people need only two or three.

Not only that, but how and how often you wash your skin can be as important as what you use. "Many people overwash. That dries out skin, making it itchy, flaky, and rough, which doesn't look too nice," Dr. Kenet says.

Follow this basic daily skin-care program and watch your skin regain its youthful glow.

Morning Routine

■ Take a 2- to 3-minute shower. Using cool to room-temperature water, get wet, then step out of the shower stream. Lather yourself up with a mild soap such as Dove, Basis, or Cetaphil.

Stay out of the water stream as much as possible. Do not use a loofah or abrasive washcloth that will scratch and dry out the skin. Rinse off and step out of the shower, Dr. Kenet says. Pat your skin dry with a towel.

■ Moisturize your body while your skin is still damp, so it traps the moisture. For full-body moisturizers, inexpensive products work just as well as expensive ones, says Dr. Kenet. And if you're really on a budget, even olive oil or vegetable shortening can do the job. He suggests avoiding heavily fragrant moisturizers.

■ Apply a sunscreen with an SPF of 15 to the areas that will be exposed.

■ If you are just washing your face, use a soap-free cleanser, such as Cetaphil Gentle Skin Cleanser for dry skin or Neutrogena Oil-Free Acne Wash for oily skin. Regular soap may dry out your skin and accentuate wrinkles.

Dampen your face with tepid water. Evenly apply a quarter-size amount of the cleanser to your face and massage gently with your fingertips. Rinse with tepid water and then pat dry.

■ Apply an SPF 15 sunscreen to your face every day. Use a combination sunscreen and moisturizer to save a step in the process.

■ You usually would use Retin-A or an AHA product at night, but if you are using both, apply your AHA in the morning. Just be sure to check with your dermatologist first. If you get the go-ahead, apply your AHA at least 10 minutes after using your cleanser. (Moisture on the skin can dilute the effects of the AHA product.)

Night Routine

■ If you have dry skin, you may not need to wash your face every night, Dr. Kenet says. Excessive washing will dry it out even further.

■ If you decide to wash your face, use the same technique as you did for your morning wash.

■ Apply either an AHA or a Retin-A/Renova product, waiting at least 10 minutes after using your cleanser.

Makeup: Take Off Years—And Pounds

As they get older, many women succumb to the notion that they must wear more makeup to cover up the signs of age.

But it's really just the opposite. "A flawless and as natural a look as possible appeals to women over 40. You want to enhance the beauty that is already there instead of wearing too much to try to offset what you don't like," says Julie Mollo, a professional Hollywood makeup artist and creator of the video *Makeup Secrets Uncovered.*

No longer must you feel intimidated by the women in white lab coats at the cosmetics counter. Mollo, who has been applying makeup to Hollywood stars for more than 10 years, says that you can get the look you want with a trip to the drugstore.

"I know I can always go to the drugstore and get what I need at half the price. The quality of makeup is usually comparable. At the cosmetic counters, 9 out of 10 times you are paying for the brand name more than just the makeup," Mollo says.

With makeup, you can take years and even some pounds off your face. The key is to remember the three basic rules.

1. Forget trends. Makeup trends and fads are for the hordes of 20-year-olds, not you. And that's a good thing.

"I looked in a magazine once and saw this woman with black smeared all over her eyes. I thought to myself that somebody out there thinks this is supposed to be cool. It looked absurd," Mollo says.

While fads may look hip on the very young, nothing makes a woman appear older than desperately trying to look like a kid again. Instead, you want a timeless, natural look that won't change much from year to year.

As a bonus, you won't find yourself smearing black across your eyes.

2. Update your look. Although you should ignore the trend of the month, if you are still wearing false eyelashes and thick liquid liner, it's time for a change, Mollo says. Just as trying to look too hip will age you, sticking with the makeup styles of the distant past will date you like a poodle skirt.

3. Go toward the light. Your natural inclination may be to wear more makeup to hide wrinkles and age spots, but that will actually highlight them. "You need a slightly lighter touch than what was done in your early years," Mollo says.

To keep a younger look, choose natural and lighter colors, use less makeup than before and apply it with a softer and lighter touch, she says.

Looking Younger

Used correctly, makeup can help peel years off your face. Here's how.

Base. The one step most women like to skip is the one that Mollo says is the most important. A proper base evens out your skin tone, hiding signs of age such as darkness around the eyes and red blemishes around the nose.

When buying a base, look for a yellow tone. Over her years of experience, Mollo says that she has learned that a yellow-tone base works best on a large majority of women.

When testing a base color in the store, put it on your cheek or on the inside of your arm. Mollo recommends Max Factor Lasting Performance, Almay Amazing Lasting Makeup, and L'Oréal Color Endure as good bases with yellow tones that can be easily found in drugstores.

The secret to perfect base application is stippling, Mollo says. With stippling, you blend in the base using short, frequent strokes with a sponge. When you apply base using long, wide strokes, you end up with a streaky look.

Concealer. If you have a small blemish or spot, cover it up with a base product that's one or two times lighter than your normal shade. But for more visible signs of aging such as broken blood vessels, age spots, sun damage, and darkness under the eyes, you'll need a concealer.

Certain concealer colors cover up specific signs of aging. Yellow concealer takes out red, such as broken blood vessels, blemishes, and red skin tones. Orange concealer blocks out blue and brown problems, such as age spots, freckles, sun damage, veins, and darkness under the eyes.

Try using Physicians Formula Neutralizer Color Corrective Primer in yellow as well as Revlon's New Complexion in sand beige (for yellow) and in natural beige (for orange). They both are good choices that can be found in drugstores, says Mollo.

To apply the concealer, use a small brush, much like a tiny paintbrush. Place some of the concealer on the brush, then rub the tip of the brush on the back of your hand to wipe off the excess. Apply a thin film to the area you want to cover up. Blend it in by dabbing the concealer. Don't wipe it in—you'll only wipe it off, Mollo says. After the base and concealer, apply a light coating of translucent powder.

Eye products. As women age, their eyes tend to droop a bit, making them appear smaller. And crow's-feet also take away from your eyes' natural impact. But makeup can open them up for the world to see, Mollo says.

First, choose the right eye-shadow colors. Mollo picks what she calls her foolproof colors for eyes: matte gold, mauve, peach, brown, and ivory. Most women get a great natural look with these shades.

The secret to perfect base application is stippling.

Using a small, fluffy brush, apply a lighter color to the upper lid closest to your lashes and to the brow bone, which will "open up" your eyes. If you have darkness around the inside corner of your eye, apply some lighter eye shadow there as well. Fill in the rest of the eyelid with a slightly darker color, Mollo says.

Choose a medium to light brown eye pencil with gold or red tones. Apply along the lash lines of your eyelids, starting from the inside and moving outward. Here's another eye-opening trick from Mollo: Don't follow the natural downward slant of your eye. Instead, when you get toward the outside end of your eye, draw the line slightly upward. Using a cotton swab, blend the eyeliner until it looks smudged. If you keep the eyeliner solid, it doesn't give the eye a deep and soft look. Then apply your mascara, she says.

Blush. When it comes to cheeks, Mollo says that less is more. Cheeks should be soft and warm and shouldn't take away from the real focus of your face—your eyes and lips. As for "foolproof" blushes, Mollo recommends shades of pink, mauve, and peach. Buy yourself a big, fluffy blush brush because the ones that usually come with blush aren't big enough, Mollo says. Apply a very soft layer to the "apples" of your cheekbones and the hollows of your cheeks.

Lip products. Another sign of aging is that lips lose their shape and definition. Reverse that process with a little lip liner, Mollo says. You can choose from many lip colors and shades, so have fun trying ones that you like. But always start with lip liner, she says. Fill in your entire lip with the liner. This will ensure that your lipstick stays on longer. Then apply a glossy clear lip balm or a lipstick shade on top.

Looking Thinner

You don't have to actually drop all of the weight you want before you start looking thinner. The right makeup techniques can take off pounds as well as years. Here's how.

Use some shading. To play down a double chin or a full face, create some shadow, Mollo says. Buy a powder that is a shade darker than your face. In fact, Mollo recommends buying a taupê *eye shadow,* which is a perfect shading color for many women. After putting on your base and concealer, apply the powder directly underneath your jawbone with a big, fluffy brush.

To get a little shading around your cheekbones, apply the powder in the recess just underneath the cheekbone. "It will look more sculpted," she says. Mollo warns that both techniques require a good bit of practice.

Go easy on the blush. Heavy blush will bring attention to a full face, Mollo says. Instead, layer translucent shades of blush onto your cheeks. It's easier to add more blush than it is to take some off.

Highlight your eyes or lips. Enhance your lips and eyes when you have a full face. "Makeup allows us to draw attention to what you like and take attention away from what you don't like. If you love your eyes, play down everything else. If you love your mouth, treat yourself to a really great lipstick," Mollo says.

Week Four

A New You Each Day

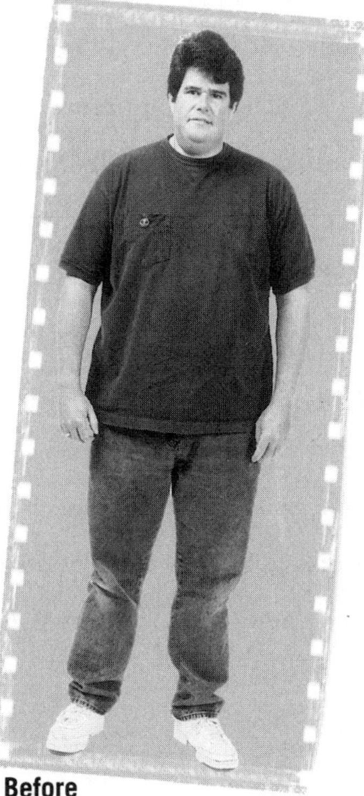
Before

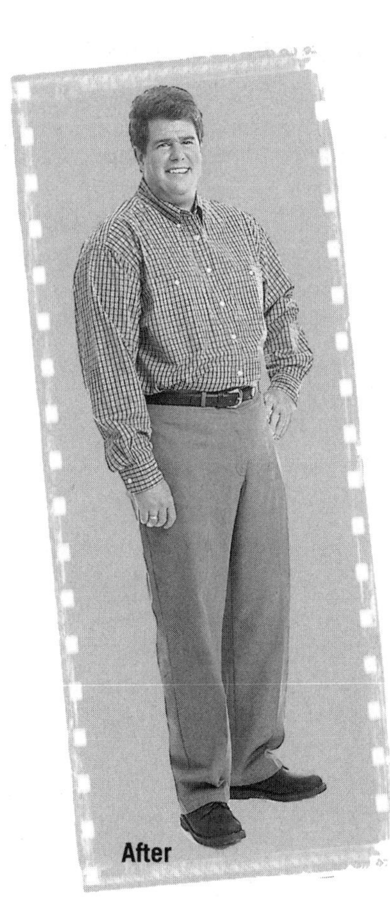
After

ANNE AND I KNEW THAT IF WE WANTED TO LOSE WEIGHT, WE HAD TO STOP MAKING TWO DINNERS. PLUS, IT WOULDN'T HURT OUR KIDS TO EAT HEALTHY—IN FACT, IT WOULD HELP THEM.

—Dave Harbove

Week Four

You're already starting the fourth week of The *Prevention* Get Thin, Get Young Plan. When you look back and compare your life today to your life when your started, you probably will notice that you're more active and you're eating more healthfully—and you're seeing some positive results. The small lifestyle adjustments that you're making each week are resulting in a new you.

This week, you'll learn how to short-circuit the impulse to skip workouts or overeat. And you'll find strategies for dealing with hectic schedules and temptations from family and friends. If you've had trouble some days finding a block of time to fit in exercise, you'll learn how to gain the same benefits by squeezing in a few short bouts during the day. Plus, you'll get tips for choosing a new hairstyle that will immediately give you a more youthful, attractive appearance.

Taking Your Cue—And Changing It

DURING THE HECTIC AND UNSTABLE TIME OF WORLD WAR I, WOMEN IN GERMANY BEGAN TO PUT ON WEIGHT. AS EXPERTS LOOKED INTO THIS PHENOMENON, THEY DISCOVERED THAT THESE WOMEN—WHOSE WAR-TORN WORLDS WERE UNPREDICTABLE AND FILLED WITH FEAR, STRESS, AND OTHER EMOTIONAL TRAUMA—TURNED TO FOOD FOR COMFORT.

To describe these women, experts used the German term *Kummerspeck,* meaning "fat of sorrow."

As many people have discovered from their own experiences, successful weight loss requires more than just exercising and eating well. Experts now know that people must learn to react properly when certain emotions and situations compel them to overeat and skip workouts.

When faced with one of these "cues"—your boss tears apart your report, the sweet aroma of freshly baked bread wafts to your nose, you're speeding to your next appointment—you automatically respond by eating whatever is in sight. Indeed, all these unnecessary and often unhealthy calories add pounds and years to your body.

"In many cases, we have learned it. We saw our parents doing the same thing. And certainly, we all have different coping mechanisms. Some react to certain situations by having a cigarette; some put on their sneakers and go for a run. Other people may eat," says Ross Andersen, Ph.D., assistant professor of medicine at Johns Hopkins University School of Medicine in Baltimore and one of the nation's leading researchers on lifestyle activity and weight loss.

To lose weight and keep it off, you need to rein in these triggers. You can diet and exercise down to a certain weight, but if you haven't changed those core behaviors that send you to the cookie jar or leave you lying lethargically on the couch, it may be in vain. As soon as you finish dieting, you'll probably slip right back into your old habits, and the weight will return.

The good news is that you can break out of these old habits. Not only can you thwart these troublesome cues, you also can transform them into triggers that work for you and your weight-loss program.

In other words, you can replace negative habits with positive ones, Dr. Andersen says.

Three Steps to Stop Any Cue

Get 10 people in a room, and you'll discover that they have at least 10 different cues. Even with very common triggers, each person develops his own version. Stress might be a universal cue, but it can send one person into an endless potato chip binge, while it puts another into such a funk that putting one foot in front of the other seems entirely out of the question.

Despite the individual nature of cues, everyone can use the same process to find and eliminate them, says Raymond C. Baker, Ph.D., a clinical psychologist and director of the Center for Wellness and Counseling at Bradley University in Peoria, Illinois.

Try this three-part method to banish your triggers.

Identify the cue. To stop a cue, first you have to learn what it is. The best way to do so is to write about your eating and exercise habits. That's one of the reasons it's so important to keep a weight-loss diary. (For more on diaries, see Dear Diary: The Key to Self-Evaluation on page 27.) Your diary allows you to study your behaviors and identify your cues, Dr. Baker says. If you see that midafternoon meetings send you off on a vending machine attack, you've identified a cue.

Brainstorm alternatives. Once you identify your cue, devise alternative ways you can react to it. "This is the time to think: 'What could I do instead?'" Dr. Baker says. As you brainstorm solutions, write them down. If boredom prompts you to raid your fridge, come up with a list of things that you can do instead of eating.

The choices are endless: Read, take a walk, write an e-mail to a good friend, or balance your checkbook. The next time you find yourself en route to the kitchen because you're bored, look at your list, pick an activity, and do it.

Prepare. Have your healthy alternatives ready so that when a cue pops up, you can immediately counteract it. If you come home from work hungry and wanting to eat an entire bag of Oreos, banish these troublemakers from the house and have healthier food ready to eat instead. By being prepared, you're more likely to be successful against a trigger, Dr. Baker says.

The Four Types of Cues

As individual as they can be, cues tend to fall into one of four categories. Some people may have problems with only one type of cue, while others feel the pressure from all four. Find which type of cues you identify with and try some of the suggested solutions.

Emotional cues. By far, emotions rank as the top overeating cue, Dr. Andersen says. Dealing with emotions and their underlying causes never seems as enticing as losing yourself in a hot-fudge sundae. Anger, sadness, stress, and even jubilation cause many people to overeat or skip exercise. The next time you feel the rush of emotions overwhelming your healthy habits, try one of the following:

- Take a 5-minute walk. Exercise squashes stress and other negative feelings.
- Breathe deeply for a minute. This will help calm you down.
- Write your feelings down. Expressing yourself on paper may help release your emotions.

Habitual cues. You always uphold your membership in the "clean plate club." You always munch on corn chips while watching television. You always eat so fast that you often forget that you actually ate. Habitual cues are those that you do just because you always have—and perhaps you don't know why or how you even got started. But just because you always have done something doesn't mean you always have to.

- Try not to eat and do something else at the same time, such as talk on

Living Proof
PANEL

Our Friday Night Ritual

Delma A. Gordon

Friday nights have always meant no-cook nights. Pizza and wine while watching *Friends* reruns is how we unwind after a stressful week.

So even though I was trying to eat differently, I knew there was no way I was going to give up that end-of-the-week ritual. Instead, I found a way to make the pizza healthier.

Now, my husband and I gorge ourselves on white pizza with spinach and anchovies—getting a valuable leafy green vegetable and extra fiber, not to mention the omega-3 fatty acids found in the anchovies.

The guy at the pizza place says that I'm the only woman he's ever met who likes anchovies. And he's so used to our Friday night order that he automatically gets it going even before we call it in.

the phone or watch TV. By focusing on what you eat, you'll stop eating unconsciously and actually taste and enjoy your food.

■ Eat at set times and at the dinner table. That will prevent you from gobbling on the run or eating over the sink.

■ Keep busy with hobbies, activities, and socializing. Fill your spare time with these habits instead of filling up the blank space with food.

Environmental cues. You're driving down the highway at 6:00 P.M. when you see those ever-present golden arches looming ahead. "We know there is a drive-through window waiting for us. That certainly is a cue," Dr. Andersen says. Other environmental cues: A full bag of potato chips lures you to eat your way to the bottom; a buffet offers a variety of tasty treats; you unconsciously reach for the chocolate candy on a coworker's desk. Environmental cues are the sights, smells, and location triggers that often haul you in. Change the environment, and you'll change the reaction.

■ Take a different route. If you always pass by a particularly enticing fast-food joint or a bakery on your normal driving route, find an alternate way.

■ Take what you want—then put it away. If you want a few chips, then take a few—but put them on a plate and put away the bag. That'll keep you from devouring the whole thing.

■ At a buffet, take a spoonful of each food. Once you are done, don't go back for more. This way, you'll get to taste it all without overeating.

■ Before you put something in your mouth, say "Stop." Think about why you are eating. Do you really want it? Even if you do, wait a few minutes. The craving may pass.

Cues of omission. How can there be such a thing? How about when you're so tired that you skip your workout and opt for the "exercise" of channel surfing? Or you get so caught up in your schedule that you forget to buy fruits and vegetables, so at dinnertime you call the pizza place? These are the cues that lead you to forgo a healthy habit. To break out of this pattern, leave yourself positive cues—signs that remind or motivate you to do the right thing. Here's how.

■ Leave your sneakers at the end of your bed or by the front door. That will prompt you to exercise as soon as you wake up or come home from work.

■ Make an exercise date with a buddy. You're more likely to exercise if you have a friend waiting for you.

■ Designate a "food planning night." On this night, map out how you will eat and what meals you'll prepare for the coming week. Make a list of what you'll need and go to the grocery store. Prepare what you can that night, such as making casseroles and cutting up fruits or vegetables for snacks.

How Much Exercise Is Enough?

IT'S EASY TO UNDERESTIMATE THE POWER OF A SINGLE STEP. BUT WHEN YOU'RE STARTING TO EXERCISE, THOSE STEPS ADD UP IN SOME IMPRESSIVE WAYS. CONSIDER THIS: JUST 3 HOURS OF BRISK WALKING EACH WEEK IS ENOUGH TO CUT YOUR RISK FOR HEART ATTACK BY UP TO 40 PERCENT. IS LEISURELY STROLLING MORE YOUR SPEED? NO PROBLEM. EVEN CASUAL TREKS THROUGH THE NEIGHBORHOOD CAN REDUCE YOUR RISK FOR HEART ATTACK AND STROKE BY UP TO 25 PERCENT, AS LONG AS THEY ADD UP TO A TOTAL OF 3 HOURS WEEKLY.

In fact, that same amount of exercise may be enough to turn back the clock and reduce the risk for serious illnesses of all kinds. Researchers in the Honolulu Heart Program followed a group of retired men in Hawaii who walked a total of 2 miles a day. They found that the men were half as likely to die from *all* causes over a 12-year period compared to men who walked less than a mile.

What does this mean for you? It means that if you have a few free minutes a couple of times a day, you can get fit, feel younger, and live longer. Don't worry if you can't carve out a large block of time to exercise. All

Living Proof PANEL

Little Steps for the Long Run

I would love to be able to take an hour to exercise every day. I enjoy walking and riding my bike and playing tennis. The problem is time. I have a long commute to work. I work long hours, so I don't get home until 9:00 or 10:00 P.M. And I teach classes, so I have a lot of extra work to do when I get home.

As a result, I always thought I couldn't do any kind of exercise—and I've been battling extra weight for years. This program has taught me a whole different way of thinking.

Now I know that even if I walk for only 10 minutes, that makes a difference over time. All of those little things—like parking farther away from work, taking the stairs, and getting up from my desk to take short walks around the building—have really helped me. Even during weeks when I couldn't do any other kind of exercise, I still maintained my weight loss.

Losing weight through these little steps isn't as fast as making huge lifestyle changes. I can live with that, however, because I know I can stick with these little changes for the rest of my life. That'll make a big difference in the long run.

the new research suggests that a less rigid approach works just as well. So you can feel comfortable just grabbing a 10-minute jaunt when it fits into your life.

Still unconvinced that every step counts? How about this: "If every day at work you were to take 2 minutes every hour and walk down the hall to talk to someone instead of spending those 2 minutes every hour sending an e-mail, you could save yourself 11 pounds over 10 years," says Joyce A. Hanna, associate director of the health improvement program at Stanford

University and an exercise physiologist in Palo Alto, California. "And that's just 2 minutes every hour."

A New Approach to Exercise

Health experts used to believe that in order to improve your cardiovascular health through exercise, you had to do at least 20 minutes of sustained, moderate-to-hard aerobic activity three to five times a week. The usual recommendation was to spend 10 minutes warming up, 20 minutes in your target heart range, and 10 minutes cooling down—adding up to 40 minutes all together.

That's not bad advice. But we have something even better. For folks who have a hard time finding 40 minutes for vigorous activity—and let's face it, by the time you've changed your clothes and showered, it's more like an hour—there's another approach that may work just as well.

If you can take two or three short breaks during the day and take a quick walk around the block, you'll get the same fat-burning and cardiovascular benefits that you would by exercising longer, says fitness researcher Marie H. Murphy, Ph.D., an exercise physiologist at the University of Ulster at Jordanstown, Northern Ireland. For losing weight, in fact, the short bouts might even be better.

"Your metabolism remains raised for a period after you have finished exercising. So you're still burning calories and receiving benefits even after you stop," says Dr. Murphy. Exercising several times for short periods may increase your total after-exercise burn time, she explains. "So you could actually burn more calories."

Here are a few quick ways to take advantage of this unique afterburn.

Get up 10 minutes earlier. If you avoid hitting that snooze button one last time in the morning, you can sneak in one-third to one-half of your exercise for the entire day, says personal trainer Michelle Edwards, a certified personal trainer and a health educator for the Cooper Institute for Aerobics Research in Dallas. "If you can take 10 to 15 minutes in the morning and 10 to 15 minutes after work and use them to take a brisk walk, you'll not only get your daily exercise in a manageable way but also begin and end the workday with a calmer, clearer head."

When you think it, do it. One reason people aren't more active is that they spend too much time thinking about what they need to do and not enough time actually doing it, says Al Secunda, author of *Ultimate Tennis* and *The 15-Second Principle*. "Instead of planning ahead like you do when you're going to do a 30- or 40-minute exercise session, just seize the moment when it occurs. As soon as you hit a little lull and think, 'I could take a break,' head out for a walk."

Write it down to make it a habit. It takes a few months for your brain to form new habits, so you have work a little harder at first to make exercise part of your routine, says running coach Michael Gilewski, Ph.D., a clinical psychologist for post-acute care services at Cedars-Sinai Medical Center in Los Angeles. "If you're having trouble remembering to take your walks, simply jot two or three short breaks into your day planner," he suggests. "Put them in at the same times each day. Before you know it, your brain will register it automatically."

Smart Strategies for Daily Living

YOU'VE MADE YOUR VOW TO SHAPE UP AND LOSE WEIGHT. YOU'RE TRYING TO DEVOTE YOUR MEALS TO HEALTHY EATING, AND YOU'VE BUILT UP YOUR RESISTANCE TO THE CUES THAT TRIGGER YOU TO EAT POORLY. NOW, IF YOU COULD JUST GET YOUR FRIENDS, FAMILY, AND THE REST OF THE WORLD TO STOP TEMPTING YOU, THE JOURNEY WOULD BE A LOT EASIER.

If there's one thing you can count on, it's that events don't always turn out as you've planned, especially when you're trying to lose weight.

But that's okay, says weight-loss expert Dr. Ross Andersen of Johns Hopkins University School of Medicine. When you create a strategy to deal with the unexpected, you'll improve your chances of weight-loss success.

When Time Is Not on Your Side

Experts agree that a lack of time is the biggest challenge to healthy eating. When a hectic schedule tempts you to turn to fast food, try these timesaving techniques.

Keep it simple. A busy weeknight probably isn't the best occasion to make low-fat lobster bisque and a high-fiber plum tart. Instead, keep your meals simple during the week and save the complicated dishes for when you have more time, suggests Joyce Nelsen, R.D., nutrition instructor at the Culinary Institute of America in Hyde Park, New York.

Stop chopping. From lettuce to cheese, it's easier than ever to stock up on ready-made products that will cut your cooking time in half and, as a result, keep you on track.

"All my meals take 20 minutes or less to cook," says Tammy Baker, R.D., a registered dietitian in Cave Creek, Arizona, and a spokesperson for the American Dietetic Association. She zips through the kitchen with shredded low-fat cheese, precut and washed lettuce, canned soup, frozen vegetables, and ready-made spaghetti sauce as she whips up low-fat tostadas, chef salad, soup, and pasta.

Make meaty meals fast. Extra-lean ground beef isn't just good for you—it's also one of the quickest-cooking types of beef, along with flank steak and stew meat. Looking for a speedy poultry dish? Use boneless, skinless chicken or turkey breasts, turkey tenderloin, or ground chicken or turkey breast. Among the fastest-cooking seafood meals are fish fillets, scallops, shrimp, crab, clams, and mussels.

Add some family fun. Get your dinner routine down to a science and get your family to help with the experiment. For example, let your kids set the table, stir the sauce, and measure ingredients, Baker suggests. You'll sneak in family togetherness while getting dinner on the table in record time.

Lunch on leftovers. Bring dinner leftovers back for encore presentations as fast lunches throughout the week. Put your vegetable lasagna in small microwaveable containers and heat them as you need them. Or use leftover meat loaf and baked chicken in tasty sandwiches, Baker suggests.

When Your Next Meal Is Hours Away

When you take your body through long stretches between meals, those high-fat snacks can seem to almost walk up and leap into your mouth, despite your best intentions. Plan beforehand so that you always have a tasty, healthy alternative on hand instead.

Schedule a snack. Since you're bound to get hungry every 4 hours between meals, keep apples, oranges, bananas, fig bars, pretzels, baked tortilla chips, air-popped popcorn, raisins, low-fat crackers, or granola bars

A Toast to Weight Loss

Marilyn Monroe liked champagne so much that she once took a bath in it—350 bottles' worth.

It may make an unusual bathing habit, but if you're trying to lose pounds, that's the only easy way to enjoy champagne—or any other kind of alcohol—while watching your weight.

While alcohol is typically fat-free, it's extremely high in calories, says John P. Foreyt, Ph.D., director of the Behavioral Medicine Research Center at Baylor College of Medicine in Houston and coauthor of *Living without Dieting.*

For example, bread and other carbohydrates have 4 calories per gram, while peach schnapps has about 7 calories per gram, as does any other form of alcohol, including the amount found in wine and beer. That translates into 168 calories for a 12-ounce serving of beer—the equivalent of a few handfuls of greasy potato chips.

Here's another eye-opener: Calories from alcohol don't burn as fast as those from other food. "If you ate a Twinkie and drank a glass of beer, you'd burn the carbohydrate calories from the Twinkie first," Dr. Foreyt says.

What's more, alcohol lowers your inhibitions, making you more likely to overeat. All these reasons add up to a pretty convincing case for staying away from liquor

handy, says Dominique Adair, R.D., a registered dietitian in New York City.

Play hide and seek. When you hit the kitchen starving and see a jar of chocolate chip cookies on the counter, it should surprise no one when you help yourself to a handful. One of the best ways to keep yourself from indulging in high-fat goodies is to keep them out of sight, Adair says. Or better yet, don't buy them at all.

Snack on nutrients. If the high-fat fare isn't handy, what is? Make sure that you have low-fat snacks where you can get to them quickly. Leave a platter of cut-up bell peppers, carrots, and broccoli and low-fat dip in your refrigerator to munch on, suggests Jyl Steinback, a personal trainer in Scottsdale, Arizona, and author of *The Fat-Free Living Cookbook* series. Or keep a bowl of grapes or sliced melon handy.

while you're trying to lose weight, says weight-loss expert Dr. Ross Andersen of Johns Hopkins University School of Medicine.

But if you still feel the need for an occasional drink, try these suggestions.

Stick to two. You'll keep those empty calories to a minimum by having no more than two drinks a day, suggests Dr. Foreyt. Keep in mind that one drink equals 12 ounces of beer, a shot (1 ounce) of liquor, or 4 ounces of wine.

Staying below two not only will help you stay lean but also may help keep your heart healthy and strong. Men who drank no more than two to six drinks a week in the large-scale Physicians' Health Study lowered their risk of sudden cardiac death by up to 79 percent.

Spring for a spritzer. They're not just for holiday parties. Add some calorie-free club soda to your wine, and you'll slash your calories.

Go light. If you don't want a wine spritzer, choose other low-calorie drinks, such as 4 ounces of champagne for 84 calories, a 6-ounce Bloody Mary for 87 calories, or 6 ounces of white wine for 121 calories.

Lose the umbrella. The next time you're tempted to order a piña colada, think about a different order. It has a hefty 330 calories and 10.8 grams of fat in only 6 ounces. Steer away from rum toddies, too. They have 334 calories and 11.4 grams of fat in a 10-ounce glass. And White Russians have 295 calories and 3.6 grams of fat in just 4 ounces.

When Your Kids Don't Want It

If you're watching your kids gobble hot dogs and french fries while you're lifting forkfuls of Brussels sprouts from your plate, guess whose meal is going to look better? Instead, wean your kids onto healthier fare, which will improve their eating habits, save you from cooking two meals, and keep you out of temptation's way at the dinner table.

Start a new "night." Instead of ditching their old favorites entirely, make a special night with a whole new healthy entrée. Introduce low-fat tacos or fajitas on "Mexican night" and black beans and rice on "Caribbean night," Nelsen suggests.

Or have "picnic night" and munch on fresh salad, sandwiches, and melon, all while you stretch out on a checkered blanket on the living room floor.

Living Proof
PANEL

No More Wrinkled Noses

David Harlow Our typical dinner routine always involved cooking two meals, like macaroni and cheese for our four kids and chicken and rice for my wife, Anne, and me. Unfortunately, I found myself often finishing off the leftovers from my kids' plates—sometimes even eating as much of their food as my own.

Anne and I knew that if we wanted to lose weight, we had to stop making two dinners. Plus, it wouldn't hurt our kids to eat healthy—in fact, it would help them.

We decided to make the change one day without looking back. We served broiled chicken, couscous, and stir-fried mushrooms and told our kids this was all they were getting for dinner.

For about a week, they refused to eat much of their meals, but Anne and I wouldn't budge on our new rule. Then my oldest daughter took the plunge and ate some broiled fish and mushrooms. I think the others felt sibling pressure, and soon they were all eating the healthy dinners we served—and I wasn't filling up on macaroni and cheese anymore.

Start with a few replacements. If your family usually eats macaroni and cheese, you may trigger a revolt if you suddenly drop a dinner of stir-fried vegetables, brown rice, and tofu on them. But if you make the transition to healthier eating slowly, they may not even notice the change, Nelsen says. For example, use low-fat Cheddar and fat-free milk in that macaroni and cheese.

Slip in some health. You can probably cut up vegetables small enough and slip them into your kids' food without them even noticing. Chop or shred spinach and put it in chili. Sneak slices of onion into tomato sauce. Turn up the flavor of an omelette with peppers and scallions.

Bring it in on the side. Adding a few carrots to your kids' plates isn't exactly a nutritional revolution, but it does bring you one step closer to the long-awaited vegetable stir-fry, Dr. Andersen says. Instead of cake for dessert, try slices of apple or a berry cup topped with vanilla yogurt.

When Your Spouse Wants Junk Food

Your kids may not be the only ones wrinkling their noses at healthy fare. What do you do when your mate insists on high-calorie meals and snacks?

Cook it healthier. If your spouse is not about to abandon burgers, simply buy the leanest cuts of meat you can get, such as ground round instead of ground chuck, suggests Marsha Hudnall, R.D., director of nutrition programs at Green Mountain, a weight-loss program for women in Ludlow, Vermont. Or even slip ground turkey into chili and tacos instead of using ground beef, and your scheme may go unnoticed.

When you're making steak fries, cook them in the oven instead of in a deep fryer. When you're making mashed potatoes, if you lose the butter and cream and add chicken broth and garlic, a potentially fattening side dish becomes healthy and flavorful.

Get a taste of fat. Drizzle or brush a little olive oil onto salads, tortilla crisps, and baked french fries so that fat is the first thing your spouse—and you—will taste. Adding a touch of oil, butter, or cheese to your first bite can make your whole meal taste richer in fat than it really is.

Add flavor without fat. The next time you're simmering a soup or stew, pump up the flavor by adding a few slices of a mild or hot pepper, such as an Anaheim, jalapeño, or pequín, to your entrée while it cooks. Remove them before you serve.

Keep temptation down. If your spouse brings home sweets that you can't resist, have a heart-to-heart discussion about it, says Dr. Andersen.

Say something like, "I know you don't do it intentionally, but when you come home with cookies, it feels like you're not being supportive." Then set a ground rule: No sweets in the house for the next few weeks, or until you feel comfortable enough with your eating habits that you won't splurge.

When You Don't See It Coming

Sometimes, no matter how prepared you are for daily obstacles, you'll suddenly find yourself face to face with temptation.

Simply refuse. You're at your neighbor's house in the afternoon, and she offers you a piece of fresh-baked coffee cake. It feels rude to say no.

So what do you do? Simply say, "Thank you, but I'm not hungry," Nelsen says.

If you're afraid of hurting her feelings, tell her that you had a late lunch but you'll take a piece home with you for later—and then give it to your family. If that doesn't work, then be a little more blunt, Nelsen suggests. Say, "It looks delicious, but my skirts are getting a little tight, so I'm cutting out the sweets."

Get preoccupied. What do you do when you're confronted with a box of glazed doughnuts at your first meeting of the day, and your will is weak at such an early hour? To keep from reaching for a doughnut, find something else to do with your hands, Adair suggests.

Fix yourself some coffee or tea, or pour some water or juice. Keep the cup in your hands until the snacks are gone. This is another reason to make sure that you eat breakfast every morning. You'll be less likely to get blindsided by fattening choices.

Keep your distance. If you find yourself in a meeting or other situation where there are sweets on the table, take a seat where you can't see or smell them. At the very least, stay more than an arm's length away.

Split it with someone. If seeing your friends nibbling on pastries is just too much to bear without indulging yourself, ask someone to share one with you, she suggests. Or cut yourself one-fourth of it to get a taste without all the calories.

Go With the Grain

ON-SCREEN OR OFF, IN THE 1960S, FEW COULD COMPETE WITH THE EXOTIC BEAUTY OF SULTRY ITALIAN ACTRESS SOPHIA LOREN. DECADES LATER, THE MEDIA WERE STILL CALLING THE SIXTYSOMETHING ACTRESS ONE OF THE SEXIEST WOMEN OF THE CENTURY. WHAT'S HER SECRET?

"Everything you see, I owe to spaghetti," Loren told an interviewer.

Sound like another Hollywood story? Though this buxom brunette likely owes thanks to genetics, too, science suggests that eating spaghetti does have a beauty payoff—if it's made from whole grains.

That's right. Unrefined grains, such as whole wheat, brown rice, oats, corn, and rye, are nature's own "beauty cream," full of wrinkle-preventing nutrients that you won't find behind any cosmetics counter. They also hold appetite-suppressing fiber that's unavailable at any drugstore.

Unfortunately, many Americans choose refined grains, such as white bread, and miss out on these benefits. To give your body a beauty boost both inside and out, increase your intake of whole grains to six servings a day. (A serving is about one slice of bread, an ounce of cereal, or ½ cup of cooked grain.)

As you pile these whole grains on your plate, you can peel off the pounds and turn back the clock. And best of all, they add flavor and pleasure to your meals.

"They taste good. If you're going to stick with any type of weight-loss plan,

Living Proof
PANEL

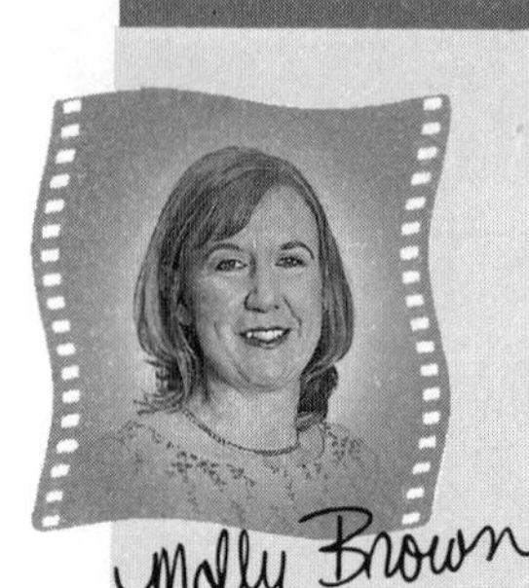

Getting the Kids to Try Something New

When it comes to new taste experiences, my husband and I are up for the adventure. But, like most kids, my daughters aren't exactly culinary Indiana Joneses. I knew that new whole grains, with their unfamiliar texture and taste, would be a huge turnoff to my kids' tastebuds. Fortunately, I've discovered a simple trick to get new foods on the table: masquerade them as familiar foods.

For example, I made my kids one of their favorites: pasta with marinara sauce. Only this time, the macaroni was made with whole corn flour rather than regular low-fiber white flour. I prepared the meal the usual way but used extra of their favorite brand of tomato sauce and Parmesan cheese.

The whole family loved it, especially my 15-year-old, Nicole. Out of all the new whole grains we've tried (ranging from seven-grain breakfast cereal to herbed quinoa), she gave corn pasta the highest rating. Now that she's familiar with the taste, she won't hesitate to eat it. So next time I serve it, I'll let her decide how much cheese to add.

the food has to taste good," says Melanie Polk, R.D., director of nutrition education at the American Institute for Cancer Research in Washington, D.C.

Get Thin

In the battle of the bulge, whole grains are a hardworking first line of defense. They ward off hunger by stretching your stomach, quickly sending the "I'm full" signal to your brain. They slow digestion, too, so you feel full longer, which means fewer snack attacks during the day.

But those aren't the only ways that whole grains defend your waistline. Their fiber traps fat in your food, preventing you from storing it on your thighs and stomach.

Since whole grains also slow digestion of foods that you eat along with them, they help limit surges in blood sugar and the following bombardment of insulin that tells your body to start stocking fat.

Get Young

How can brown rice or whole wheat bread offer a greater benefit to your appearance than your Oil of Olay? Simple. Whole grains are loaded with antioxidants, such as vitamin E and selenium, and lots of phytochemicals, which are components that aren't nutrients but have a protective effect in your body.

These free-radical fighters may reduce the risk of mutations to your DNA, leaving you with the beauty benefit of fewer wrinkles.

The benefits may be even more beautiful on the inside. That DNA-shielding action may also help prevent cancer. In fact, according to the American Institute for Cancer Research, whole grains may lower your risk for cancer of the breasts, pancreas, colon, and stomach. Moving on through your body, soluble fiber found in grains also protects your ticker by lowering your cholesterol, says the American Heart Association.

And let's not forget your bones. Whole grains, especially amaranth, also have calcium. Just 1 cup of this cooked grain contains 10 percent of the Daily Value of calcium. So adding it to your meals may also lower your risk for osteoporosis.

Remember, though, "grains" means *whole* grains. Roughly 50 to 80 percent of 23 body-friendly nutrients are lost when grains are refined—and those are just the ones the experts know about.

"There is a wide array of beneficial phytochemicals lost during milling that researchers are just beginning to identify, like lignan, phenols, and phytic acid," says Greg Hottinger, R.D., a specialist in whole foods and a registered dietitian with the Duke University Diet and Fitness Center in Durham, North Carolina.

Enriching the grains doesn't help much. Manufacturers only add back five nutrients: thiamin, riboflavin, niacin, folic acid, and iron. Along with the permanent loss of phytochemicals, many micronutrients disappear, too, such as chromium and magnesium, which are important for controlling blood sugar. That may be one reason why the famous Nurses' Health Study found that diabetes was less common among women who ate a lot of whole grains.

Go for the Goal

Obviously, there are many reasons to let these whole grains work their magic in your body. Fortunately, you can pick from a multitude of choices—from familiar to exotic—so you'll never run out of ways to enjoy them.

When you're looking for whole grains, you'll often find sparse pickings at supermarkets, with options seemingly limited to brown rice and microwave popcorn. (Though with some persistence and a lot of label reading, you may unearth a loaf of whole-wheat bread, too.)

For better options, head to your local health food store and get ready for a culinary adventure. You'll find dozens of whole grains there. If you don't know how to pronounce quinoa or triticale—let alone how to cook them—read on. It's time to meet the kernel.

Here are 11 whole grains found at nearly all health food stores, along with suggested uses and cooking directions.

Amaranth. This is a tiny grain that looks like sand and tastes like a pungent cross between oatmeal and toasted sesame seeds. It contains very little gluten, an elastic substance found in wheat and some other grains, so it's a great alternative for those who are wheat-sensitive. If you're allergic to ragweed, stay clear of amaranth, however, since it's in the same family.

When cooked, amaranth softens relatively quickly but retains a slight grit. In fact, you can prepare it like grits or oatmeal. Try adding a cup to vegetable or bean soup. Or season it with garlic, ginger, onions, and other assertive flavors.

Use amaranth flour in place of wheat flour to coat eggplant Parmesan. Along with calcium, amaranth supplies protein, riboflavin, vitamin B_6, folate, pantothenic acid, copper, magnesium, phosphorus, potassium, and zinc.

Cooking basics: Simmer 1 cup of amaranth in 3 cups of water, broth, or other cooking liquid for 25 to 30 minutes.

Yield: 2½ cups, or five servings

Barley. This tastes like oatmeal, only chewier and more flavorful. Most grocery stores carry pearled barley, a refined grain. You want the whole grain *hulled* barley found in most health food stores and upscale supermarkets.

Add a cup to soup at the same time you pour in the broth. Mix with rice in pilafs. Simmer with milk, cinnamon, and raisins and serve as a high-protein oatmeal alternative.

Cooking basics: Simmer 1 cup of barley in 3 cups of liquid for 90 minutes.

Like tofu, millet picks up the flavor of whatever it is cooked with.

Yield: 4 cups, or eight servings

Buckwheat. Although buckwheat is not a true grain, it's packed with nutrients like iron, magnesium, potassium, and zinc. Untoasted buckwheat has a delicate flavor and makes a great alternative to white rice. Toasted buckwheat, called kasha, has a stronger taste. Add the kernels to soups, or mix buckwheat flour into bread dough or pancake batter for a nutty-flavored fiber boost.

Cooking basics: Simmer 1 cup of buckwheat in 2 cups of liquid for 15 minutes.

Yield: 2 cups, or four servings

Bulgur. Bulgur is uncooked wheat that has been steamed, dried, and crushed. This nutty grain comes in three varieties: coarse, used in pilafs and stuffings; medium, used in cold salads, like tabbouleh; and fine, typically used in bread and some desserts. To extend bulgur's shelf life and to keep bugs at bay, keep it refrigerated.

Cooking basics: Pour 2 cups of boiling water over 1 cup of bulgur. Let it soak for 30 minutes. For fluffier grain with a slight crunch, soak bulgur in cold water for 2 to 3 hours before cooking.

Yield: 3 cups, or six servings

Irish oatmeal. The quicker the oatmeal cooks, the more refined it is. For the true whole grain oat, try Irish oatmeal, also known as Scotch oats or steel-cut oats. You can also use it to stretch bread crumbs and add extra flavor to meat loaf and stuffings.

Cooking basics: Add 1 cup of Irish oatmeal to 3½ cups of boiling water. Simmer for 20 minutes, then let stand covered for 5 minutes.

Yield: 2 cups, or four servings

Millet. This is a very smooth, slightly sweet and crunchy food. It makes a great hot cereal that's not as thick as oatmeal or as loose as rice. Like tofu, millet picks up the flavor of whatever it is cooked with.

If you bake, add millet flour to bread or muffins to add protein, fiber, thiamin, riboflavin, niacin, vitamin B_6, folate, copper, magnesium, phosphorus, and zinc. Or pick up a loaf of millet bread for your next turkey sandwich.

Cooking basics: Simmer 1 cup of millet in 3 cups of water for about 25 minutes.

Yield: 4½ cups, or nine servings

Quinoa. It's not a true grain but rather a fruit, so it's low in gluten, making it another tasty wheat substitute for people who are gluten-sensitive. Quinoa (pronounced KEEN-wa) cooks up like rice but in half the time.

It contains fiber, thiamin, riboflavin, niacin, vitamin B_6, folate, pantothenic acid, vitamin E, and many vital minerals.

You can use it in soups, stews, and salads; mix it with beans; or top it with a stir-fry or peanut sauce for an Asian spin. You may be able to find preseasoned quinoa mixes. They cost about as much as boxed rice or couscous mix.

Cooking basics: Simmer 1 cup of quinoa with 2 cups of water for about 15 minutes.

Yield: 3½ cups, or seven servings

Spelt. This grain can be put to work in all sorts of dishes. You may find that spelt flakes at breakfast taste like Wheaties. Mix ½ cup of the flakes with ½ cup of granola, and you'll get just enough fat and fiber to fill you up without weighing you down.

Or, if you want to convert to whole grain pastas, try starting with spelt spaghetti. It's not as soft as white pasta or as chewy as whole wheat pasta. Spelt bread also tastes great with turkey or tuna.

Cooking basics: Simmer 1 cup of spelt kernels with 3 cups of water for about 2 hours.

Yield: 2¼ cups, or five servings

Triticale. This combination of wheat and rye is the world's first hybrid grain. Use triticale (pronounced trit-ih-KAY-lee) flour or kernels in dough for sweeter bread.

Cooking basics: Simmer 1 cup of triticale with 2 cups of water for about 15 minutes.

Yield: 3½ cups, or seven servings

Wheat berries. When these berries are ground up, the result is called whole wheat flour—the flavor behind many breads, granola, and pasta. You can top wheat berries with a marinara sauce or add them to soups, pilafs, or cold salads.

Cooking basics: Soak berries in water overnight, then drain. Simmer 1 cup of wheat berries in 3 cups of water for approximately an hour, or until tender and sticky. If you skip the presoak, the berries can take as long as 2 hours to cook.

Yield: 3 cups, or six servings

Whole wheat couscous. You might be surprised to learn that regular couscous is a refined grain product. To get the whole grain payoff, use whole wheat couscous. Like any other pasta, whole wheat couscous has a stronger flavor and chewier texture than its white-flour cousin. Use it the same way you would regular couscous.

Cooking basics: Add 2 cups of boiling water to 1 cup of couscous.

Yield: 2 cups, or four servings

Hair That Shines

WHEN KAREN KLUESNER OF NEW VIENNA, IOWA, LOST 25 POUNDS, SHE WASN'T ALONE IN HER JOURNEY. NOT ONLY DID HER SISTERS AND NEIGHBORS DIET WITH HER, LOSING A COMBINED 3,560 POUNDS IN A PROGRAM SPONSORED BY NEARBY TOTAL FITNESS RECREATION CENTER AND MERCY HEALTH CENTER, BUT WHEN SHE EMERGED FROM A LOCAL SALON WITH A NEW HAIR STYLE TO MATCH HER SLIMMER FIGURE, THEY CHEERED.

Kluesner is making the most of her new look, and she's feeling great about herself.

"People tell me I look younger now," she says, and her hairdresser agrees. Verla Tegeler, co-owner of the Head Shed in nearby Dyersville, gave Kluesner a cut that complements her neckline. "When you lose weight, you feel more confident about wearing different clothes, so you also feel more confident about changing your hairstyle," she says.

Even if you don't have a whole town cheering you on as you lose your extra pounds, you can still feel as fabulous as Kluesner after a trip to the hairdresser.

Getting the right hairstyle can do more than give you a youthful, attractive reflection in the mirror—it can be a way to express yourself, too. Let your hairstyle help your slimmer physique send the message that you feel more confident, daring, and younger.

Sending the Right Message

"Everything about our bodies, including our hair, is like this neon sign saying, 'Here is who I am,'" says Marietta Baba, Ph.D., professor and chairperson of the anthropology department at Wayne State University in Detroit. Without your hair, you'd be missing a valuable way to express your identity, she says.

So how do you send the world the right message? First, get to know your hair. You have about 100,000 strands of it on your head. Each strand is a protein made of microscopic fibers coiled together, growing out of a hair follicle that's buried beneath the skin.

Though we all have different hair textures, they fall into the categories of fine, medium, and coarse, says Kenneth Battelle, owner and master stylist of Kenneth's Salon in New York City. Each type has its own handling characteristics, he says: Fine hair is soft and tends to get oily; medium hair tends to have a shine and is easy to style; and coarse hair has a lot of body, which can be hard to manage. As a result, the texture of your hair helps determine how you can wear it, Battelle says.

Nick Berardi agrees. As senior creative director at Vidal Sassoon in New York City, he says that the first thing he looks at before styling a head of hair is its texture.

"It's like if you're building a house, you need to know what kind of wood you're going to use," he says. Once you know what kind of look your hair texture will allow, focus on finding a style that accentuates your slimmer figure and youthful attitude.

Fine hair becomes too weak if it's layered, so Berardi suggests giving it a heavier shape, with a bob or a really short cut that's only a couple of inches long.

Or try a chin-length blunt cut, in which the hair is cut straight across as if you put a ruler to the ends, Battelle says.

Since medium hair is easy to style, women with this type can wear it long or short in their choice of styles. "You can do anything with it," Berardi says. Layer it, cut it one length, curl it, straighten it. Take your pick, and it should look good.

Coarse hair, on the other hand, often requires a lot of work. You can tame it by having it layered with the ends tapered, and do your part in the shower to soften it with conditioner every time you shampoo, Battelle suggests.

An Investment Worth Keeping

When you invest in a new hairstyle, be sure to maintain it with regular haircuts and, if needed, color touch-ups.

We've all stretched the time between haircuts to its limits, racing to the salon when our hair becomes unmanageable. When people wait too long to get a cut or color touch-up, however, they tend to look older, says Richard Cordoba of Sam Wong Hair Salon. If you have short hair, he suggests going in for a cut every 4 to 6 weeks. If your hair is long, you can have it done every 8 to 10 weeks. When one of his clients comes in with a grown-out cut, she usually leaves looking years younger.

Keeping a fresh look that complements your hair texture, face shape, and body shape will help you maintain a well-kept and youthful appearance every day.

If you don't want to spend a lot of time styling it in the morning, get it cut very short. But if you prefer a longer hairstyle, let it hang past your chin. A chin-length cut will get very wide and round, Berardi says, so wear it longer and let its own weight drag it down a bit.

A Hairstyle That Complements Your Body

So what happens when your hair looks great in the bathroom mirror, but when you back up and look at your hair *and* your body, they just don't match?

"I think the reason people get the wrong haircut is because stylists sit them down, cover up their bodies, and try to fix some sort of problem with the face," says Laurie Krauz, an image consultant in New York City. She suggests that you look at the whole picture instead.

Stand tall. Your height should play a role in how you wear your hair. If you're short, don't wear your hair very long. You'll only look shorter if your hair covers up your neck and body, Berardi says.

Trust your lines. Let your hairstyle complement the shape of your body. Check a full-length mirror to gauge your body's lines, Krauz says. When you look at yourself head-on, is the line that starts from under your shoulder and extends to your hip straight or curvy? Are your arms and legs angular or soft? If you have a straight body, get an angular, blunt cut. If your body is curvy, let your hair look soft and flowing.

Give your hair a little height. A little height and width can make all the difference when you're trying to balance out a not-so-small body. "If you wear your hair flat or straight around your face, you'll look heavier," Battelle says.

Watch out for super-short haircuts, too. "The shorter it is, the heavier you look," he adds.

Wear It Well

While hair texture and body shape are important when choosing a new style, don't forget to consider the shape of your face, too. When you create a balance between your face, body, and hair, you let people know that you're in charge and in style. Take some advice from the experts on how to achieve the look you want.

Take a measure. The key to looking great is proportion, according to Catherine Schuller, a fashion retail editor of *Mode* magazine and author of the *Ultimate Plus-Size Modeling Guide.* While hair with a little height is important for balancing out a fuller-figured body, make sure that you add height in proportion to your face and overall size. Don't get the height you need by teasing, either. Instead, add texture and volume with layers for a softer, easier lift at the crown.

"Simple is best," Schuller says. "It's much more modern and clean looking to allow the cut to determine the way the hair falls rather than teasing and spraying the hair into place."

While standing in half-profile to your mirror, measure the distance from the bottom of your chin to the top of your ear. Then measure the distance from the top of your ear to the top of your hair. Both measurements should be the same. If your hair is higher, take it down to match the distance from chin to ear.

Notice the shape of things. By breaking your look down into shapes, you can create balance. "I'm like an artist playing with shapes and trying to make sense out of them," says Richard Cordoba, a hair-care specialist at Sam Wong Hair Salon in New York City. "When you put them together, some things are going to feel as though they have more balance."

An oval face is the easiest to work with because most shapes look good on it, Cordoba says. But keep in mind that long, straight hair will make an

Living Proof
PANEL

A Hairstyle That Pleases

Molly Brown

After one bad haircut, I needed years to ease myself away from a one-length style. In college, a body wave and a short haircut made me look matronly, exactly when I wanted to look the opposite.

"Why did you cut your hair?" my new boyfriend asked . . . before canceling our next date.

That was the end of our relationship and the beginning of my obsession with a safe hairstyle: a one-length cut that fell a few inches past my shoulders, with wispy bangs. I wore it for the next 18 years.

As I approached 40, I wanted a shorter, more sophisticated style without looking older. My solution was a trim that left my hair a little above my shoulders, with blonde highlights to brighten my face. As I began losing weight, I wanted an even fresher look, so I layered it.

Because I'm tall with an oval face, the layers at my jawline keep my face from looking too long, and the soft style of the cut complements the curves of my body.

This time my new style drew applause from the man in my life. My husband loves it.

oval face look too long. To complement this shape, get your hair cut in layers, especially around your face.

But if your jaw is wide, put a round shape on your style. Don't put a bob line at the jaw because it will accentuate your jaw's square shape, Berardi says.

Instead, add bangs and layers that start at the cheekbone and go down to give your face a round frame that will offset your jaw, Cordoba says.

And if your face is round, complement it with a longer, layered cut. Keep your hair one length in the back and put layers around your face that start either at your cheekbone or jawline and go down. Remember that long hair makes your face look longer and rounder cuts make your face look rounder.

A Hairstyle to Dye For?

Now that you have a style that matches the rest of you, what action do you take on those hairs that have decided to turn gray? Maybe it's just a few hairs here and there that have made the change, or maybe each and every one has paled. How do you decide whether to color or not? Easy. Go with what makes you comfortable, Cordoba says.

"If people feel good about their gray hair, I encourage them to go that way," he says.

If you decide to keep your hair gray, use shampoos that are specially made for it. Cigarette smoke and the elements can give gray hair a yellowish tint. Use a color-maintenance shampoo with a blue-violet base to get rid of the yellow, Cordoba says. It will whiten the hair and make it shiny.

If you're not comfortable having gray hair, then coloring it may be the way to go. But coloring your hair doesn't necessarily mean that you'll look younger or better than wearing your hair gray. Try these tricks to ensure that your color is doing its job.

Regress. The best way to look younger is to choose a shade that is a little lighter than what you had when you were a child, according to Brad Johns, artistic director of the Avon Centre in New York City. "The lighter you go, as long as you don't get to white, the more youthful the appearance." If you were dark brown as a kid, choose medium brown. If you were light brown, choose dark blonde. And if you were blonde, stay blonde.

"The darker the color, the older you will look," he adds.

Go multicolor. Get your hair fully colored and then put highlights near your face. Stick with lighter and warmer colors for a youthful look. A dark frame around your face will only make you look older because the dark hair throws shadows that define lines.

Though it depends on how fast your hair grows, once you start covering your gray, expect to recolor the roots every 4 to 6 weeks, says Johns.

Keeping Your Hair Healthy

Now your look is set. Your new style flatters your new figure as well as your personality. So how do you avoid damage and keep it looking good?

"We're lucky because our hair is very strong," Battelle says. "You have to go a long way to really hurt it, yet people damage their hair every day."

Find the right shampoo. Choose your shampoo according to your hair type and then use it daily. Fine hair benefits from a clarifying shampoo, which is clear when you pour it into your hand. Coarse hair needs a hydrating shampoo, which is creamy. If you can't tell if it's creamy or clear, check the ingredients, Cordoba says. Citrus and eucalyptus are good for fine hair because they're uplifting and cleansing, while emollient oils help moisturize coarse hair.

Rinse with apple cider vinegar. No matter what type of hair you have, rinsing with apple cider vinegar after shampooing is a natural way to keep your hair shiny and healthy, according to Shatoiya de la Tour, an herbalist and owner and director of education at Dry Creek Herb Farm and Learning Center in Auburn, California.

Mix 1 tablespoon of apple cider vinegar into 1 quart of cool water and take it into the shower. After you shampoo and rinse, pour it over your head, taking care not to get it in your eyes, and let it absorb into your skin. You don't need to rinse again. The vinegar will make your hair shiny and balance out the pH level of your scalp, helping to avoid dandruff. Use it as often as you like.

Don't overlap color. If you get your hair color touched up, make sure that the stylist is adding new color only to the roots. Putting new chemicals on hair that is already treated will damage it, Battelle says.

Avoid overstyling. You already know that too much blow-drying, straightening, and curling will damage hair, but how do you know when your morning routine is too much? Time it. If it's taking you longer than 20 minutes to style your hair in the morning, you're probably overdoing it, says Berardi.

"The more you fight the natural texture of your hair, the more you're going to damage your hair," he adds. If you need a long time to style in the morning, your style probably doesn't agree with your hair texture.

Week Five

Feeling Free to Have Fun

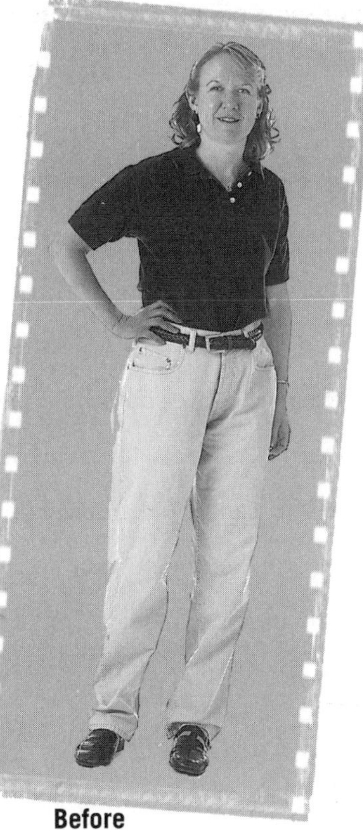

Before

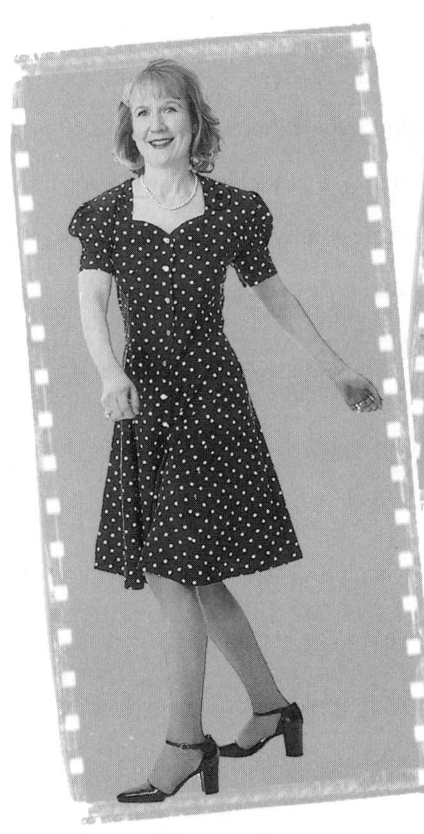

After

I'VE ALWAYS THOUGHT THAT IN ORDER TO GROW, YOU HAVE TO STEP OUT OF YOUR COMFORT ZONE.

—*Molly Brown*

Week Five

For some people, the easiest way to approach a weight-loss program is to have a schedule, to exercise at the same time and place every day, and to eat the same food week after week. If they're not careful, however, this rigid approach can turn into a rut. You've been on the program for 5 weeks, and if you find that boredom is creeping in, deal with it now; otherwise, it could sabotage your weight-loss efforts.

So maybe it's time to add some adventure. Read the suggestions within these pages and give yourself permission to try different activities and foods. You'll learn about the latest workout trends that have staying power and resources that can help you select new fitness activities. And this week's quiz will help you determine your personality type—and choose clothes, a hairstyle, and makeup to complement you. The key is to create your own individual style.

An Adventurous Attitude: The Key to Lasting Weight Loss

YOU HAVE EMBARKED ON A GREAT ADVENTURE.

THAT'S RIGHT, YOUR PATH TO WEIGHT LOSS SHOULD BE FILLED WITH FUN, EXCITEMENT, AND NEW EXPERIENCES.

Not exactly what you expected to hear, is it? Typical weight-loss efforts usually entail complete uniformity. Eat the same foods the same way every day for months. Exercise the same way in the same place at the same time.

That rigid approach, which is often sold as the path to weight loss, actually leads straight to apathy. "Everything can get pretty boring if everything I eat, every activity I do is the same," says Dana G. Cable, Ph.D., professor of psychology at Hood College in Frederick, Maryland. And once you get bored, you want to stop. That's the reason that so many well-intentioned weight-loss efforts fail.

After years of being told that trying to lose weight requires deprivation, limitations, and forced requirements, now you're discovering the truth. The key to lasting weight loss is the exact opposite: The best way to shed pounds

Living Proof
PANEL

Swinging Into Adventure

Molly Brown

When we were younger, my husband and I would go out dancing a lot. Nothing really fancy, but we had fun. In college, we did a 24-hour dance marathon together, and I had done one in high school. Over a 4- to 5-year period, we counted that we went to 33 weddings. Think of all the dancing you do at weddings, and you know we were dancing a lot!

As time went on, we didn't dance as much. But awhile back, our friends started to talk about taking swing dance lessons. We thought it would be a lot of fun, and that a bunch of us could go out to dinner on Friday nights and then go dancing afterward. But when the time came to sign up, our friends backed out. I've always thought that in order to grow, you have to step out of your comfort zone. So even though they weren't going to take lessons, I signed my husband and me up anyway.

I've really enjoyed it, and it's great that I get to spend quality time with my husband. It's been quite an adventure, learning the steps and dancing with everyone in class. We've been taught the East Coast swing, which involves a lot of turning and twisting. Although we don't work up a sweat, it keeps us moving. I can't wait to try out our new moves at the next wedding we're invited to!

is by experimenting with new foods, trying new activities, and seeking different ways of accomplishing your goals, says Dr. Cable.

You need an adventurous attitude.

Developing a sense of adventure in all areas of your life—not just with your weight-loss efforts—will turn back the clock as well.

"As long as you know that there are new things on the horizon, you will still feel young. That is true whether you are 30 or 90. The people who age the most successfully are those with adventurous attitudes. They are the ones who see themselves as having a lot of things to do in life," says Dr. Cable.

Regaining Your Sense of Adventure

As a child, you had an innate sense of adventure. You wanted to try new things, see new places, explore. But as you got older and responsibilities mounted, you took refuge in the familiar. As safe as that may feel, doing the same thing without being open to new experiences only deadens your youth and vigor.

"If we are not open-minded and not willing to try new things, we find ourselves very unhappy. If we keep doing it the way we have done it before, pretty soon we lose that zest for living," Dr. Cable says.

Being an adventurous person doesn't mean that you have to climb Mount Everest, travel through the jungles of the Amazon, or bungee-jump off a bridge. "It is an adventure as long as it is something out of the ordinary. It can be as simple as walking into a new restaurant and trying a different food," he adds.

Many people fear adventure because they think it means they have to permanently change. Not so, Dr. Cable says. "You can always go back to what you were doing before. You can say, 'I am just trying this.'"

By making simple, small changes, you can add adventure to your daily life. Here's how to find the everyday adventurer in you—and some suggestions on how to become an explorer of new experiences.

Take it slow. While you should actively look for new experiences, don't try to do it all in one day. "Start out slowly, doing the little things. If you change too quickly, you won't like it and then won't try it again," Dr. Cable says. Find something small in your routine to change. Once you've become accustomed to that, experiment with something else.

Seek one small adventure every day. Each day provides an opportunity for adventure. "You can look at almost any part of your life and see some ways you can make changes," he says. Pick one aspect of your day—what you have for breakfast, for example, or what restaurant you eat at or how you dress—and change it.

Change your direction. Just altering your normal traveling patterns can become an adventure, Dr. Cable says. Try a new route to work, to the supermarket, to school. Walk a different place each night. If you usually follow a certain pattern when walking around in a mall, reverse direction.

Expand your reading and viewing horizons. Thanks to the pleasure of books, magazines, television, and the Internet, you can go on a new adventure every day. Read, watch, and learn about different cultures, different ideas, and different people. Also, be sure to read and watch genres other than the ones you normally enjoy. That alone will expand your world, he says.

Stop procrastinating. Dr. Cable works with a lot of people near the end of their lives, many of whom have regrets. "You hear a lot of, 'One of these days . . .' We keep putting it off until it is too late," he says.

Take stock of the one thing you have always wanted to do—and do it *now*. Whether it's going back to school or learning to ski, start working on your adventurous goals today.

Try Something New

IF THERE'S ONE GOLDEN RULE OF EXERCISE, IT'S THIS: IF YOU'RE NOT EXCITED ABOUT IT, YOU WON'T DO IT.

Fifty percent of new exercisers who begin fitness programs drop out by the end of the first 6 months. And boredom is a big reason why. During those first couple of weeks, your routine feels fresh and new. By the 3rd or 4th month, it can feel dull and repetitive. By the 5th or 6th month, you're beating yourself up for lacking motivation when what you're really lacking is fun.

"I train NFL linemen, and even these guys who love to work out can get into a rut with the same routine," says John Yetter, M.D., medical director at SSM Rehab Sports Medicine in St. Louis. "It's important to incorporate an aspect of play into your routine, to shake things up a little, to try new things, and most of all, to have fun."

It all comes down to keeping your brain as excited about exercise as your body, says running coach Michael Gilewski, Ph.D., a clinical psychologist for post-acute care services at Cedars-Sinai Medical Center in Los Angeles.

"Your brain thrives on new experiences. Trying new activities puts you back in a childlike state where you're experiencing life through your body again and your brain is busily working to build new pathways to help you master this new activity," Dr. Gilewski says.

That's the key to keeping boredom at bay: keeping your brain stimulated.

It doesn't have to be as drastic as switching from fitness walking to sea kayaking, though that would certainly do the trick. Breaking out of a rut can be as simple as using medicine balls instead of dumbbells for your weight training or just finding a different exercise tape. As long as it's something new to you.

In Search of Stimulation

Eager to try something new but at a loss for what that something might be? It's understandable. There are so many options in the world of fitness, you can get analysis paralysis trying to decide what would be right for you, especially if you're new to exercise. Thankfully, there are plenty of resources that can help.

Introductory classes. Trying a new fitness class used to be trial by fire. You walked into a roomful of people who already knew what they were doing, and you desperately tried to follow along. No more. Now most gyms offer introductory classes for curious newbies.

You can get formal instruction in the activity, learn the rudimentary moves, get comfortable with the class, and decide if you like it before moving into the real thing.

"These classes are the ideal way to get your feet wet and experiment with new activities," says exercise physiologist and certified personal trainer Ann Marie Miller, fitness director of the New York Sports Clubs in Manhattan. "They're a safe, instructional environment where you're surrounded by people who are learning, just like you." Check with your local gym for a class schedule.

Specialty magazines. If there's an activity you can try, there's a magazine to tell you all about it. From bicycling to yoga, you can read up on what the activity is about, why people like it, what kind of equipment or clothing you need, and where you can do it.

Though many of these magazines cater to folks already deep into the sport, they are great ways to get the flavor of an activity. They also provide motivation and training tips as well as directories of upcoming events and competitions, says Miller.

Next time you're browsing at your local bookstore or newsstand, take a walk down the sports and outdoor activity magazine aisles. It could open up a whole new world, says Dr. Gilewski.

Sporting goods stores. Reluctant to try a new "gear-based" activity like hiking because you don't want to lay down the cash for something you may not enjoy? Rent the gear instead. Many sporting goods stores, such as Eastern

Mountain Sports (EMS) and Recreational Equipment Incorporated (REI), rent sporting equipment of all kinds to get people started in a new activity. As a bonus, they also run free clinics, so you can learn what you need to know from an expert before you try it out, says Dr. Gilewski.

Multisport vacations. Thanks to a booming interest in outdoor recreation like kayaking and horseback riding, there are now travel companies solely dedicated to giving you a taste of a wide variety of activities all in one vacation. You can try hiking, mountain biking, horseback riding, sea kayaking, snowshoeing, cross-country skiing, rafting, and even dogsledding on these trips.

A personal trainer can help you match your likes and dislikes to fitness activities.

They provide all the equipment and instruction. You provide the willingness to have a good time. There's zero pressure to do anything you don't like. And there are guides to accommodate people of all skill levels.

Planning a multisport vacation also can provide motivation for your workouts and keep your training focused in preparation for your upcoming adventure. Several reputable companies to investigate are Adventures Plus, The World Outside, Backroads, and GORPtravel. Look them up on the Internet and see the world of fun you can have on your next trip, says Miller.

Personal trainers. Personal trainers can do more than show you how to do a biceps curl correctly. They're fabulous resources for matching your exercise likes and dislikes to fitness activities.

"Trainers are a wealth of information about all the different ways you can work out," says certified personal trainer Jana Angelakis, founder of PEx Personalized Exercise in New York City. "Just sign up for a few consultations with a trainer. Tell her what you like to do or think you might like to do, and she can find places for you to try those things in a safe, fun environment. She may even be able to connect you with other people interested in those activities, so you can try them out together."

Aiming to Please

If you think you get bored using the same equipment, watching the same videos, and taking the same exercise classes over and over again, imagine how the fitness professionals who are in the gym instructing, teaching, and

Living Proof
PANEL

A New Way to Shape Up

Molly Brown

For 18 years, my husband had tried to persuade me to do strength training. "It'll cure anything that ails you," he used to tell me. But I was resistant to trying it because the only strength training I'd seen was the heavy-duty kind that guys used to put muscles on their arms. I also thought it would take a long time to see results, so I never bothered.

Then a personal trainer introduced me to a whole new way to strength train. Instead of doing boring, repetitive motions with barbells and dumbbells, I started doing full-body motions with weighted medicine balls.

I love the exercises. They are simple, yet very effective. I've had great results in toning up all my muscles, and it happened much faster than I would have ever believed.

Sometimes, it's just a matter of trying something new.

working out with the same equipment and in the same classes feel. That's why they're always so eager to bring in new equipment and promote new classes. The result has been an explosion of fitness possibilities that literally offers something for everyone.

"The fitness marketers have been ingenious the past few years," says Dr. Yetter. "They're learning how to combine all the fun parts of sports and activities and turn them into a great workout. Equipment has improved, too, with more options to suit everyone's needs."

Here are a few trends that are here to stay. Try some on for size.

Martial arts aerobics. Classes that combine martial arts moves to an aerobics beat are wildly popular. Tae-Bo, cardio kickboxing, and other boxing and kicking aerobics classes are fun and less "dancy" than traditional aerobics classes. Plus, they're a great workout. Try them out at your local gym, or buy some videotapes to work out at home, says Miller.

Personal trainers. Paying a pro to teach you the ropes and provide inspiration is not just for the Hollywood set anymore. Personal trainers have become affordable to everyone. Many also now offer group training for up to eight people to diffuse the costs while still maintaining an intimate, hands-on training atmosphere. Ask at your local gym if they offer sessions with credentialed personal trainers. It's a great way to get started and to learn new activities, says Angelakis.

Cardio-strengthening classes. New body-shaping aerobics classes offer all the benefits of aerobic exercise and resistance training rolled into one class, as you do aerobic and strength-training exercises set to music.

"Women really love these classes because they're social, and they allow you to do your strength training without sitting in the weight room by yourself," says Michael Bourque, certified personal trainer and personal training coordinator for the Center for Health and Wellness of the Central Florida YMCA in Oviedo.

Group equipment classes. First there was Spinning, the group exercise class set on stationary bikes. Then there was Trekking, a group treadmill workout. Now there's even a group class for the stairclimbing machines. If you can't take the monotony of spending 45 minutes on one of these machines by yourself, these classes could be just what you need. They'll also give you great ideas for how to breathe more life into your solo workouts, says Angelakis.

Mind/body workouts. Yoga and tai chi have become mainstream. These classes focus on activating your mind as well as your muscles and promoting a greater sense of wellness. Sign up for a few and find out for yourself, says Angelakis.

Low-impact machines. "One of the most popular pieces of fitness equipment in recent years has been the elliptical trainer," says exercise physiologist Robert Brosmer, vice president of health and wellness at the Central Florida YMCA in Orlando and coauthor of *Health and High Performance.*

These machines, which are a cross between a treadmill and a stair-climbing machine, offer the benefits of running on a treadmill without the jarring impact. They also incline and decline to simulate hiking or cross-country skiing. And they burn tons of calories (500 to 600 per hour). You can even buy personal-use models for your home.

GOAL

Learn to Lean on Protein

TO LOSE WEIGHT AND PRESERVE YOUR HEART HEALTH, YOU MAY THINK THAT YOU HAVE TO GIVE BEEF THE BOOT AND MAKE *365 WAYS TO COOK CHICKEN* YOUR NEW KITCHEN COMPANION. BUT THAT'S NOT TRUE.

There are more than 250 different sources of lean protein. And those are just the whole foods, like chicken and soybeans. Add in some of their products, like veggie burgers, tempeh, and tofu, and you could prepare a different type of lean protein for a year and never eat exactly the same thing twice.

You don't even have to exclude beef: Studies show that lean cuts of red meat can be as low in fat and as heart-healthy as chicken.

Why do you need protein? This body-friendly nutrient is vital for healing wounds, building strong bones and muscles, and replenishing energy. Choosing lean sources not only cuts down on fat but also helps you feel full on fewer calories.

GET THIN

When you choose lean protein, such as low-fat yogurt or grilled rainbow trout, over its more corpulent cousins (whole-milk yogurt or deep-fried fish sticks), you can lose up to half the fat without shrinking your portion size. That means fewer calories per bite.

It gets better. Make protein part of your breakfast, and it not only will help prevent overeating at that meal but also may make you less hungry at lunch, says Barbara Rolls, Ph.D., professor of nutrition at Pennsylvania State University in University Park and author of *Volumetrics.* That's because protein, like fiber, is a satiety trigger, helping you say no to seconds. And because it is digested somewhat more slowly than simple carbohydrates, you feel full longer.

Combining protein with carbohydrates at every meal may also cut down on your cravings for sweets, says Franca Alphin, R.D., a registered dietitian and administrative director of the Duke University Diet and Fitness Center in Durham, North Carolina.

Protein may help diminish that dramatic jump in blood sugar that occurs when you eat simple carbohydrates, such as doughnuts and a cup of coffee with sugar. These sudden jumps in blood sugar are quickly followed by crashes that leave you low in pep and craving more sweets to boost your energy.

Get Young

There is evidence that eating protein-rich foods may help keep you mentally sharp, especially during periods of the day or evening when you must mentally exert yourself. It doesn't take much. For most people, 5 to 6 ounces (two to three servings) of high-protein foods a day is all you need to maintain your brainpower, says Judith Wurtman, Ph.D., a research scientist at the Massachusetts Institute of Technology in Cambridge.

You also need protein to maintain your basic health. Without daily deliveries of this essential nutrient, wounds wouldn't heal, bones would break, and you would have a tough time defending yourself against typically harmless viruses such as the flu, says Robert Wildman, R.D., Ph.D., assistant professor of nutrition at the University of Louisiana at Lafayette. There's nothing like frail bones and an unshakable fever to make you feel like you're 90. Fortunately, you can easily avoid these problems by getting two to three servings of protein a day—for instance, a peanut butter sandwich and a cup of milk.

And as a bonus, protein may help you find your smile. A study in France found that people feel happier after a meal with protein than they do after one without.

Go for the Goal

Shoot for two to three servings of lean high-protein foods a day, with at least one serving coming from plants. Of course, that doesn't mean that you can't have a little extra protein some days, only that at the end of the week it should average out to no more than three servings a day.

So, if you have a 12-ounce sirloin (four servings of protein) one night, compensate the next day by eating a low-protein lunch, like spaghetti with meatless marinara or a pita stuffed with vegetables, lightly sprinkled with cheese, says Alphin.

Where do you find protein? Beef and chicken are obvious sources. You'll also find it in dairy products, fish, beans, and whole grains. Here are some ways to add physique-friendly, protein-rich foods to your menu.

Beans and Lentils

There are at least 25 types of beans and lentils available in the United States. All provide significant amounts of protein, with soy leading the pack. Unlike most plants, soy is well-stocked with amino acids (the building blocks of protein)—meaning its protein is complete and as high-quality as beef.

Stir-fry soy. When it comes to great sources of protein, tofu and tempeh (both made from soy) are right up there with sirloin steak and chicken breast. Tempeh is the top of the crop, however. Made by fermenting ground soybeans, it's higher in protein and easier to digest than regular soybeans and other soy products. Chunky, and with a nutty flavor, tempeh can be grilled or stir-fried like tofu. It should always be cooked before eating, says Greg Hottinger, R.D., a specialist in whole foods and a registered dietitian with the Duke University Diet and Fitness Center.

One thing you should know: Like blue cheese, tempeh contains some active cultures, so don't be alarmed when you open a package of this low-fat meat alternative and see splotches of blue staring back at you. It's supposed to look like that.

Add a can of beans. Although the protein in lentils, kidney beans, and other legumes is not "complete," they still are all good sources of protein. Back in the 1970s, vegetarians were told to combine plant proteins at every meal to ensure that they consumed all the essential amino acids. Now nutritionists know that if vegetarians eat a variety of foods (beans, rice, whole grains) over the course of a day, they'll get all the amino acids their bodies need to assemble complete, high-quality protein, says Hottinger. So heat up a can of black beans as a side dish or add white beans, chickpeas, or red beans to soups, chili, pilafs, rice dishes, stir-fries, or salads.

Find the hidden beans. Dining out? Scanning the menu, you may not realize that these items have beans: hummus (bean dip), hoppin' John (warm bean side dish), veggie burgers (frequently made of soybeans), cassoulet (bean and meat casserole), and pasta e fagioli (pasta and bean soup). Except for the veggie burgers, all of these foods are high in fat, so be careful how much you dish out. One-quarter cup of hummus (3 to 4 slightly mounded soup spoons), ½ cup of hoppin' John, and 1½ cups of cassoulet or pasta e fagioli count as one serving, says Alphin.

Whole Grains

There are nearly 20 different kinds of whole grains and rice. Grocery stores typically have 4 of them: whole wheat, corn, oatmeal, and brown rice. For more variety and a little culinary adventure, take a trip to your local health food store. (For more information on whole grains, see Go With the Grain on page 227.)

Some whole grains are good sources of protein. Here are some suggestions on how to prepare the three highest in protein, says Hottinger.

Say *sayonara* to white rice. Like soybeans, quinoa (pronounced KEEN-wa) is a complete protein. One of the most nutritious grains, it is also one of the fastest cooking—ready in 20 minutes. With more than five times as much protein as in white rice, quinoa makes a delicious bed for stir-fries.

Try a taste of amaranth. Add amaranth to soup when you add the broth. Or cook it and mix with vegetables and curry for a taste of India.

Go nuts with millet. This staple tastes great topped with a spicy peanut sauce and vegetables.

Dairy Products and Eggs

As a food group that is known for its high calcium content and is independent of the meat, fish, and grain groups, it's easy to forget that dairy products, as well as eggs, also provide some protein.

Go for the cup. Fill up fast on the low-calorie, high-energy combo: protein and carbohydrates. Grab a cup of low-fat yogurt (protein) along with your 2- to 3-ounce morning bagel (carbohydrate), says Alphin.

Get milk. Milk and milk-based drinks, such as fat-free milk, breakfast smoothies, or low-fat milkshakes, help people feel full and eat less at the next meal, says Dr. Rolls.

What's more, 3 cups of low-fat or fat-free milk supply a day's worth of protein and calcium. So pour a cup over cereal. Wash down your afternoon snack with a glass. Or, for an energy boost, mix a cup with your favorite fruit about an hour before working out.

Say cheese. To add protein to a salad, sprinkle on ¼ cup of shredded part-skim mozzarella cheese. Or to curb midafternoon snack attacks, toss six dice-size cubes of Monterey Jack cheese in a plastic sandwich bag, along with a handful of baby carrots. Serving for serving, cheese contains 60 percent less protein than beef, making it a great option for balancing out your protein the day after a big meat meal, says Alphin.

Fish may be the best satiety trigger for meat lovers.

Refuel with eggs. To gain some control over low blood sugar and hunger, reenergize at midmorning with a hard-boiled egg. Toss the yolk, and all the fat goes with it, Alphin suggests.

Double up on the whites. For a quick, medium-fat, high-protein dinner, scramble two egg whites in 1 to 2 teaspoons of olive oil. Top with tomato and a thin slice of Colby cheese and slide it between two slices of whole grain bread. Bonus: This meal provides one serving of healthful fat (olive oil), says Alphin.

Seafood

There are more than 125 kinds of fish and shellfish sold in markets. Though most are seasonal, you'll always find a variety to choose from year-round.

Fill up on fish. Fish may be the best satiety trigger for meat lovers. In one Australian study, the protein in fish consistently made participants feel fuller than when they ate beef or chicken. While some fish are high in fat (halibut, mackerel, and salmon), all are safe bets as long as you limit your portions to one to two servings (about the size of one to two decks of cards), says Dr. Rolls. Bonus: Cold-water fish such as salmon are highest in heart-friendly omega-3 fatty acids.

Pop some shrimp. When it comes to losing weight, shrimp is a big catch, says Alphin. Although a 3-ounce serving of shrimp packs about as much protein as salmon, it contains fewer calories than a cup of orange juice. (If you have really high cholesterol, limit your shellfish consumption to no more than two or three times per week.) Here's a helpful serving tip: Three ounces isn't much to look at, so cut the shrimp lengthwise to give the illusion of more in your dish.

Play with shells. Mussels, clams, and oysters are the other forgotten homes of protein. For a subtle taste of the sea, mix one of them in your favorite marinara sauce. (Cook over medium heat for 3 to 5 minutes, or until the shells open.) For seafood lovers, try topping a homemade pizza with clams from a can and seasoning it with Old Bay, says Alphin.

Poultry

It's quick, easy, and low in fat. Compared to beans and seafood, your selection of white meat is limited, but its culinary uses are infinite, Alphin says.

Wrap it up. Rotisserie chicken from your local supermarket makes not only a quick and easy dinner but also a high-energy breakfast. Place a cup of cut-up leftover chicken in a whole wheat tortilla wrap. This protein-carbohydrate breakfast combo supplies a steady stream of energy and curbs hunger all morning.

Mix in ground turkey. With one-third less fat than extra-lean ground beef, ground turkey breast makes a tasty lean substitute for beef. It doesn't taste exactly like beef, however, so don't expect to substitute turkey burgers for beef burgers without your dinner guests knowing. Your best bet is to mix it in a sauce (marinara, chili, or sloppy joes).

Duck, duck—goose! With an extra layer of blubber to keep them buoyant, ducks and geese are naturally high in fat. But that doesn't mean waterfowl are off-limits. The fat is not marbled into the meat, so it's easy to deflate the fat factor. Simply remove the skin and poke holes in the meat with a fork before cooking so that the fat can drain out.

Beef and Game Meat

There's no need to exclude red meat. You just have to know how to choose lean cuts of beef, pork, and lamb. And if you're feeling adventurous, some game meats are naturally lower in fat, says Alphin.

Sizzle lean. Anything with *loin* or *round* in the name signals a lean cut of beef. As a bonus, studies show that eating lean beef is just as effective at lowering your bad low-density lipoprotein (LDL) cholesterol and raising your good high-density lipoprotein (HDL) cholesterol as eating skinless chicken.

Improve your grades. Make your lean cuts leaner. Choose "select" and "choice" grades of beef, such as choice sirloin. They contain less fat than meats stamped "prime."

Head for the plains. Game meats, such as bison and beefalo (a cross breed between buffalo and cattle), are becoming regulars on many restaurant menus. With less than half the fat of select sirloin, bison makes a lean, tasty alternative to beef. Beefalo has the same amount of fat as sirloin but over one-third less cholesterol.

Grab this little piggy. It's okay to ham it up once in a while, as long as it's lean. Ham, along with pork chops, can be part of your weight-loss program provided you choose lean meat and trim off the fatty outer layers. Loin and leg are the leanest cuts of pork.

Go on the lamb. Like pork, lamb can be a low-fat option if you choose lean cuts, such as loin or shoulder arm, and remove all visible fat.

Try a different red meat. For an exotic meat that doesn't taste like chicken, try ostrich, emu, or rhea. Although they are birds, their meat is classified as red meat, not white. That's because their flesh has a similar pH to beef. When cooked, it looks like beef and tastes like it, too, only sweeter. And best of all, it has about one-third less fat than beef.

Factor in the Fun

Play is as important as love. Why live?
Why live longer? Why lose weight
if you're not having fun?

—Patch Adams

Swimming in a pool full of spaghetti. Midnight balloon safaris. Mooning his entire graduating class. Physician and professional clown Patch Adams, M.D., immortalized on the big screen by actor Robin Williams, certainly knows a thing or two about how to have fun—even when losing weight.

Although *fun* may be the last word that enters your mind when you think of dropping pounds, when it comes to losing inches and keeping them off, a good laugh can be almost as important to success as cutting back on calories.

Dr. Adams believes that humor also helps keep things, including weight loss, in proper perspective.

"My goal is peace and justice," says Dr. Adams, director of the Gesundheit! Institute in Arlington, Virginia. "But if I die and there are still wars and injustice, I'm not going to punish myself. (Partially because I'm dead and I can't.) I try. I make my goal a quest."

So if your quest is to lose weight, don't punish yourself or give up if you slip one day and eat enough fried chicken to make the Colonel blush. Start fresh the next day. Sit down for a finger-lickin' good-for-you meal with people who make you happy. Here's why.

Play with Your Food

Dinnertime *is* playtime—contrary to what you heard as a child. After all, if play has a home in the cancer ward, why shouldn't the kitchen be fair game? It certainly is to Dr. Patch Adams of the Gesundheit! Institute.

"We used to have 'trough meals' at the hospital," Dr. Adams says. "The food was served in a *real* trough, and you had to root for your meal. Everyone ate less."

Their favorite: spaghetti, tossed salad, and watermelon. Not mixed together. They weren't raised in a barn. "Ah, no, we had classy troughs. Spaghetti in one area, watermelon in another," he says. "We've had trough meals for 30. Everybody ate out of the same bin. Hands behind the back, or you didn't eat. No dissenting. People loved it."

That's just one idea. Make mealtime as outrageous as you like. "The suggestions are infinite," Dr. Adams says.

Here are some of his favorites.

- Take a string bean and put it in your ear.
- Be repulsively competitive. TV chefs are always talking about spicing food to taste good—how about spicing it to taste horrible? Or overcook it. Have two meals a week where you really try to outdo your roommate, spouse, or children at making a repulsive dinner.
- Eat naked. "That's my favorite," he says. "It can make you put your fork down or make you think, 'Hey, I'm not so bad.'"

Though your idea of fun may involve a few more articles of clothing, always remember, says Dr. Adams, that play, like love, is appropriate at even the most inappropriate times.

Get Thin

Laughter is similar in some ways to aerobic exercise. In fact, like running and rowing, a deep belly laugh works nearly every muscle in your body and hikes up your heart rate—doubling your ticker's tempo within a minute or two.

"It takes about 10 minutes on a rowing machine or 15 minutes on a treadmill to get that same effect," says psychiatrist and laughter researcher William F. Fry, M.D., associate clinical professor emeritus at Stanford University School of Medicine. Deep belly laughs also improve your circulation, increase your breathing rate, and accelerate your metabolism—so you burn more calories.

But those are just the immediate effects. In the long run, a little mealtime merriment improves your odds of sticking with your weight-loss program, says Ross Andersen, Ph.D., assistant professor of medicine at Johns Hopkins University School of Medicine in Baltimore and one of the nation's leading researchers on lifestyle activity and weight loss.

Get Young

Children laugh 400 times a day on average. Adults, on the other hand, laugh only 15 times daily. So one of the fastest, most fun ways to feel younger is to simply laugh more.

A good belly jiggler is a battery for your brain, energizing you and waking up your mind. "When you feel energetic, enthusiastic, and alert, you feel more alive. You feel younger," says Dr. Fry.

But mirthful laughter not only keeps your mind young, it may also prevent your relationships from getting old. One study of 50 married couples found that humor accounted for 70 percent of the difference between blissful couples and unhappier ones.

Singles benefit from a sense of humor, too. A study from the University of Louisville found that without a sense of humor, beautiful people are no more desirable than anyone else. We should all aim for a healthy dose of laughter each day.

Go for the Goal

Mealtime is one opportunity to become a kid again and bring more laughter into your life. According to Dr. Andersen, there are two ways to do it.

First, choose healthful foods that make you salivate. Brussels sprouts and oatmeal can be real killjoys if you don't like them, so eat low-fat Mexican food if that's what you enjoy. Just choose more bean and whole grain dishes, and substitute healthful fats for lard and butter.

Second, alter your atmosphere. Awaken the child within and create a zany dining environment. The possibilities are limitless. Here are 10 to get you started.

Turn off the tube. Dr. Adams recommends that you turn off the television and turn on the conversation. You're less likely to overeat when the TV is off and more likely to laugh when gabbing with friends and family.

Why? Laughter's infectious, especially if you're comfortable with your dinner companions. "One person starts, and everyone joins in, so your meal will be much more enjoyable," Dr. Fry says.

Host a potluck party. Have a theme, such as "dips and sticks night," where all appetizers, entrées, and desserts must be served on a stick (an opportunity to finally use your fondue pot). "It's not just a night of entertaining conversation and contagious laughter, it's also an opportunity to learn new recipes and try unfamiliar produce and grains," notes Dr. Fry.

Be a cutup. You can use cookie cutters to make festive croutons for soups and salads or to create seasonal sandwiches, suggests Regina Ragone, R.D., a registered dietitian and food editor for *Prevention* magazine.

Dress up the table. Once a week, liven up your table with vibrant table linens. Better yet, unleash the Martha Stewart within and design something for the table, like personalized place mats, conversation-starting table runners, or silly centerpieces, Dr. Fry suggests. (This is also a great way to keep kids occupied while you're preparing dinner.)

Be an artist. Ragone offers this idea: Paint your plate with nature's colors: red peppers, orange carrots, leafy greens, black beans. Create a visual masterpiece that would make Jackson Pollock weep. If you have kids or a niece and nephew on loan for the day, let them handle plate presentation. You'll be amazed at what a child can create with a tuna sandwich and a few baby carrots.

Go off-road. It's hard to enjoy anything, including a meal, when you're trapped in traffic or dodging an SUV fueled with road rage. So get out of your car when it's time to eat, Dr. Andersen suggests. If the weather's kind, find a park bench to relax on.

Find a restaurant buddy. Seek out someone with a taste for adventure, Dr. Andersen suggests. Once a month, try a new eatery (Korean, Greek, or vegetarian) and a new dish, like namool (Korean assorted vegetables), pasta e fagioli (pasta and bean soup), or tabbouleh (a Middle Eastern grain dish).

Put romance on the menu. For a romantic meal with your honey, pick up a bottle of red wine, a baguette, some shrimp, green olives, cherries or exotic fruits, or anything that has a pungent flavor and doesn't require silverware, Ragone suggests. (Sugar-Free Cherry Jell-O Jigglers work, too.) Set one rule: You can't feed yourself. Other than that, anything goes.

Have an indoor picnic. Don't let the weather or lack of green acreage prevent you from having a picnic. Unearth your kitchen table. Replace the unpaid bills and laundry with a picnic blanket and your derriere. If your table has seen sturdier days, set up your summery buffet on the family room floor, but keep the TV turned off.

Pick a prize. Reward yourself for accomplishing one of your food goals with a nonfood prize. For example, for every serving of whole grains you eat, you earn a dollar toward a babysitter and a night on the town. You could even save up for a weekend getaway.

Quiz

Are You a Cher or an Oprah?

We all know women who look great all the time—whether they're working out, lounging on the couch, or dressed up for dinner at a fancy restaurant. Whatever they throw on seems to belong on them.

What's their secret? They have an eye for styles, textures, and colors that look good on them.

But if everything you pull over your head just doesn't seem right—or if you want to touch up the style you already have—take this quiz, developed by writer Bridget Doherty and Anna Wildermuth, a corporate and individual image consultant and owner of Personal Images in Elmhurst, Illinois. It will help you choose the clothes, hairstyle, and makeup that fit just right with your personality.

Circle one answer per question.

1. What's your favorite color to wear?
   a. Red
   b. Bright colors
   c. Earthy tones, like brown and beige
   d. Black

2. If you had your choice, what would you wear every day?
   a. Clingy tops and skirts
   b. Jeans and sweaters
   c. Long dresses
   d. Fitted suits

3. When you sit in a chair, do you:
   a. Cross your legs at the knee
   b. Set one ankle on your opposite knee
   c. Dangle your arm over the back of the chair
   d. Cross your legs at the ankle

4. The skirts and dresses in your closet:
   a. Are shorter than some of your tops—miniskirts are your passion
   b. Are in the back of your closet—you hardly wear them

c. Are so long that they almost touch the floor
d. Are tailored, lined, and pressed, and they hang with a matching blazer or sweater set

5. Before you leave your house, do you:
a. Bend over and spritz your hair with hair spray so it looks full
b. Simply run your fingers through your hair
c. Spend a minimum amount of time curling and styling
d. Make sure that every strand on your head is in its proper place

6. Your makeup bag contains:
a. Dramatic colors, such as dark gray eye shadow and garnet lipstick
b. Just the basics: concealer, eyeliner, and lipstick
c. Conservative as well as dark colors: cream eye shadow for work and hunter green for weekends
d. Only conservative colors: brown eyeliner, ivory eye shadow, and berry lipstick

Score Yourself

IF YOU CIRCLED . . .

Mostly *as*

Your personality type is: Cher. You may not want a group of sailors leering at you while you're wearing thong underwear, but you like to call attention to yourself. Now it's time to think about which parts of your body you want people to notice.

If you like your chest, wear low V-neck tops, necklaces, or clingy shirts with Lycra to bring attention to it. If you're more proud of your legs, wear skirts that fall above your knees, high-heel shoes and sandals, and slim-cut pants.

Choose different shades of your favorite color: red. It commands attention. If you want to know if a particular shade will look good on you, hold it next to your face. You'll be able to tell immediately if it's a good shade for you.

And whether your hair is thick and curly or thin and straight, choose a style that makes people notice you, such as out-of-control curls or a dramatic short cut.

Make a statement with the colors you choose to wear on your face, too, but be careful not to overdo it. If you make your lips ultradark, then go light on the eye shadow, and vice versa.

(continued)

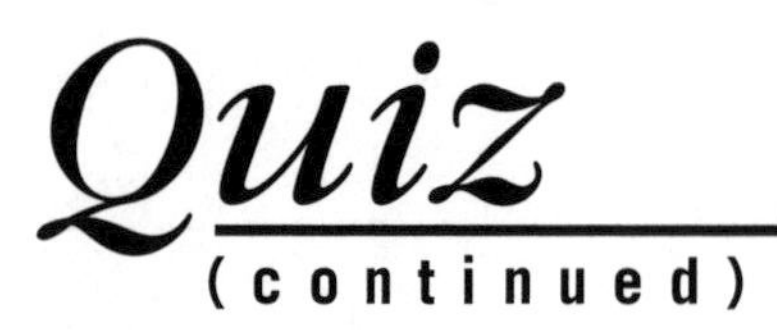

Mostly *b*s

Your personality type is: Meg Ryan. You're a kid at heart, and you gravitate toward a youthful look, so stick with bright, fun colors, such as pink and sky blue. They'll brighten your face and make you look younger. Choose sweater sets made of soft, thin fabrics—such as cotton, silk, and wool—with A-line skirts. Or buy playful capri pants. If your calves are wide, choose a length that falls above your ankles. But if your legs are thinner, wear capri pants that fall just above your calves.

You don't want to spend a lot of time on your hair, so choose a style that doesn't require a lot of upkeep, whether it's a one-length cut with bangs or short and tousled. And keep light colors in your makeup bag, such as soft pinks and blues.

Mostly *c*s

Your personality type is: Oprah Winfrey. Your individual style is a mix of professional and fun. You might wear a tailored pair of pants with a white blouse just as easily as you would put on a long, comfortable cotton dress. On the days you want to look authoritative, wear dark gray, and on the days you want to look more approachable, go for beige.

If your body shape is more curvy than it is angular, choose soft, flowing fabrics, such as thin wools, cotton jerseys, and lightweight silks. If you have a straighter, more angular body type, choose crisp cottons and stiffer silks.

Your hairstyle is versatile, too. You can either wear it down in a classic layered style, pull it back, or curl it for a softer look.

When you choose your makeup, complement the variety in your wardrobe with different colors, such as deep brown and pink lipstick and navy and cream eye shadow.

Mostly *d*s

Your personality type is: Diane Sawyer. You're a professional, no-nonsense woman, and you want to make the best impression with your wardrobe. Wear tailored suits in colors like black, dark gray, and dark brown. They all hold power and authority, while navy communicates trust. To look slimmer in your suits, choose long blazers with thin pockets.

Wear your hair layered or one length. And keep your makeup simple and sophisticated, with brown or black eyeliner, brown eye shadow, and light lipstick.

Creating Your Own Individual Style

DAWN BOEHMER GREW UP IN THE WEST INDIES, WHERE SLIM FIGURES ARE CONSIDERED FAR FROM BEAUTIFUL. THIN AND WHITE, SHE WAS DIFFERENT FROM THE OTHER CHILDREN IN HER COMMUNITY AND WAS TEASED FOR IT. FOR DECADES, SHE WORE GRAY, BROWN, AND BLACK CLOTHES THAT HELPED HER FADE INTO THE WOODWORK.

It wasn't until she turned 40 and was a designer of her own clothing line, Moda Madonna in Mount Kisco, New York, that Boehmer finally discovered her own individual style. She dumped the dark clothes for pink capri pants and a menswear-inspired suit with rhinestone buttons.

"It took a little longer for me to realize that I am who I am regardless of how anyone perceives me," she says.

Pink pants and rhinestones may not be for you, but as you lose weight, you may realize that you haven't found your individual style either. The key to developing your own style is to be true to yourself.

"Every woman's body shape and personality is different, just like our fingerprints," Boehmer says. Here's how to find what's right for you.

Find a fashion maven. One of the best ways to start your style search is to cut out pictures of women with whom you share features and body shape and whose style you would like to mirror, suggests image consultant Anna Wildermuth of Personal Images.

If you're losing weight now, collect pictures of women who look the way you will eventually. Can't see yourself 10 pounds thinner? Trust your instincts. "A person gravitates to certain styles because they fit her body shape and coloring," Wildermuth says.

If you have a friend or a coworker who has a style you love, ask her how she pulls it off, suggests Margaret Voelker-Ferrier, associate professor of fashion design at the University of Cincinnati. Then ask her for advice on your own look.

Get tickled pink or green or blue . . . One of the first questions Boehmer asks her clients is, "What is your favorite color?" Once you've figured that out, *wear* your favorite color in shades that complement you.

In general, primary colors such as blue, red, green, and yellow look good on women with dark features, while pastel colors such as pink, baby blue, and soft greens look good on women with light features. Try it out for yourself. Put different-color fabrics next to your face.

"You'll be able to tell immediately if the color looks good on you," Wildermuth says. "If it adds life and color to your skin, it will look good on you. If it drains color from your skin, don't wear it."

Stick with colors that express you. Do you prefer to look powerful or casual? Choose a color that matches your personality. "Everything you put on communicates something about you," Voelker-Ferrier says. Whether you want to command attention or look trustworthy, there is a color that speaks for you.

■ Black connotes power.

■ Dark gray holds authority.

■ Dark brown communicates control.

■ Navy inspires security and trust.

■ Red commands attention. Wear it if you're giving a speech.

■ White has authority when it's worn at the right time. In the summer, white looks cool and refreshing, but in the winter, black looks more comfortable.

■ Beige is soothing. "They say that if you're going to fire somebody, wear beige," Voelker-Ferrier says, because it doesn't look as harsh.

■ Bright colors bring attention to your face. Frame your face and brighten it with a scarf or sweater tied around your neck, or add a gold or silver necklace.

Personalize Your Dress Code at Work

The workplace isn't exactly the best place to show your fashion individuality, especially if you have a dress code or you wear a uniform. But you do have some opportunities, so take advantage of them with style and accessories.

Choose style or color for a look all your own. Dressing for work is a dance between style and taste. Dressing tastefully means dressing appropriately for your environment while still being true to yourself.

If you have wide-open body language and prefer looser clothes, wear an unstructured business suit in a conservative color, such as black or brown. The unstructured style matches your personality, while the color looks professional.

If you feel comfortable in a more form-fitting tailored suit, show your personality by choosing a unique color, such as mauve. You'll look professional while expressing your personality through color.

Wear it on your lapel. Wearing accessories is another great way to strut your style at work. If you have a hobby, accessorize it, says fashion expert Margaret Voelker-Ferrier of the University of Cincinnati. She collects Barbie dolls, so she wears Barbie pins. If you have a creative bent, bring a unique bag to work. If you're an Elvis Presley fan, hang a dancing Elvis clock on your wall.

As you lose weight, you can also use accessories to accent your new figure. If you have a great waist, wear an interesting belt, developing it into your signature piece, says Georgette Braadt, an image and communications consultant in Allentown, Pennsylvania. Or wear earrings to show off your slimmer face. If you want to keep attention away from your waist, wear a pin on your shoulder to bring people's focus up instead of down.

Pair up. Pairing colors also has an effect on how people react to you. Do you like to make people sit up straight when you're around? Wear a dark suit with a white blouse. The contrast conveys authority.

As contrast fades, approachability increases. To achieve a more accessible business look, wear a color under your dark blazer to soften your appearance, says Diana Kilgour, an independent wardrobe and image consultant in Vancouver, Canada. Natural colors, such as beige and brown, along with more textured fabrics, such as brushed silk, tell people you're approachable.

Stay comfortable. Since the whole idea of finding your individual style is to look comfortable in your clothes, don't force yourself to wear a wardrobe that isn't right for you.

"If you're going to put a dress on someone who never wears dresses, she'll carry her body in a way that will make it look wrong," says Claudia Kaneb, wardrobe head at NBC's *Today* show.

Also, choose a style that fits your body language. Do you lounge in your chair or do you sit up straight? Your answer makes the difference between wearing a relaxed or tailored outfit.

If you sit with your left ankle on your right knee and your elbow dangling over the back of your chair, you have wide-open body language, Kilgour says.

"You can't wear clothes that are too narrow or too tight," she says. You need room to express yourself, so wear loose pantsuits.

If you're more composed, you'll be comfortable in a tailored suit buttoned up to your neck because your body language is more modified. You sit calmly without fidgeting and keep your hands in your lap. "Your body posture is such that the suit fits well on you," Kilgour says.

Look slimmer. Wear tights, skirts, and shirts of the same color to look thinner. Voelker-Ferrier wears long skirts and turtlenecks to lengthen the effect. "The more color from head to toe, the thinner and taller you look," she says.

Listen to your heart. Your best bet in finding your personal style is to listen to intuition. "What does your heart say?" Boehmer asks. "By the time you turn 40 or 50, way down deep you know your style. If you pay attention, if you listen, you know who you are."

Wear it every day. Once you find your look, be consistent. It's the key to having a personal style. If you can't afford to be consistent in your whole wardrobe, get one piece of clothing or an accessory that perfectly communicates your personal style, such as a sweater, a purse, jewelry, or even makeup.

If you wear only red lipstick, that's your signature. When your look is consistent, people will talk about you in a favorable way. When people say, "She always wears those great shoes," you'll know you've found an individual style.

Week Six

All in the Family

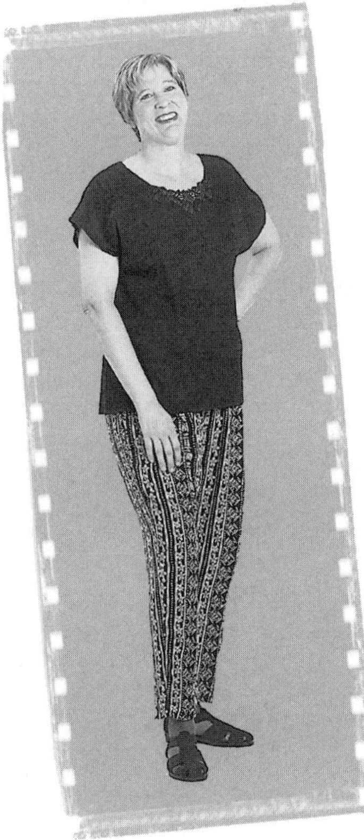

After

Before

OUR WALKS TOGETHER WHILE A BABYSITTER WATCHES THE KIDS ARE THE ONLY TIMES WE GET A CHANCE TO TALK UNINTERRUPTED, ENJOY EACH OTHER'S COMPANY, AND WORK OUT FAMILY ISSUES.

—Ann Harbove

Week Six

For the past few weeks, you've been busy creating a thinner, younger, and healthier you. If you're lucky, your family and friends have been supportive. Changes are, though, that you're getting some resistance. No one really likes change. And maybe some of that resistance is coming from within, from guilt you feel for focusing on yourself rather than on your family and other obligations.

This week, you'll learn strategies to move you beyond these motivational blocks. You'll find ways to help carve out some guilt-free time for yourself—and to get your family to rally around you with encourgement. Having some type of social support is key to staying motivated. So read the advice on how to find an exercise buddy or start your own support group. And if you must go it alone, know that you can still get support from nonexercising friends and family members.

Making Time for Yourself

AS A CHILD, YOU HAD ALL THE TIME IN THE WORLD: PLAYTIME, NAP TIME, READING TIME, BEDTIME, AND MAYBE EVEN TIME-OUTS. BUT AS YOU GOT OLDER, YOUR RESPONSIBILITIES INCREASED ALONG WITH YOUR AGE, CHIPPING AWAY AT ALL THAT PRECIOUS TIME MEANT FOR FUN AND PLAY. NOW IT SEEMS AS THOUGH EVERYTHING AND EVERYONE GETS YOUR TIME BUT *YOU*. IT'S TIME TO TAKE BACK SOME OF THAT TIME.

As careers, children, parents, and other obligations pile up, the first thing that always vanishes is what you want and need.

"We neglect ourselves because we feel that we have to take care of each other. We have to be in control at all times, and we can't let others see us stop or rest," says Sharon Keys Seal, a professional business coach and owner of Coaching Concepts in Baltimore.

But here are four very important reasons to make time for yourself.

You need it to lose weight. When you make a commitment to lose weight, you also commit to setting time aside to exercise and eat right. But in addition to those reasons, time for yourself—even if it doesn't directly involve weight loss—builds self-esteem and self-confidence, which in turn increase your chances of slimming down.

You need it to stay young. Activities, interests, hobbies, and friendships that

Here Come the Television Tubbies

When it comes to sabotaging weight-loss efforts, your television may pose more of a threat than your refrigerator. Consider the following:

- Television erodes free time. According to the book *Time for Life* by John P. Robinson and Geoffrey Godbey, Americans have more than 40 hours a week in free time. Yet they feel as though they have less than ever. One of the culprits? Television. Americans lose 15 hours of free time a week watching the box.
- Many studies have linked television watching with weight gain and obesity. Studies have shown that men who spend more time watching TV are more sedentary, eat more snacks, and are generally more obese. A study at the University of Minnesota found that television viewing predicted weight gain in women.

"Television has become a distraction," says Carla Wolper, R.D., a nutritionist and clinical coordinator at the Obesity Research Center at St. Luke's/Roosevelt Hospital Center in New York City.

It zaps away time that could be better spent fulfilling other needs such as exercise, hobbies, or even just quiet time with yourself, she adds. For many people, watching the tube sends them on more trips to the refrigerator as well.

This doesn't mean that you have to throw out the TV. Choose the programs you want to watch beforehand and watch only those instead of having the set on all the time. Keep hobby materials, books, and exercise equipment out and ready so that you can easily pick them up instead of turning on the television, she says.

And if you do want the TV on, do something productive while you watch, such as paying bills or knitting.

are all your own provide the basis of a young, active lifestyle, no matter what your age, says Dana G. Cable, Ph.D., professor of psychology at Hood College in Frederick, Maryland.

Though you may be too busy with your job and family to see it now, setting aside time for yourself today will keep you younger for years to come.

Someday, the kids will move out and you'll retire, leaving you with plenty of free time. Developing interests and activities will ensure that you remain active when you're older.

You need to take care of yourself first. Giving your all to others may seem like the ultimate sacrifice, but you aren't doing them any favors. Eventually, you'll burn out, and your performance will suffer, whether it shows in doing your job or taking care of your children. Taking time for yourself gives you the chance to recharge.

"You'll be better at everything you do," says Cathleen Gray, Ph.D., associate professor of social work at the Catholic University of America in Washington, D.C.

You're worth it. You merit your own time and interests. "We deserve it. It reflects and strengthens our self-love and self-worth. It is showing ourselves that we are indeed worthy," Seal says.

The Five-Step Make-Time-for-Yourself Program

With all you have to do, how can you make time for yourself? Easy. Planning is the key to getting what you want while also handling your responsibilities, says Barry Miller, Ph.D., a career counselor and associate professor of management at the Lubin School of Business of Pace University in New York City.

To make time for yourself, follow these five simple steps.

1. Figure out what do you want to do. When Dr. Gray asks people this question, they often ignore her or don't have an answer. We are so well programmed to think of the wants and needs of others that we never even consider our own desires. So the first part of making time for yourself is to decide what you want to do with that time.

As a start, consider your weight-loss needs. Do you want to exercise every day? Do you want to keep Sunday afternoons open for food shopping? Then, think about your other wants: Do you want a few minutes a day to read a book? Do you want to see the sun rise each morning? Do you want to take a class, start a hobby, or volunteer for an organization? Do you want to eat lunch with your best friend every week? Do you want to get a facial or massage?

2. Schedule it. Once you have determined what you want to do, calculate how much time you need each day or each week to do it. Write it down in your planner or calendar. For example, if you want 5 minutes a day to just relax, mark that down. If you want to take a walk every day at lunch, write it down—in ink.

"You need to work out a plan for what you want," Dr. Miller says. Then plan the rest of your day or week around your personal time, not vice versa.

3. Prepare. Your free time needs preparation and structure just like your workday does. "Quality time needs structure to it. If you didn't structure your job, you'd be fired. But people don't put that same energy into their own time," Dr. Miller says.

Without that structure, it's very easy to fritter away your time, Seal adds.

Have what you need ready to go: Put your sneakers by the door for your walk. Leave your book ready and waiting for you. Have your craft or hobby items out when you get home. Make reservations for lunch or a massage several days before. Call and ask for membership materials for organizations or groups you want to join.

4. Stick to it. Life can get hectic, but avoid the urge to sacrifice your personal time, Dr. Gray says. This time for you is just as important as a big meeting or your child's school play. Perceive this time as a goal or a prescription, she adds. That way, you're more inclined to see it as something that needs to be done instead of an easily discarded luxury.

5. Lay down the law. "You need to let other people know that this is not the time to bother you," Dr. Miller says. Make it clear to everyone—family, friends, coworkers—that this is *your* time. If they violate your boundaries, look them straight in the eye and say, "I'm busy right now, you'll have to wait until later."

Busting the Time Busters

Even though you have a plan to ensure that you carve out time for yourself, you probably still have a hectic schedule. So in addition to the five-step plan, take simple steps to pare down the stuff that steals away your time. These easy moves will cut back some of your responsibilities and allow you to get more done in less time. They'll also give you more time to spend working on a thinner and younger you.

Set up phone rules. Answering and talking on the phone wastes time. To keep phone time in control, set up phone rules. If possible, don't answer the phone, and let your answering machine or voice mail take messages, Dr. Gray suggests.

Living Proof
PANEL

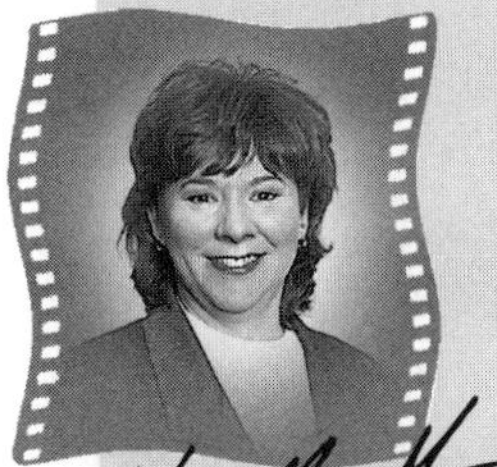

Reclaiming the Lunch Hour

Busy? Try this: I have a full-time job, I teach design classes at a local college two nights a week, and I take a studio class one night a week. On top of this, I have undertaken the daunting task of single-handedly renovating my home. So, yes, I am very busy.

That's why this program appealed to me. It's based on small lifestyle changes that I could glide into instead of having to set aside huge chunks of time for aerobics classes. But in order for the program to work, I still needed to figure out how to fit those changes into my hectic schedule. My first challenge was finding time for a healthy dinner. Typically, I get home around 10:00 P.M. I was eating too late and didn't have the energy to prepare a healthy meal.

My solution? Lunch has become the biggest meal of the day for me. Because I have access to healthy fare at work, I make that my main meal, and then I can burn it off as the day goes on. When I get home late, I'll have a small salad and some fruit.

Since I have an hour for lunch, I use half of it for my daily walk. I go outside and get away from my desk, which enables me to fit in my exercise. And I really do believe that I am more productive in the afternoon because of it.

So even though practically every hour of my day is booked, I have found the time I need rather easily. And I am seeing great results. Better yet, these schedule changes have now become habit. I don't even think about them as part of my program anymore. It's just what I do every day.

Designate a certain time of day to listen to the messages, and return those calls that you deem important. Also, set up specific friend and family chat times. For example, let your family know that you are available to talk on Sundays after 7:00 P.M.

Ban office chitchat. Countless hours are lost talking by the coffeepot or in your office, Dr. Miller says. While chatting can be fun, it can also take you away from your work, which then eats into your free time.

If someone walks into your office to talk, tell them you're busy and you can't chat right now. If cornered by the coffeepot, smile and say, "Sorry. Can't talk right now." Or close your office door and put up a Do Not Disturb sign.

Take stock of your commitments. Every 6 months or so, review all your activities, says Patricia Liehr, R.N., Ph.D., associate professor of systems and technology at the University of Texas School of Nursing in Houston. She lists her activities in order of importance. If she has too much on her plate, she starts writing a few "resignation letters" to the ones at the bottom of the list.

"I don't really need to be doing it all," she says. If you are pulled in too many directions, figure out the obligations you want to keep and the ones you want to unload. Break free from the lesser commitments and use that time for yourself.

Delegate jobs. Find tasks and responsibilities to pass on to others. The best way to do this is to give people jobs that you hate but they enjoy. For instance, Seal has her friend's teenage son fix and keep her computer running smoothly. She hates it, he loves it. They are both happy.

Stop doing it. Seal has a game she plays: She chooses a task, such as washing her car, and just stops doing it. Then she waits to see how long it takes people to notice that she has stopped. More often than not, no one does. If no one notices the chores that you have neglected, drop them.

The Benefits of a Buddy

IF IT WEREN'T FOR HER WORKOUT BUDDY, PAM, HELENE WAGNER OF ALLENTOWN, PENNSYLVANIA, WOULD STILL DO SOME EXERCISE. "BUT I SURE WOULDN'T DO NEARLY AS MUCH," SHE CONFESSES. "PAM KEEPS ME HONEST. AND MORE IMPORTANT, SHE MAKES IT FUN."

It's a simple yet often overlooked fact: Exercise is more fun with a friend. "It's human nature to want to do things with other people, especially exercise," says Deborah Saint-Phard, M.D., an exercise physiatrist for the Women's Sports Medicine Center at the Hospital for Special Surgery in New York City.

When you were a kid, you'd knock on every door in the neighborhood to find someone to come out and play with you. "When you finally found someone to come out, you'd play until dark," says Dr. Saint-Phard. "But if no one was around, you'd go back home and watch TV. Why should we feel any differently as adults?"

Aside from being fun, exercise is simply more effective when you do it with a friend.

"If you find a partner who likes to do the same things as you and has similar abilities, you'll be less likely to quit exercising and more likely to make it a regular habit, have fun, and see results," says certified international lifestyle fitness expert Lynne Brick, owner of Brick Bodies Health Clubs in Baltimore.

Say, "I Do!"

For married folks, your best training partner may be your partner for life. People who start fitness programs with their spouses are much more likely to exercise regularly—and much less likely to drop out entirely—than those who start exercising solo. The reason? Researchers speculate that the support and camaraderie people feel when working out with loved ones keep them going past the point where many solitary exercisers throw in the towel.

"Couples who exercise together achieve what I call active intimacy," says Walter Bortz II, M.D., clinical associate professor of medicine at Stanford University School of Medicine and author of *Dare to Be 100*. "There's a sense of fun, like going out to play with a best friend. They grow closer and get in great shape while spending quality time together. As a result, they can end up living longer, happier, healthier lives."

Not sure how to get your spouse moving? Perhaps these suggestions can help.

Trade eating for exercise. You and your spouse already enjoy some leisure time together. The problem is, for lots of people that time is spent with food rather than exercise. The next time the two of you head out the door together, try the tennis courts instead of the food courts. This can be a great way for you and your spouse to enjoy your leisure time, says Michelle Edwards, a certified personal trainer and a health educator for the Cooper Institute for Aerobics Research in Dallas.

"What couples sometimes do not realize is that becoming more physically active together can be easier than you think," she says. There are a variety of fun activities that couples can do together. For example, instead of simply going out to eat for recreation, add a little physical activity to your plans, such as taking a brisk walk together, playing a quick game of tennis or racquetball, or even dancing.

For some couples, the ideal "joint activity" would be joining a health club together. All of these suggestions are great ways to become more physically active and spend some quality time together, Edwards says. The object of the game is to get up and get moving.

Recruit your kids. Couples with small children often sacrifice exercising together because they don't have anyone to watch the kids. Well, a better alternative to taking turns exercising alone is to take the kids along, says Brick. "Technology today has made exercising even with small children easier than

Five Ways to Find a Workout Buddy

It's great when you have someone to exercise with, but what do you do when you don't know *anyone* who's willing to join you? Here are five easy ways to get some company.

1. Join a club. Most community centers have exercise clubs for all kinds of activities. Do you like walking? Join a hiking club. Play tennis? Join a round-robin tournament. You're bound to meet someone with similar interests.

2. Check out the stores. Major sporting goods stores like Eastern Mountain Sports (EMS), as well as bike shops and running stores, usually conduct regular outings. Find out when the next one is and tag along.

3. Read the classifieds. Almost every community has groups that meet for active trips, like dayhiking or park walks. These groups are great places to meet other people who are also trying to stay active.

4. Look online. Many gyms have Web sites with message boards, where you can post a note looking for a workout buddy. This way, you can also get to know each other a little through e-mail before you actually meet.

5. Ask around. Talk to your neighbors or to people at church or anywhere else that you socialize. Chances are that there's someone just like you who's looking for a friend to work out with.

ever," she says. "There are baby joggers, bike trailers, and special harnesses for hiking. If your kids are old enough, there's no reason that you can't hike or bike together. Let them pick the activity sometimes. That way, it's more fun for everyone."

Divvy up the chores. Your kids want time to play. You and your spouse want time to play. Maybe you're all playing together. So who's taking care of the housework? There are two ways you can approach this chore and get some health benefits from it as well, says Edwards.

First, try increasing the intensity of doing your household chores. Vacuuming is a good example. Instead of vacuuming at a leisurely pace, pump it up a bit by keeping time to your favorite upbeat tunes. You can use the same approach for dusting the furniture or even washing the car, she says. If that approach doesn't grab you, try dividing up the chores so that everything that needs to get done gets done and everyone in the family has more time to go out and be active.

Girl Talk

Between family and work responsibilities, it's hard for women to catch up with their friends as often as they would like. One way to change that is to work out with your friends, says Michael Bourque, certified personal trainer and personal training coordinator for the Center for Health and Wellness of the Central Florida YMCA in Oviedo. "That way, you're meeting two of your priorities at once," he says. "You're keeping up with your girlfriends, and you're getting regular physical activity."

Working out with friends has some of the same benefits as working out with your spouse: You'll be more likely to stick with your exercise program in the long run. Research shows that the most important factor for sticking with a workout program for the first year is having the support of friends and family. "There's no better support than actually having a friend right there with you," says Bourque.

To ensure that your exercise sessions work best for both of you, here are some things you may want to try.

Take new classes. One of the biggest exercise obstacles people face is going to a new exercise class and feeling as though they're the only ones there who don't know what the heck they're doing, says Bourque. "If you sign up with a buddy, that fear is gone," he says. "You'll feel calmer going into it and have more fun once you're there. By taking turns picking classes that interest you, you'll also get a chance to try some potentially fun activities that you might otherwise overlook."

Be good mentors. One of the best parts about working out with a buddy is that you can learn a lot from each other and grow, says Paul Konstanty, clinical supervisor and exercise therapist at the University of California OrthoMed Spine and Joint Conditioning Center in San Diego. "Maybe your partner has a great tennis serve, and you're a strong swimmer. You can each improve tenfold just by watching the other's form and picking up some pointers."

Be cheerleaders. "No, you don't have to don a skirt and shake pom-poms,

Living Proof
PANEL

It's a Family Affair

My husband, Dave, and I have four young children at home. He travels extensively for his job, so we don't have much time together, especially during the week. Needless to say, life is crazy and hectic most of the time.

Our walks together while a babysitter watches the kids are the only times we get a chance to talk uninterrupted, enjoy each other's company, and work out family issues. We also walk longer and farther when we walk with each other than when we have to go alone.

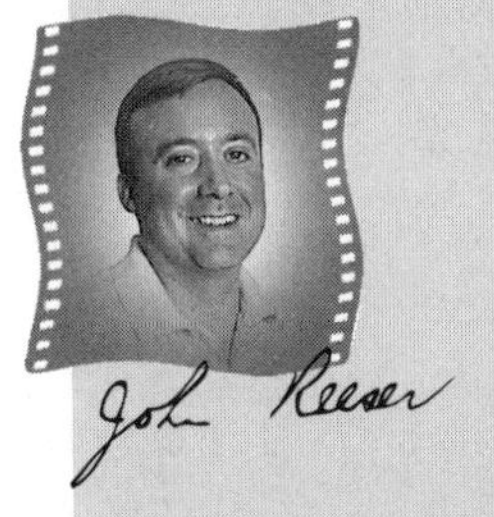

My wife, Ana, and I are pleased with our progress. Working together to start a healthier lifestyle has really helped. Ana has been an especially good motivator for me. She's been getting up early to do her walks and weight routine. We eat out less and at home more, serving lots of fruits and vegetables at every meal.

I'll admit that I can be lazy sometimes. But seeing Ana put in so much effort gets me moving. We've even invested in a treadmill so that we can exercise during the winter and on days when the weather is bad. I would have never put forth so much effort by myself.

My 11-year-old daughter and I have started working out together. We've been walking and doing aerobics together. It's really wonderful to be able to spend that kind of quality time with her instead of doing things separately or doing something like watching television. And she really looks forward to it, so she's developing healthy habits.

but encouraging even the small accomplishments of your partner, such as losing 2 to 3 pounds, can mean a lot," says Edwards. That's where having a buddy can help. Cheer each other on and compliment one another's progress. That can help you both stay motivated to reach your fitness goals.

Add a little peer pressure. No matter how much you like what you're doing, and no matter how much you like who you're doing it with, there's going to come a day when you just don't want to exercise. "That will be the day when having a buddy is the best thing for you," says John Yetter, M.D., medical director at SSM Rehab Sports Medicine in St. Louis. "We complained about peer pressure as kids. But as adults, it can be a big help. I know plenty of folks who wouldn't get off their couches most days if they didn't have a good friend waiting for them at the gym. It's a great motivator for both of you."

Forming Your Own Support Group

As you progress into your weight-loss program, you may be thinking of all the changes that come with it: the decisions you have to make, the foods you eat, the exercises you do. The key word here is *you,* because losing weight is often considered to be a lonely, solitary process. And that may be part of the problem.

You can't do it alone. In fact, the more you involve others, the more likely you are to be successful. "When you are trying to lose weight, you are talking about a lot of changes in your life. You need the support of other people," says Ellen Parham, R.D., Ph.D., professor and coordinator of dietetics, nutrition, and food systems at Northern Illinois University in De Kalb.

Along with physical activity, healthy eating, and self-monitoring, social support is one of the basic ingredients of successful weight-loss programs. And this support remains crucial for keeping weight off once you've lost it, says Dr. Parham. It's easy to make changes for a short amount of time, but you need the help of others to turn those changes into lifetime habits.

A study at the University of Pittsburgh analyzed two groups of weight-loss subjects: those who joined a program along with three friends and family members and received social support, and those who joined alone and didn't have social support.

Of those who joined with friends and had social support, 95 percent completed treatment, and 66 percent maintained their weight loss. Of those who didn't join with friends or have social support, 76 percent lost weight, but only 24 percent maintained it.

Form a Band

Call it a support group, a friendly gathering, or a weekly get-together. Whatever you label it, surrounding yourself with other people who are trying to lose weight is a source of comfort, knowledge, and refuge.

"It helps by letting people share their experiences," Dr. Parham says.

While friends and family often want to support you, many times they may not understand what you're going through. That's when a support group helps. Because you are all trying to achieve the same type of goal, you know firsthand the joys and obstacles of weight loss.

In a group of caring friends, you realize that you are not alone. "A lot of people think that they are the only overweight person in the world, that their problems are unique. When people get together as a group, they find themselves saying, 'That happens to me, too,'" says Ross Andersen, Ph.D., assistant professor of medicine at Johns Hopkins University School of Medicine in Baltimore and one of the nation's leading researchers on lifestyle activity and weight loss.

Getting together with others who are trying to lose weight also can help you find answers to problems that you all face. For example, if you're having trouble finding time to exercise, seek a solution from the group, and you may be amazed at all the ways others have dealt with the same problem.

While the advantages of having a support group may be clear, figuring out how to find people to take this journey with you may not be. Here's how.

Start your own. If you want to start a support group, look around you. Colleagues, friends, family, neighbors, parents of your children's friends, people you see walking every night—chances are that they are trying to lose

Living Proof
PANEL

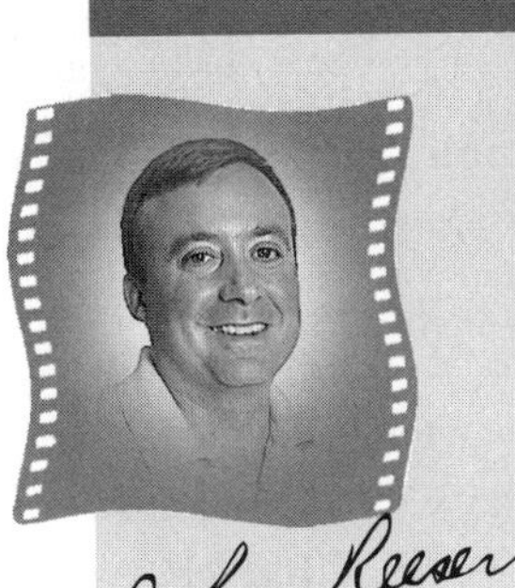

Losing Weight—Married Style

John Reeser

The variable in our weight-loss program is Sam, our 4-year-old son. We can't just say, "Let's both go out for a jog." One can't take off to exercise without asking the other. We have to cooperate and be supportive of each other to make it happen.

I've helped my wife, Ana, by giving her the time to exercise. She tells me when she wants to do it—mornings, weekends, whenever. And I put aside whatever I am doing to watch Sam so that she can run. Helping each other works both ways, though.

In previous weight-loss tries, Ana would tell me when I shouldn't eat something, and that would only make me want it more. This time, she hasn't been bugging me or making comments. If I say that I want ice cream, she simply says that I don't want it. Or she tells me that she isn't going to have any. That's enough to trigger my internal "stop" mechanism.

Our latest joint decision is a treadmill. I've been against it for years. If I wanted to run, I figured I'd just run outside. I didn't see the point of the expense. But Ana has wanted one for a while. She wanted a place where she could run inside as it got darker and colder outside.

So I finally broke down and agreed to buy one. Now I wonder why we didn't buy this years ago. It's wonderful because it helps us fit exercise into our busy schedules. Ana mostly uses it when Sam takes his afternoon nap, and I run on it around 8:30 to 9:00 P.M., after Sam's gone to bed for the night.

weight just like you, Dr. Andersen says. Explain what you want to do: Come together to help each other and have fun, too.

Meet once a week. To get the most out of being part of the group, come together about once a week, Dr. Parham says. Schedule the meeting at the same time to establish a routine. If people start to get bored, take a field trip or change the location every few weeks.

Pick a comfortable, private place. When you decide on a meeting place, make sure that people can speak without fear of others outside the group hearing or intruding.

"It needs to be private, a place where people feel secure," Dr. Parham says. While a house can be a good meeting spot, choose a room where other family members can't walk in and out. Also, have comfortable chairs and a seating arrangement that allows the group to see and talk among others freely.

People may translate your decision to lose weight as a comment on them personally.

Set the ground rules. Before you get started, clearly explain group regulations. Some basic rules: All conversation is to remain confidential; treat each other with respect; do not judge or criticize; and everyone gets a chance to speak. If you want other rules, such as how much time a person gets or how to set an agenda, that's up to you, Dr. Parham says. But make them clear from the beginning.

Keep the agenda positive. A support group will only be helpful when it convenes for the right purpose. Getting together to simply complain about how useless it is to try to lose weight will not help your cause. "They can't be a group of enablers," says Daniel Stettner, Ph.D., director of psychology for the Beaumont Hospital Weight Control Center in Royal Oak, Michigan. Set the tone that your support group is to be positive and encouraging.

Meet for exercise. Perhaps your support group can talk and walk at the same time. Dr. Andersen suggests that pairing up with others increases the chances that you'll maintain your exercise program, since you're more likely to keep your appointment when someone is waiting for you. And exercising with a friend gives you a chance to talk.

Join an existing group. If starting a group is more than you want to take on, just find a weight-loss support program that has already begun, recommends Dr. Stettner. Contact local hospitals (many of which have weight-loss centers), ask your doctor for tips, or inquire at health clubs. You can also troll the Internet for like-minded people.

Have a friend on call. In addition to your weekly meetings, use the phone or e-mail to provide during-the-week support. "Call each other and see how you are doing. Ask, for example, 'How did you handle that party?'" Dr. Andersen says.

Find a group member to call for emergency times when you need someone to talk to right away, Dr. Stettner adds.

Dealing with Family and Friends

When you undertake any important effort, you hope you can count on the people closest to you for support. But despite everyone's good intentions, it isn't always that simple. "People don't always anticipate problems with social support. They assume there will be support. But we've found that it may break down," Dr. Stettner says.

When you make the lifestyle changes needed to lose weight, you also inadvertently make changes in the lives of those around you. Those changes may make others feel put upon and lead them to resist your efforts. In other cases, friends and family may think they are helpful, but they actually make the process harder by nagging you.

But with your help, your family and friends will rally around to give you the encouragement you need. You just have to show them how.

Get them in your corner. Before you embark on your weight-loss program, gather your close friends and family and tell them what you intend to do. "It frequently helps to talk to people and explain what you are doing," Dr. Stettner says. List the reasons why you want to lose weight and why this change is important to you.

Use "I" statements. In some cases, people translate your decision to lose weight as a comment on them personally. So they may undermine your efforts or withhold their support. To deflect this, use "I" statements when explaining your situation, Dr. Stettner says. Say things such as "I want to lose weight because of my health" or "I'd like to buy healthier food so that eating is easier for me."

Be specific with your needs. Tell your loved ones exactly what you need from them. "The more precise you can be, the more likely it will work," Dr. Stettner says.

Don't just say, "I need your support." Instead say, "Eating at night in front of the television is a problem for me, so I'd like you to not to bring food in from the kitchen."

Living Proof
PANEL

Setting an Example

From the first day that my son, Sam, was able to eat solid foods, I always made sure that he had plenty of fruits and vegetables in his diet. He was probably 3 years old before he ever had any candy. So I was probably more conscious of what he ate than I was about my own dietary habits.

Now I realize that it is very important for me to set a good example for him about eating well and exercising. In many ways, this program has helped me get back in touch with the examples my parents set for me as a child. My parents were always very healthy. They've had their own ups and downs with their weight. But my dad has always exercised, and my mom always made sure that we had good, healthy food.

As a mother myself now, I think the example we set for our children really does make a difference.

Also, tell them precisely what you don't want. For example, inform them that nagging you every time you put something in your mouth is not what you consider support.

Point out that you are a team. If your immediate family members aren't being helpful, remind them of all the things you do for them. "Tell them, 'You guys count on me. Now I am asking you to be sensitive to a few of my needs,'" Dr. Stettner says. Don't try to elicit guilt, he adds, but highlight that they indeed owe you this courtesy. Ask that you all be in this together.

Assert yourself. If your friends or family aren't willing to be supportive, be clear that you're going to do this anyway. "Tell them, 'If you are not going to be supportive, don't get in the way. Don't judge; don't make comments.' Even a sense of toleration can be helpful," Dr. Stettner says.

Start Living It Up

People trying to lose weight sometimes place their social lives in a perpetual holding pattern: "When I lose weight, I'll go back to school." "When I reach my goal, I'll go out more often." "When I can fit into a size 10, I'll take up a hobby . . ."

Get your life off hold now.

"I have people tell me that they aren't going to meet people until they lose 50 pounds. That is nuts. Get on with living. Don't just focus on your weight," says John P. Foreyt, Ph.D., director of the Behavioral Medicine Research Center at Baylor College of Medicine in Houston and coauthor of *Living without Dieting*.

Even though it may not directly affect weight loss, enjoying life is a form of social support. You feel good about yourself, and you realize that your worth is not defined by your weight. The friends you make and the good times you enjoy will strengthen your resolve to succeed. So get up and get out.

Enroll in school. Sign up for arts and crafts classes or academic classes at a local college, Dr. Foreyt says. Developing a skill and working your intellect makes you feel good about yourself. Once you develop an interest, you realize that there is a lot more to you than your weight—and others think so, too.

Get involved. What do you like to do? What are your hobbies? What civic organizations interest you? Answer these questions, then get involved, Dr. Foreyt suggests. Being active improves your self-esteem and introduces you to others who will support you.

"It leads people to make lifestyle changes. And you'll feel better about yourself," Dr. Andersen adds.

Go out. Don't let your weight turn you into a social hermit. "Many people cut themselves off from doing things like going out with friends after work," Dr. Andersen says. Get out there and have fun. Closing yourself off to all social events will only make you feel more isolated.

Exercising on Your Own

OF THE MORE THAN 195 MILLION ADULTS LIVING IN THE UNITED STATES, 6 OUT OF 10 DON'T EXERCISE ONE IOTA. WHAT'S MORE, ONLY 1 IN 10 ARE ACTIVE ENOUGH TO BE PHYSICALLY FIT. WITH THAT MANY SEDENTARY FOLKS HANGING AROUND, ODDS ARE THAT YOU KNOW A FEW YOURSELF.

Heck, there's a pretty good chance that those are the only people you know. And that can be the highest hurdle for new exercisers who are trying to make activity a daily part of their lives: finding the motivation and discipline to go it alone.

"Lots of women find themselves without an exercise partner, especially as they get older and have more family and job responsibilities to tie up their time," says weight-loss expert Dr. Ross Andersen of Johns Hopkins University School of Medicine.

"And many of their friends are becoming increasingly busy and sedentary as well," he adds. "Not having a buddy can definitely make it harder to exercise on days when you don't feel like it. But you can be just as successful exercising on your own if you set up the same motivation and support systems for yourself as you would have with a good partner."

Here are several ways to make your solo efforts work for you.

Find a friend. "When we look at all the factors that predict whether people will be successful at losing weight, outside support is always one of the most important things they need," Dr. Andersen says. That support doesn't have to come from a fellow exerciser. Rather, it can be anyone who takes an interest in what you're doing.

"Find a close friend or coworker who will ask how things are going, who will encourage you when you're feeling low, and who will give you a pat on the back when you make progress," he advises.

Ask for family assistance. Your husband and kids don't have to join you on your daily walks, but if you want to be successful, you're going to need their help, says Dr. Andersen.

"Women often have trouble asking for assistance because they're used to being the caretakers. But it's essential," he says.

Tell them your goals and how you need their help. If you don't have enough time to work out, delegate a couple of the chores that you usually do. If you can't resist certain foods, ask that they not be brought into the house.

"And don't feel guilty about it. They all have their needs. You deserve yours. Your family will easily adjust," Dr. Andersen says.

Make some music. "Researchers find that people who exercise to music exercise longer and feel as if time goes more quickly," says Joyce A. Hanna, associate director of the health improvement program at Stanford University and an exercise physiologist in Palo Alto, California.

Music also helps you maintain a brisk, steady pace. And it lifts your mood even before you start exercising. You can buy special music to exercise to, like the kind aerobics instructors use. Even better, make a couple of tapes of songs you find upbeat and inspiring. Just keep the headset off when you're walking in potentially unsafe areas, like along a road.

Work out your problems. Solo exercisers often have trouble pulling themselves away from their work to exercise, Hanna says. To make it easier, pick one particularly perplexing dilemma and set it aside to ponder during your workout hour.

"Exercising gets your blood flowing, clears your mind, and brings you clarity. Solutions come to you more quickly when you're out walking than when you're behind your desk pulling out your hair," she says. Just take along a pad and pen to make notes.

Plan your progress. Part of the fun of working out with other people is that you challenge each other, Hanna says. And without someone to push you, it's easy to fall into a rut without making much progress.

"To combat this, write down some goals and keep track of their progress," she says. "Let's say you're walking an 18-minute mile right now.

Living Proof
PANEL

O Solo Mio

I live alone and have a long commute to work, where I put in long days, so I'm pretty much on my own when it comes to eating better and working out.

In terms of nutrition, going it alone is helpful because I'm in charge of what food is and isn't in the house. I keep lots of high-fiber fruits, vegetables, and grains around, and I don't buy any junk foods. The exercise part is harder. It works best for me to use exercise as a way to start my morning and as stress breaks during the day.

I get up and ride my bike on the indoor trainer for 10 to 15 minutes in the morning. It's a great way to wake up, and I don't have to get up that much earlier to squeeze it in. Then I try to take two 10-minute walking breaks during the day or fit in a longer walk on my lunch hour.

Sometimes I can get a coworker to join me. Sometimes I'll take a quick walk alone to clear my head. Either way, by the end of the day, I've exercised 30 to 40 minutes without needing to be disciplined enough to schedule a big block of time to work out on my own.

Set a goal to be able to walk a 14-minute mile in a couple of months. Find a long hill and set a goal to make it to the top without stopping. It's motivating to set goals, and it's satisfying to reach them."

Find a league of your own. Playing games like volleyball or softball can provide much-needed exercise and make you feel like a kid again.

"Almost every town has adult leagues for people who love to play sports but have no one to play with. Just check the local activities listing in your newspaper or try the town's Web site for contact information," says Laura Senft, a registered physical therapist at the Kessler Institute for Rehabilitation in West Orange, New Jersey.

Not into sports? Look into local walking or hiking clubs for less competitive organized activity.

Become a regular. You can get the benefits of working out with a buddy by simply joining a workout class, says personal trainer Michael Bourque of the Center for Health and Wellness of the Central Florida YMCA.

"Exercise classes don't just make working out more fun, they provide a sense of belonging for solo exercisers," he says. "You get to know other people who come regularly, and they come to expect you there, which gives you a sense of accountability."

Make it a great escape. "For many busy women, their workout time is the only time they have to gather their thoughts without interruption," says John D. McPhail, senior health educator at the Michigan Public Health Institute in Okemos.

To make exercise feel more like a treat than a chore, try scheduling it on your calendar as a mental health break. That way, you're less likely to feel as if you're going out to exercise alone and more likely to feel as if you're pampering yourself with some stress-busting solo time.

Start a rewards program. It won't be as hard to get yourself going if you know you're going to reward yourself for your hard work, says exercise therapist Paul Konstanty of the University of California OrthoMed Spine and Joint Conditioning Center.

"Start an exercise log, and build in rewards at various intervals. After accumulating 50 miles of walking, for instance, treat yourself to tickets to a show," he suggests. Map out the rewards in advance, and you'll have prizes to look forward to for months to come.

Exercise altruism. Having trouble exercising for yourself, by yourself? Pick a charity and do it for others, suggests exercise physiologist and certified personal trainer Ann Marie Miller, fitness director of the New York Sports Clubs in Manhattan.

"Sign up for charity walks, runs, or bike rides. It'll give you something to work for, and you'll feel good about helping a cause that's important to you," Miller says.

GOAL

Choose the Right Fats

A BOWL OF FRESH-FROM-THE-GARDEN VEGETABLES DRIZZLED WITH OLIVE OIL, A SPLASH OF VINEGAR, A SPRINKLING OF FETA CHEESE, AND A HANDFUL OF CALAMATA OLIVES. TENDER SEA BASS SEASONED WITH VIRGIN OLIVE OIL, PINE NUTS, AND GARLIC. ALL SERVED WITH A FRESH, CRUSTY BAGUETTE AND A GLASS OF MERLOT.

On the Greek island of Crete, where this is a typical lunch, it's no surprise that residents eat a diet containing a flavorful 40 percent fat. What's shocking is that, on average, Americans consume 6 percent less fat but suffer about 24 times as many heart attacks a year. Wine was the tasty staple originally praised for providing this heart protection. But a deeper investigation revealed that olive oil, nuts, and fish, which are as prominent on Cretan tables as pasta in Italian restaurants, are the Greeks' buddies, too.

Why? These foods provide health-promoting nutrients, two of which may strike you as unlikely: monounsaturated fats and omega-3 fatty acids. That's right, fats that are actually *good* for your health and that can help with weight control.

So how can you use this strategy to stay trim and live longer if you don't happen to call the Mediterranean your home? "Rearrange your choice of fat," says Mary Flynn, R.D., Ph.D., assistant professor of medicine at Brown University in Providence, Rhode Island, and coauthor of *Low-Fat Lies, High-Fat Frauds, and the Healthiest Diet in the World.*

In other words, cutting back on fat isn't as important as choosing the right sources. So eat more foods high in monounsaturates and omega-3's—like olive oil, canola oil, nuts, and fish—and cut back on those high in saturated fats, omega-6's, and trans fatty acids—like meat, soybean oil, and processed foods, recommends Dr. Flynn.

Get Thin

Contrary to what you've probably heard, you don't have to cut out every last bit of fat if you want to lose weight. Fat doesn't make you fat. Excess calories do. So you can enjoy the full-fat Italian dressing and still lose weight if you limit your portion sizes.

Here's how: Fat can help minimize your urge for the munchies. That's why some people on low-fat diets feel constantly hungry, and that's why many diets fail. With less fat, dieters take longer to feel full while eating, so they eat more. They also get hungrier more quickly after a meal with no fat than after a meal containing some fat. Having a little of this natural appetite suppressant at each meal satiates you longer.

Fat adds flavor. Taste—or rather, the lack of it—is another one of the main reasons that people quit weight-loss diets. "Eating a moderate-fat, portion-controlled meal not only tastes better, it increases your odds of sticking to your weight-loss program," Dr. Flynn says.

Get Young

Eating a little bit of fat—of any kind—is good for you and can help slow the aging process. After all, every cell in your body needs fat to function properly. And having a little fat with your vegetables helps your body absorb those all-important fat-soluble vitamins and phytochemicals that protect you from cancer-causing, artery-damaging free radicals.

Problems occur when you get too much of certain types—namely, saturated fat, omega-6's, and trans fats. That's when you start bumping up your risk of heart disease and other chronic illnesses. But studies show that you can prolong your healthy, active years by keeping those fats to a minimum and increasing your daily doses of monounsaturates and omega-3's. Here's how these healthful fats can help you.

Healthy Fats

BENEFITS	MONOUNSATURATES	OMEGA-3'S	FOOD SOURCE TESTED
Keep Your Heart Young			
Lower total cholesterol	X		Olive oil, almonds
Lower triglycerides	X		Olive oil
Lower bad cholesterol (LDL)	X		Olive oil, walnuts, almonds
Raise good cholesterol (HDL)	X		Olive oil
Lower heart attack risk	X	X	Salmon, olive oil, peanut butter
Keep Your Life Long			
Prevent stomach ulcers		X	Olive oil, fish oil, sunflower oil
Prevent breast cancer	X		Canola, nut, and olive oils
Keep Your Brain Happy			
Reduce depression		X	Fish oil

Go for the Goal

So how can you boost your intake of monounsaturates and omega-3's without going overboard on calories? Two words: portion control. Shoot for one to three servings of these body-friendly fats a day. A serving is about 1 tablespoon of olive oil or salad dressing, or 2 tablespoons of peanut butter.

Here are more recommendations from Dr. Flynn on how to fill up on these healthful fats and stay young.

Go fish. Eat fish, preferably cold-water varieties like salmon or halibut, at least two times a week. Substituting these tasty treats from the deep for chicken or beef will not only increase your omega-3's but also lower your daily dose of saturated fat. Be sure to think pink. The pinker the fish, the more brain-friendly omega-3's it contains.

See red. The less white you see in a piece of red meat, the less fat it contains. Best buys are cuts of red meat with the words *loin* or *round* in the name. They contain not only less total fat but also fewer grams of saturated fat.

Shake things up. Most bottled salad dressings contain your heart's archenemy: polyunsaturated fats. Watch for them on the ingredient label. Better yet, make your own salad dressing by combining olive oil and your favorite vinegar with herbs or a packet of salad spices. This not only eliminates the polyunsaturated fats but also increases your daily dose of monounsaturated fat.

Go nuts. Add walnuts, flaxseed, or Brazil nuts (which are sources of omega-3's) or pistachios, pecans, or almonds (which contain monounsaturates) to oatmeal, pancakes, breakfast cereal, yogurt, pasta sauces, salads, or stir-fries. But avoid nuts roasted in hydrogenated fats, because they are packing the trans fatty acids that you don't want.

Say "hello" to full fat. What's the skinny on reduced-fat foods? Most are less tasty and contain as many calories as their full-fat siblings, so you may as well go with the real deal. An exception to the rule is low-fat dairy products. Choose dairy foods like low-fat or fat-free milk and yogurt, and low-fat cheese. They'll provide a little bit of fat to help you feel full, but they are lower in saturated fat than regular dairy products.

Look for the white flag. Most foods contain a combination of saturated and unsaturated fat. How can you tell which one predominantly presides in your meal? Saturated fats become a white solid at room temperature, whereas mono- and polyunsaturated fats remain liquid. That's why a cup of beef juices, which is chock-full of saturated fat, hardens when left out on your countertop, but a homemade vinaigrette, made mostly of unsaturated fat, remains liquid. This trick also helps you avoid partially hydrogenated fats and the trans fatty acids they contain.

Get baked. When dining out, choose a baked potato or rice instead of french fries. Most restaurants cook fries in hydrogenated shortening or vegetable oil loaded with trans fatty acids. Also, you can't control the amount of fat that goes into fried foods—another reason to avoid them.

Bet on fruit. Here's one more reason to dodge vending machines. When you toss a few coins into these dietary slot machines, you'll hit a jackpot almost every time—of trans fatty acids. Almost everything in there, right down to the Nutri-Grain bars and Fig Newtons, contains them. But what do you do when your blood sugar crashes harder than Evel Knievel jumping Vegas fountains? Choose fruit. Keep some on hand so that you don't have to resort to the vending machine.

Spray on flavor. Purchase an oil sprayer, fill it with extra-virgin olive oil, and spray it on when you cook vegetables. For a little culinary diversity, try nutty oils like sesame, peanut, or walnut. Or add a few sprigs of a favorite herb, like rosemary, thyme, or basil, to olive oil—or mix ginger and soy sauce into sesame oil. They add ethnic flavor without a lot of calories.

Go for taste. Although most of the studies highlighting olive oil's benefits used extra-virgin oil, there's no point in picking up a bottle of this greenish stuff if you don't enjoy its pungent flavor. For a healthy dose of monounsaturates—with a lot less bite—try regular or flavored olive oil or canola oil.

Skip the trans. Unless you've been a shut-in without cable TV for the past 20 years, you've probably heard that both butter and margarine can be unhealthy sources of fat. But let's face it, sometimes when you're making a meal or dessert, you have to choose one. Which is better?

Butter and trans-fatty-acid–free margarines, Dr. Flynn recommends. Regular margarine is basically a stick of trans fats. But an even better topping for bread is a spritz of virgin olive oil instead of butter.

Go retro. Avocado . . . it's not just the color of countertops and telephones from the 1970s. It's also a tasty way to add monounsaturated fat to your diet. Substitute a tablespoon of mashed avocado for mayonnaise on your next turkey sandwich. You'll lose several grams of saturated fat from your meal and gain lots of fruity flavor.

Get milk. The next time you warm yourself with a mug of hot cocoa, choose a type that you stir into milk. You're more likely to find trans fatty acids in mixes made with water.

Go with the grain. Choose whole wheat bread rather than white. You'll not only increase your fiber but also eliminate a major source of trans fatty acids from your diet.

Keep it real. Try natural peanut butter. Two tablespoons supply a healthful serving of brain-friendly omega-3's and heart-protecting monounsaturates. But unlike its processed siblings, natural peanut butter doesn't contain trans fatty acids.

Week Seven

Taking Control of Your Life

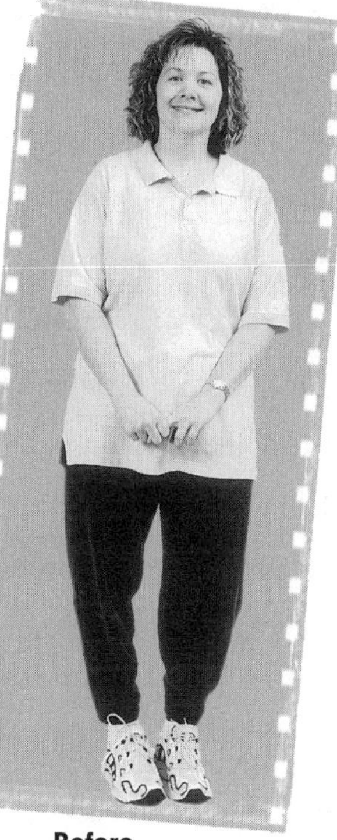

Before

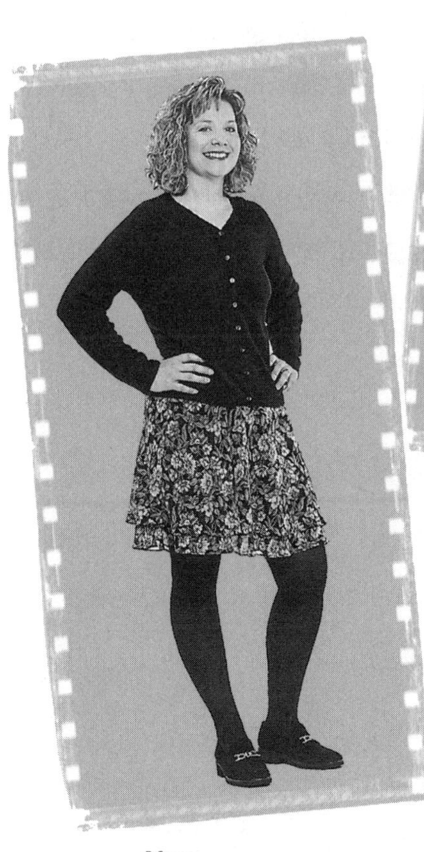

After

STRESS RELIEF HAS BEEN AN UNANTICIPATED BENEFIT OF THE PROGRAM.

—Ana Reeser

Week Seven

As you may recall, stress is a nefarious trigger that can derail your weight-loss efforts, causing you to skip exercise or crave sugar and comfort foods. It can also age you prematurely. In Week 4, you learned how to combat the triggers and react to negative emotions in healthy ways—by exercising, for example. This week, you'll learn the basics of eliminating stress at its source.

Discover how to take back control of your life and dissolve stress by using humor, relaxation techniques, and time management strategies. If you feel like you never have enough time, you can "find" time by exercising while you're doing household chores. Check the list of everyday tasks and see which ones have the best calorie-burning, fitness-enhancing benefits. Plus, you'll learn how to quell your appetite by eating several smaller meals throughout the day rather than the typical "three squares."

Destress Your Life

RESEARCHERS IN OAKLAND, CALIFORNIA, COMPARED WOMEN WHO HAD LOST WEIGHT AND KEPT IT OFF TO THOSE WHO HAD LOST AND REGAINED THE WEIGHT. OF THOSE WHO REGAINED THE WEIGHT, 70 PERCENT SAID THAT THEY ATE UNCONSCIOUSLY IN RESPONSE TO STRESS AND EMOTIONS.

Stress is the number one predictor of relapse. Stress and other emotions are major causes of overeating," says John P. Foreyt, Ph.D., director of the Behavioral Medicine Research Center at Baylor College of Medicine in Houston and coauthor of *Living without Dieting*.

Why is stress the ultimate weight-loss roadblock? Whether innate or learned, stress drives many people into the waiting arms of food. Food acts as a coping mechanism—it soothes, calms, and eases tension.

To be sure, everyone turns to food once in a while to let loose after major stress. It develops into a problem, however, when eating becomes a common sanctuary from the stresses of everyday life, says Cynthia G. Last, Ph.D., professor of psychology at Nova Southeastern University in Fort Lauderdale and author of *The Five Reasons Why We Overeat*.

For example, studies have shown that people in high-stress situations, such as firefighters and people who care for Alzheimer's patients, gain more weight than others.

Stress also robs you of your youth. Physically, chronic stress ages your heart, blood vessels, and brain. It forces your body to make more free radicals, the unstable molecules that cause signs of aging such as cataracts, gray hair, dry skin, and wrinkles. Needless to say, constant stress obliterates your vitality and vigor for life.

In today's hectic age, what can you do about stress? A lot. Obviously, you can't eliminate stress unless you hit the lottery and move to a beautiful tropical island. (But even then you'd have to worry about problems like the IRS and hurricanes and sunburn. Not to mention all the friends and relatives you never knew you had.)

Constant stress obliterates your vitality and vigor for life.

But you can reduce stress and lessen its effects on your life and your weight—all of which will help you stay on course, improve your self-esteem, and preserve your vibrant outlook on life. In the chapter Taking Your Cue—And Changing It (page 211), you learned how to immediately react to stress and negative emotions in a healthy way. Here, you will go a step further. You will learn how to use laughter, relaxation, and organization to make your life as stress-free as possible.

Laugh Away Cares—And Pounds

A grasshopper walks into a bar. The bartender says, "Hey, we have a drink named after you."

"Really?" the grasshopper says. "You have a drink called Jim?"

This joke probably made you chuckle, or at least brought a grin to your face. But inside your brain and immune system, it was doing much more.

A good laugh takes the edge off a stressful situation and actually decreases your stress hormones. Externally, it breaks tension and interjects a moment of levity. But a good chuckle also wipes out stress inside your body.

"Humor and laughter have their own ball game of neurobiology. When something makes you laugh, your biology changes substantially," says Lee S. Berk, Dr.P.H., associate director for the Center for Neuroimmunology at the Loma Linda University School of Medicine in California.

From a neuroimmunological standpoint, laughter and stress are exact opposites. That means humor and stress can't coexist. "Humor is a cross-stressor," says Dr. Berk. Like a sitcom laugh track, laughter overpowers the stress response.

Studies support the role of laughter and humor as weapons against stress. In a study at Western Carolina University in Cullowhee, North Carolina, 131 psychology students measured their stress and humor levels. Students who rated their humor low also rated their stress and anxiety levels high and said that they experienced physical stress-related symptoms.

Humor reduces stress in another way: It changes your perspective. Take, for instance, those work meetings that everyone seems to dread. You worry about what company tragedy will fall upon you next and just how the boss will humiliate you this time. (He can be very creative that way.) You can stress out about it, or you can look at it from the perspective of whoever came up with this humorous pearl of workplace wisdom: Business meetings are important. They demonstrate how many people the company can operate without.

Now you look at meetings in a whole new way. "If we can laugh at it, we can put it in perspective. It reminds you of the bigger picture in your life," says psychologist Steve Sultanoff, Ph.D., adjunct professor of psychology at Pepperdine University in Malibu, California, and president of the American Association for Therapeutic Humor. That's what humor does: It brings home the fact that many of the things you worry about are not matters of life and death.

Forget the saying "Someday, we'll look back at this and laugh." There's absolutely no reason to wait. Laugh *now*. You'll feel better. You'll look younger, too, Dr. Sultanoff says. A good sense of humor keeps you young at heart, making you look and feel younger than your years.

And the best thing about laughter as a stress reliever is that it's cheap, it's easy, and it's a heck of a lot of fun. Surround yourself with humor, and you'll find that stress will melt away. And that will make it easier to stay on course with your efforts to lose weight. Here's how.

Learn a good joke. Everyone should know at least one joke. Look for your perfect joke in books or on the Internet. We'll give you one to start:

A man and a duck are walking down the street together. Suddenly, the man notices a low-flying airplane coming right at them. So the man yells, "DUCK!!!" With an angry face, the duck yells back, "MAN!!!"

Become childlike. At some point, you got this idea that you must

Living Proof
PANEL

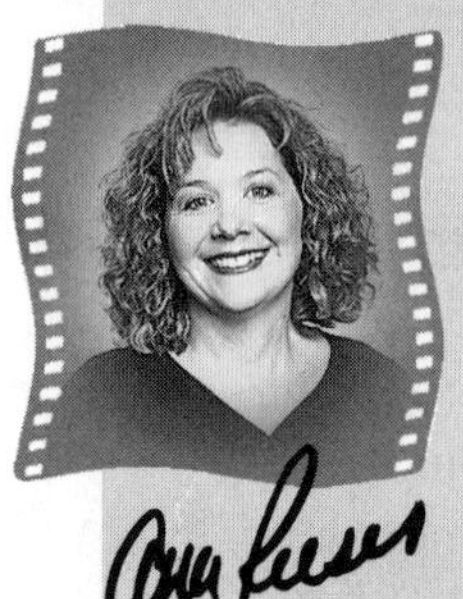

Getting Away from Stress

For me, stress relief has been an unanticipated benefit of the program. The exercises have helped me not only burn off a lot of calories but also get rid of a lot of pent-up tension.

John, my husband, has been a big help, too. He takes our son, Sam, out and does something with him for an hour or two, so I can get away and run at the track or swim laps at the pool. Just getting away and having time to myself helps a lot to lessen my stress.

act like an adult. But no one said that acting like an adult meant losing your sense of humor and playfulness. Spend time with children, Dr. Sultanoff suggests. Children haven't lost that sense of laughter and carefree spirit. Play board games, start water balloon fights, run around the yard. You'll be giggling in no time.

Wear Groucho glasses. Try being angry at a person wearing Groucho glasses. You can't. Okay, maybe you can, but you have to try really hard. Funny props like clown noses or silly ears naturally evoke laughter and general playfulness, Dr. Sultanoff says. Even looking at yourself in the mirror will crack you up. Put them on when you or those around you need a good laugh.

Play with toys. Toys aren't just for kids. Fill your home or office with basketball hoops, wind-up toys, silly action figures, or anything that grabs your fancy and tickles your funny bone, Dr. Sultanoff says.

Jot it down. If you carry around a food/activity diary, trying what Dr. Sultanoff does should be easy: Every time he sees, hears, or thinks of something funny, he writes it down in the spiral-bound notebook that he carries with him. When he needs to laugh, he reads a few passages.

Hold that funny thought. We all have a memory—whether it's from a movie, a song, a book, or that time you put the whoopee cushion on your third-grade teacher's chair—that brings us to hysterical tears just thinking about it. Find that thought and store it in your brain, Dr. Sultanoff says. Then, when you find yourself looking down the barrel of a very stressful situation, retrieve it.

Make your home "comedy central." It's been a really hard day, and the ice cream is calling. Actually, it's screaming. Drive past the supermarket to the video store, where you'll find hundreds of humorous alternatives to overeating. Laugh the cares of the day away, Dr. Sultanoff says. It may not erase the day you had, but you'll feel better without food.

Learning to Relax

The response is left over from prehistoric days: Your body goes into a natural fight-or-flight mode when faced with a stressful situation. Your muscles tense, your breathing gets shallow, your heart races, and your blood pressure inches up. Before you know it, stress takes over. Feeling powerless against this overwhelming sensation, many people turn to the comfort of food, Dr. Last says.

But you possess the power to prevent stress from overwhelming you. You don't need to buy anything or go anywhere. You just need to learn some simple relaxation techniques.

With relaxation exercises, people can train themselves to remain calm in the face of anxiety. "They have a choice. When they recognize stress, they can choose to do something about it by changing the situation or changing their attitude toward it," says Patricia Liehr, R.N., Ph.D., associate professor of systems and technology at the University of Texas School of Nursing in Houston. By changing either, you'll steer away from stress and increase your chances of staying on your path to weight loss. These techniques should be used in three ways.

As a daily exercise. The more you do relaxation techniques, the better you'll get and the more effect they will have, says Stephan Bodian, former editor of *Yoga Journal* and author of *Meditation for Dummies*. Daily relaxation calms you all day, enabling you to handle or deflect stress. Schedule 5 to 10 minutes of relaxation time in the morning and another 5 to 10 minutes before you go to sleep.

As a calming force throughout the day. Short, easy relaxation techniques interspersed with and around your activities maintains your state of calm. These little "tune-ups" keep you on an even keel, even when the pressure starts building. Decide on your own system: Use them on the hour, when the telephone rings, or during your coffee break. Or declare certain everyday activities as relaxation moments. For instance, Bodian recommends meditating during familiar functions such as washing the dishes, working at your computer, watching TV, or working out.

As an immediate reaction to stress. At that critical moment when you want to eat an entire box of chocolates or blow off exercise, relaxation techniques can save you from yourself. Even just a minute of doing a relaxation method soothes your mind so that you think before you act.

The beauty of relaxation techniques is that there are no rules, just guidelines. They shouldn't be work—they're your own fun, private oasis from stress. If one method doesn't work, try something else, says Kolleen Biel, program manager at the New Albany Health and Wellness Center in New Albany, Ohio. Using the following techniques, tailor a method that works for you, then sit back, relax, and enjoy.

Even just a minute of doing a relaxation method soothes your mind.

Deep breathing. When you stress out, your breathing naturally becomes shallow and rapid. Although it is a reaction to stress, it also compounds stress. By using your diaphragm to breathe deeply, you can slow down your breathing as well as trigger a relaxation response, Dr. Last says.

Here's how: Place your hand over your stomach below your waist. Inhale deeply and slowly. You are breathing correctly if your stomach pushes out when you inhale. Hold the breath for 3 seconds and then exhale slowly. As you exhale, say a word or phrase such as "relax" or "I am calm." Repeat 10 times or for as long as you want, Dr. Last says.

Meditation. What is meditation? As Bodian says in his book, "Just sit down, be quiet, turn your attention inward, and focus your mind. That's all there is to it." Meditation focuses you on the present moment, not the worries of the future or the regrets of the past. It triggers what Bodian calls spontaneous release—you let go of your troubling thoughts and feelings. Finally, you develop insight, allowing you to understand and possibly eliminate what causes your stress.

Meditation takes on many forms and methods, but here is Bodian's basic approach: In a quiet place, sit comfortably with your back straight. Take a few deep breaths and relax. Choose a word or phrase that has special or spiritual meaning for you. For 5 minutes or more, breathe through your nose and quietly repeat the word or phrase. If your thoughts start to wander, just come back to the repetition.

Progressive relaxation. With this technique, you tense your muscles and then consciously make them relax. Lie or sit down. Take a few deep breaths. Starting with your feet and calves, slowly tense your muscles. Hold for a few seconds, then release. Move up your body, tensing and relaxing the next group of muscles in turn—your thighs, buttocks, stomach, arms, shoulders, and neck. At the end, you'll feel lighter and calmer.

This technique also acts as a teaching tool. Because some people are always in states of stress, they can't differentiate between being relaxed and being tense. Progressive relaxation teaches you how to identify tense muscles. By becoming more aware of this, you catch yourself tensing up, Dr. Last says. And that helps you stop the stress response in its tracks.

Join the Organization

Organization frees up time and energy that you can spend on things that really matter. Not putting your glasses down in the same place, not allowing enough time to get from here to there, not saying no to another project—all of these small events add an enormous amount of stress.

Changing your outlook from "my life is out of my control, and I am under stress" to "I can manage my life and my stress" empowers you to make changes, says Jeanie Marshall, an empowerment consultant at Marshall House, an organization in Santa Monica, California, aimed at helping people and companies become more effective.

Try these simple organizational tips that will cut an enormous amount of anxiety from your life.

Set weekly and daily goals. Every Sunday night, sit down with your calendar and ask yourself, "What must I get done this week?" Make that your week's goal—everything else comes second. When you don't prioritize, you go in circles and don't get much of anything done.

"We let the urgencies of the day overrule our priorities. As we lose sight of priorities, we get into a reactive mode," says Henry Marsh, a Salt Lake City–based productivity consultant for Franklin Covey Company and author of *The Breakthrough Factor.*

Take it a step further by prioritizing your day, Marsh adds. With your week's goal in mind, each morning go over what you must get done and what you'd like to get done. Tackle what you need to do first, then handle the rest if you can. You accomplish more and feel less stress.

Learn to say no. Just because someone asks you to do something doesn't mean that you have to. In fact, the phrase "Sorry, I can't" is one of the greatest stress reducers.

"I think a lot of the things we say yes to, we don't monitor. Before you know it, we are double-booked. I don't know anyone who is calmed by that," Dr. Liehr says. If you can't take on a request—or you don't want to—politely say no.

If you need to explain, say something like, "I'm sorry I can't do that. I am very busy, and I don't feel that I could give it the attention it needs."

Be realistic. Do you give yourself 5 minutes to get from one end of town to the other? If so, your stress levels skyrocket as you speed and curse the red lights on the way there. Rationally calculate the time you need to accomplish all your tasks—and then add more time.

"There will be emergencies—computer crashes, traffic jams," says Carol Goldberg, Ph.D., a clinical psychologist and president of Getting Ahead Programs, a New York–based corporation that conducts workshops on stress management, health, and wellness. If you schedule extra time, those unexpected events won't be catastrophic.

Put things in their place. You're calm, prepared, and ready to roll when you go to look for your car keys or your glasses or important paperwork. Next thing you know, you're tearing the place apart and completely frazzled.

"It is a tremendous waste of time to have to look for things," Dr. Goldberg says. Keep items in special places: glasses on a certain table, keys in a specific drawer. File away special papers. That way, you won't waste your time or go running for high-calorie junk foods.

The Active Life

WHEN IT COMES RIGHT DOWN TO IT, EXERCISE IS TRULY A MODERN CREATION. FIFTY YEARS AGO, PEOPLE WERE TOO BUSY SCRUBBING FLOORS, CLEANING WINDOWS, AND TILLING THE GARDEN TO THINK MUCH ABOUT JOGGING AROUND THE BLOCK. AND YOU KNOW WHAT? THEY WERE A LOT THINNER.

"Technology has made our lives easier, but it has also taken a lot away from us, especially when it comes to health and fitness," says Joyce A. Hanna, associate director of the health improvement program at Stanford University and an exercise physiologist in Palo Alto, California. "Because of modern conveniences like fast foods, ATM machines, remote-control devices, home shopping, and the Internet, we burn an average of 800 calories a day less than we did just 25 years ago."

That's pretty dubious progress, considering that an extra 800 calories a day equals an additional pound every 4½ days. "This is why our waistlines keep on expanding despite how much we keep preaching about exercising," says Hanna.

There is a simple solution to this modern madness: Take a step back in time and start doing things for yourself. "You'll be surprised how doing just a few simple tasks, like making dinner or washing your car the old-fashioned way, not only is enjoyable but also can help you feel younger, healthier, and more fit," she says.

Add enough of these everyday tasks to your daily life, and you can actually get some of the same health and fitness benefits that you would get from taking a regular aerobics class or working out on the stairclimber. In a 2-year study of nearly 200 overweight, sedentary folks, researchers at the Cooper Institute for Aerobics Research in Dallas found that those who upped their daily physical activity to at least 30 minutes a day—for example, by taking the stairs at the office, walking around the soccer field during their kids' practices, or gardening—had about the same improvements in fitness, blood pressure, and body fat as did people who embarked on structured exercise programs at a gym for 20 to 60 minutes, 5 days a week. And a study at Johns Hopkins University in Baltimore actually found that women who boosted their daily activity levels were better able to maintain their weight loss than exercisers with structured programs.

Grow Your Garden, Shrink Your Belly

Digging, fertilizing, planting . . . gardening is one of Americans' favorite activities. All of this physical effort yields tons of benefits besides the fresh fruits and vegetables. "Gardening can be a healthy physical workout," says James Rippe, M.D., associate professor of medicine at Tufts University School of Medicine in Boston; director of the Center for Clinical and Lifestyle Research in Shrewsbury, Massachusetts; and author *Fit over Forty.* "But it's much more than that. There's a spiritual well-being that comes with planting seeds and watching them grow. It returns that sense of wonder about life that we have when we're young. I've seen people live long, healthy lives—a fact that I attribute largely to their love of gardening."

Plus, if you garden enough, you'll have the pleasure of enjoying the fruits of your labors while shrinking your waistline. Consider this: Mennonites, who spend most of their days working the land, eat about 500 more calories a day than most Americans, including more fat, but they are leaner and have lower blood pressure and cholesterol levels.

Are vegetables not your passion? Try flowers, ornamental hedges, or even an herb bed. Here are some ways to work out your whole body even while you're smelling the roses.

Bury your work stress. For the best fitness (and the best garden), plan on working in the garden at least three times a week for 30 minutes to an hour each time. "Try making a trip to your garden a postwork ritual," says Michelle Edwards, a certified personal trainer and a health educator for the Cooper Institute. "What better way to unwind than to drop everything,

20 Ways to Burn 150 Calories—Or More!

Even the most basic activities can be powerful weight burners—as long as you do them regularly. Here are some activities and the number of calories they burn per hour (based on a 150-pound person).

ACTIVITY	CALORIES BURNED PER HOUR
Moving furniture	408
Shoveling snow	408
Mowing the lawn (power-driven push mower)	306
Painting walls	306
Washing the car	306
Fishing	272
Planting seedlings	272
Raking leaves	272
Sweeping sidewalks	272
Grocery shopping	238
Bowling	204
Woodworking	204
Cooking	170
Croquet	170
Playing with kids	170
Pushing a baby stroller	170
Sewing (machine)	170
Vacuuming	170
Shopping at the mall	157
Ironing	156

change into some grungy clothes, and go out and play in your garden?" That nightly hour of gardening will burn off not only the day's stress but also about 340 calories.

Walk, admire, and warm up. Mulching and digging can be tough work. To avoid pulling a muscle while you're pulling weeds, take a 10-minute warmup stroll around your yard and garden. Before digging in, spend some time admiring your work and making mental notes of what needs to be done, suggests Edwards.

Hoe, rake, and pull. Gardening is a total-body workout. To give your arms, shoulders, and upper-back muscles a healthy workout, try raking leaves, hoeing the soil around your plants, pulling weeds, or turning your compost pile. Over time, you may notice your arms getting firmer and stronger from lifting and carrying buckets of dirt, tools, and produce to and from your garden, Edwards says.

A morning of housecleaning will burn more than 500 calories.

Shovel for thigh strength. Want shapely legs? Dig that flower bed a little deeper. Digging with a shovel targets and tones your derriere and upper legs. Balance the workout by operating the shovel with different feet. For a while, use your right foot to push the shovel into the ground and use your left foot for balance and support. Then switch. Always keep your knees slightly bent for better stability and back comfort, says Edwards.

Protect your back, straighten your posture. All the bending, lifting, and stretching you do in the garden can build up your back muscles, giving you a stronger, younger posture, Edwards says. But it's also important to maintain correct posture while you garden. Here's some advice from the American Council on Exercise.

- When digging with a shovel, don't twist your back. Instead, lift your front foot, point it in the direction you want to move the dirt, and turn your whole body.
- Concentrate on your breathing. Don't hold your breath, and be sure to exhale when you exert force. For example, exhale as you lift a heavy load, inhale as you lower it.
- When lifting heavy planters or wheelbarrow loads, be sure to bend your knees and lift with your legs, not your back.

Mow off pounds. Fresh grass clippings make the perfect, weed-suffocating mulch for your garden—and mowing the lawn is a great way to burn off body fat. Even if you use a power mower (the kind you push, not ride), a 150-pound person will burn more than 300 calories in an hour, says Edwards.

Stretch in the sunshine. Gardening is a labor of love, so it's easy to overdo it without even knowing it. "When you're gardening, you also tend to repeat a lot of the same motions, like squatting and pulling. It's a good idea to take short breaks, stand up, and stretch your muscles out," says Edwards. Also, remember to take a few minutes and stretch your arms, legs, and back when you're done.

A Clean House and Slim Hips

We admit it. Housework is not the sexiest of activities—or the most fun. But sweeping out the cobwebs can be cleansing for your mind and slimming for your body.

"If you take all the little routine chores you want to accomplish around the house and add them up, you have a heck of a workout," says Amy Goldwater, a certified fitness specialist and fitness advisor to the TOPS (Take Off Pounds Sensibly) Club in Milwaukee. "It's also a good chance to work out frustrations and spend some time thinking through things that are happening in your life. Plus, you have a great sense of accomplishment when it's all done—and the house looks terrific."

Do it in sets. Lots of women are so busy cooking, cleaning, and driving around that they think they don't have time to work out, says Michael Bourque, certified personal trainer and personal training coordinator for the Center for Health and Wellness of the Central Florida YMCA in Oviedo. "But if they plan their housework right, they can get as good a workout at home as they would at the gym."

For the biggest calorie burn, write down all the household chores you want to accomplish that day, then do them all without stopping. Try for a 45-minute session, suggests Bourque. "Then stop, assess your progress, and do another set." A morning of housecleaning won't just give you a clean house. After a few hours of doing chores, a 150-pound person will also burn more than 500 calories.

Work on all levels. People often divide their housework by the levels of the house, cleaning one floor at a time. But to get the best workout, going up and down the stairs makes a difference. "By alternating upstairs and downstairs chores, you've added a couple of flights of stairclimbing to your day's workout," says Goldwater. "Over time, that adds up."

Do the Hoover maneuver. Some days, you may have more energy than others. When you're feeling eager to go, and your regular housework isn't pushing your body the way you'd like, work some strength-training moves into your cleaning routine, says certified international lifestyle fitness expert Lynne Brick, owner of Brick Bodies Health Clubs in Baltimore. "A classic example is what I call the Hoover maneuver," she says. "Just take giant steps while you're vacuuming. Dip one knee down into a lunge, then stand straight as you bring the vacuum back."

Of course, you won't do that all over the house, but taking six to eight giant steps with each leg will give your hips, thighs, and butt a healthy workout. "You can do similar things while dusting or just straightening up," says Brick. "Pick up a 5- to 10-pound object and curl it 10 times with each arm. Be sure to hold your abdominals tight and keep your back erect. You can do this sitting in a chair or standing with knees slightly bent."

Pick a project. Let's face it, there are plenty of times when we don't want to do housework, no matter how good it is for us. "You do the dishes, and 2 minutes later, there are dirty dishes in the sink. That can be a drag," says Brick. On days when you don't have the energy to tackle everyday tasks, pick a pet project and start working on that. "Rearranging the living room is a super workout and lots of fun," she says. "Plus, making little changes and improvements to your environment keeps you feeling fresh and invigorated."

Better Health through Everyday Activities

Along with becoming more sedentary from all the time- and work-saving technology out there, we've also taken up sedentary pastimes, like watching television and surfing the Internet, says Hanna. "All these tiny changes don't seem like much one by one, but add them up, and they leave a huge difference between the number of calories we take in every day versus the amount that we burn."

Over time, the results of even the smallest movements can be dramatic. In one study, researchers from the Mayo Clinic in Rochester, Minnesota, gave normal-weight men and women an extra 1,000 calories a day. After 8 weeks, some people gained 3 pounds from all the extra calories. Others gained 16 pounds. Why the big difference?

Movement. People burn calories even when they're not exercising, as long as their bodies move. So instead of sitting still (the way we were told to when we were kids), go ahead and be a little childlike. Shift around. Swing your legs. Move your feet up and down. Every movement burns calories, says Hanna.

Of course, you don't need to be a chronic fidgeter to boost your metabolism. You simply want to find reasons to move a little more.

Start a hobby. Active hobbies are great ways to put a little movement in your life. "Fishing, woodworking, sewing, doing jigsaw puzzles, even playing cards are all activities that aren't necessarily strenuous, but they're nice ways to keep your body and mind young and active," says Hanna.

Stand up. It's possible to make normally sedentary activities a little more active, says Brick. "When you're talking on the phone, stand up and stroll around," she suggests. "When you're reading the newspaper, tap your foot. When you're watching TV, get up during every commercial break—maybe throw a load of laundry in the washer or just stand up and stretch. If you're mindful about moving, there are literally hundreds of opportunities every day."

Cook more. Most folks eat fewer calories at home than they do when they eat out. They also burn more because they're busy cooking. "Buying, chopping, and prepping the ingredients instead of popping something in the microwave oven is another way to burn calories," says Hanna.

Take an active position. The golden rule for burning more calories every day with only a tiny amount of extra effort is to put your body in active positions. Changes in blood pressure and heart rate, for example, occur when you change positions, so sit rather than lie down. Stand rather than sit, which will cause the muscles in your legs to contract. Walk around rather than stand still. These all require energy, which burns more calories, says Brick.

Eat Smaller Meals More Often

IMAGINE BEING ABLE TO BURN MORE CALORIES *BEFORE* YOU EVEN START EXERCISING. WELL, YOU CAN, SIMPLY BY EATING FIVE OR SIX SMALLER MEALS THROUGHOUT THE DAY INSTEAD OF SITTING DOWN TO THE TRADITIONAL THREE SQUARES.

That's because our bodies metabolize food more efficiently when we eat a little bit every few hours. And the benefits don't stop there. By supplying a steady stream of energy, smaller meals keep you invigorated all day, with no excessive highs or drowsy lows. In fact, they can lessen or even prevent the midafternoon energy slump that makes you long for a siesta—which teaches the lesson that eating more often isn't necessarily a bad thing.

GET THIN

How are you supposed to hold out for dinner when your head's throbbing from low blood sugar and a Snickers Bar is just a few coins away? When hunger strikes, it often takes control. Before you know it, you're feeding coins into the vending machine and inhaling that Snickers Bar. That helps explain why hunger is one of the main reasons that dieters regain lost weight.

"The greatest benefit of regular mini-meals is preempting hunger," says Karen Miller-Kovach, R.D., a registered dietitian and chief scientist at Weight Watchers International in Woodbury, New York. These little meals fill you up at the first sign of hunger—an empty stomach—long before your cravings turn you into Attila the Hungry.

Many people take the opposite approach when trying to lose weight: They eat one meal a day, usually skipping breakfast and lunch. By dinnertime, they are famished. They inhale their first plate of food, then reach for seconds and thirds before their stomachs can signal that they're full.

To make matters worse, research suggests that they usually overdo it on high-calorie fatty foods. Miller-Kovach says that mini-meals prevent overeating at dinnertime the same way they prevent overeating of snacks: They let you take control of hunger before it controls you. So by the end of the day, you'll actually eat less food.

Smaller meals can also rev up metabolism, which, at least in older women, can help them burn calories as fast as their younger counterparts, according to a study from Tufts University in Boston. When given 250- to 500-calorie meals, older women (average age 72) were able to burn the same number of calories as younger women (average age 25).

When they moved up to 1,000-calorie meals, however, the older women burned 60 fewer calories than the younger women. While that doesn't sound like much—it's the equivalent of just one fig bar a day—eating those extra 60 calories could sneak on 6 pounds in 1 year, which helps explain why many people gain weight as they age.

GET YOUNG

A 1960s study of factory workers in Prague found that those who ate small meals at least six times a day lived longer than others who ate three big meals.

More recent studies on diabetes patients may have discovered why. "People who eat small snacks every hour have lower levels of LDLs (the bad low-density lipoprotein cholesterol), glucose, and uric acid than those who eat the same food in three meals a day," says lead researcher David Jenkins, M.D., Ph.D., professor of nutrition and medicine at the University of Toronto in Canada. High levels of these three increase your risk for heart disease, stroke, and diabetes.

Too much uric acid also causes gout, a type of arthritis that usually attacks the joint of the big toe. So lowering uric acid levels by eating smaller meals may help keep a youthful and pain-free spring in your step.

Go for the Goal

Eating five or six mini-meals—or three smaller meals plus two healthy snacks—is a great way to keep hunger under control and lose weight if you follow a few simple guidelines.

Plan, plan, plan. By now, you've probably gotten the message that planning is one of the keys to successful weight loss. Here's another reason. To prevent overeating, you have to figure out at least a day in advance what you're going to eat, how much, and when. Pack healthful portion-controlled snacks, like bananas, 3 cups of air-popped popcorn, or lemon yogurt. Eat when you feel a little hungry but not famished, typically every 2 to 4 hours, says Miller-Kovach.

Stretch your three squares. You could cook six separate meals a day, but that's more work than you need to do. Instead, split regular meals in half or save a food group for later, Miller-Kovach suggests. For example:

- Breakfast: half a peanut butter sandwich on whole wheat bread
- Midmorning: the other half of the sandwich and a banana
- Lunch: ½ cup of grapes and half a turkey sandwich on whole wheat bread with lettuce and tomato
- Midafternoon: six baby carrots and a cup of soup or the other half of the sandwich
- Dinner: a piece of broiled fish and a salad with 2 tablespoons of vinaigrette
- Late evening: an orange and whole wheat pretzels or a small bowl of popcorn

Redefine "snacks." Many people think of snack foods as something out of the candy and chip aisle. But there are many healthy, slimming alternatives, including yogurt, fruit and vegetables, or a saved portion of an earlier meal. To avoid higher-fat foods from vending machines, store good-for-you snacks in your car and office, recommends Janis Jibrin, R.D., a registered dietitian in Washington, D.C., and author of *The Unofficial Guide to Dieting Safely*.

Join the breakfast club. To save calories, people often skip breakfast—but that doesn't work. In reality, Jibrin says, we overcompensate for the missed meal at lunch or dinner. If you have no appetite in the morning, drink a blended smoothie of fruit and yogurt to wake up your tastebuds, then have a light snack, like half of your lunch sandwich, at midmorning.

To help ensure that you feel like eating breakfast, avoid snacking late at night. Many people feel full in the morning if they eat less than 2 hours before bedtime.

Mini-meals are a great way to keep hunger under control and lose weight.

Combine grains, protein, and fat. A glass of orange juice alone doesn't have the staying power of other breakfast foods. It's a simple-sugar liquid that's quickly absorbed. Though tasty, it's not enough to fill you up and keep you energized.

Jibrin says that you should combine complex carbohydrates, lean protein, and fat to slow the absorption of food from your intestines. That way, you'll get a steady stream of energy and nutrients for several hours, rather than a sudden surge that makes you sleepy an hour later. Instead of having only a glass of orange juice, combine it with one egg, two slices of whole wheat toast, and a piece of fruit.

Personalize your plan. If you tend to be more hungry at certain times of the day, like in the evening, save your snacks for those hours. For instance, Miller-Kovach recommends that you eat two evening snacks instead of one. Eat a mini-dinner at 5:30 P.M., then have a snack at 7:00 P.M. and another at 9:00 P.M.

Carry a cooler. Are you on the road for business or traveling to visit family? Pack meals and snacks so that you don't have to stop at fast-food restaurants. "Invest in a mini-cooler," recommends Jibrin. Portion out foods like carrots and reduced-fat cheese cubes and chill them in your cooler. Put it on your backseat so you'll always have access to healthful snacks on the road.

Choose carbohydrates. During fits of hunger, one study from the University of Leeds in England suggests, people tend to overeat fatty foods, not carbohydrates. Those in the study who were allowed to eat as much as they wanted of either a high-carb or high-fat meal ate nearly double the calories when eating the high-fat meal—1,336 versus 677.

And it's not that those who ate the high-fat meal got more food. Both groups ate roughly the same amount. How's that possible? Because, per gram, fat has twice the calories of carbohydrates. So by snacking on carbohydrates, you can eat just as much and save half the calories.

Resort to fatty foods only if you're famished and there's nothing else available, says Jibrin. It's better to have some chips than to have a 5- to 7-hour stretch with no food in your stomach. Going without food for even that period of time can trigger your body's "I'm starving" signals. The result is that your metabolism slows down, your blood sugar plummets, and you wind up cranky or tired.

When you do finally get a real meal, refuel with lots of complex carbohydrates, like beans, pasta, or a whole grain bagel.

Quiz

Foods You Can't Live Without—And Foods You Can

The experts say that if you have a well-balanced diet, you won't feel cravings. But try convincing your mouth of that when it starts watering for a chocolate bar.

Let's face it, there are some foods you might not miss if they disappeared from your diet—and then there are goodies that you just don't want to give up. The good news is that you don't have to sacrifice your favorites, so long as you concentrate on fitting them into a balanced diet, says Roxanne Moore, R.D., a registered dietitian, coordinator of nutrition education at Towson University in Baltimore, and spokesperson for the American Dietetic Association.

Take this quiz to find out how to keep eating your favorite foods and still lose weight.

Circle one answer per question.

1. What's your favorite breakfast meal?
   a. Chocolate chip pancakes
   b. Breakfast sausage, bacon, and eggs
   c. Hash browns and toast
   d. Whole grain cereal with low-fat milk and fresh strawberries

2. What's in your brown-bag lunch?
   a. Always something sweet—a cupcake, cookies, or a bag of M&Ms
   b. Ham, turkey, or salami
   c. A sandwich, fruit, and pretzels
   d. A big salad

3. If you didn't have to worry about your health or how wide your hips grew, what would you eat for dinner tonight?
   a. A hot-fudge sundae with peanuts, whipped cream, and a cherry on top
   b. A hot and juicy Philadelphia cheese steak
   c. A rich, creamy dish of fettuccine Alfredo
   d. A hearty plate of stir-fried vegetables and rice

(continued)

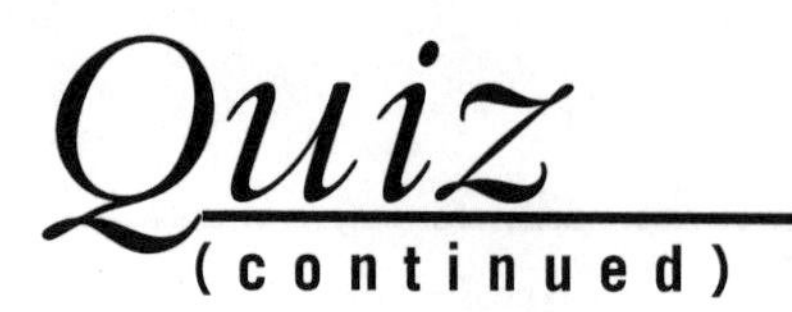

(continued)

4. Most nights, what role does meat play on the dinner table?

a. It's a small piece on my plate
b. It's the centerpiece of the meal
c. I eat it 2 or 3 days a week
d. I don't eat meat

5. When you feel a craving for an after-dinner snack, what do you automatically grab?

a. A candy bar
b. A piece of chicken left over from dinner
c. Crackers and potato chips
d. A piece of fruit

6. What is your favorite dish from your mother's dinner table?

a. A dessert, like strawberry shortcake, chocolate cake, or cherry pie
b. A thick slab of meat loaf
c. Homemade macaroni and cheese
d. Green bean casserole, glazed carrots, and her famous spaghetti squash

7. What's your attitude toward dessert?

a. Dinner isn't complete without it
b. I have it once in a while
c. I feel guilty eating it, so I fill up on other snack foods, like crackers
d. Fruit is the best dessert

8. What's your attitude toward vegetables?

a. A few servings a week is my limit
b. They're great as a side dish
c. I eat them on top of pizza and in pasta dishes
d. They make up most of my meals

9. What's your favorite fast-food fare?

a. An apple pie
b. A burger
c. French fries
d. Soup and salad

Score Yourself

IF YOU CIRCLED . . .

Mostly *a*s

You can't imagine life without chocolate and other sweets, so don't give them up completely. Eating small portions of your favorite dessert once or twice a week with balanced meals and snacks means that your diet will be healthy and satisfying, Moore says.

Round out your meals as much as possible with green salads, steamed carrots, and other vegetable side dishes; chicken without the skin, ground turkey, and lean types of beef and pork like loin or round cuts; and pineapple, bananas, and other fruit for snacks and desserts.

You need to realize that you can't make dessert a large portion of your meal. If you do, you'll lose out on nutrients and consume too many calories and grams of fat. The key to losing weight while splurging is to keep your sugar portions small.

Mostly *b*s

Meat most likely takes center stage on your dinner table, so make sure that you're buying the leanest cuts you can, like skinless chicken, ground turkey breast, and loin or round cuts of beef and pork. Keep an eye on your portions, too.

One portion of meat is the size of a deck of cards. (For more information on portions, see Goal: Master Portion Control on page 120.) Eating more than 6 ounces of protein a day could result in consuming extra calories, cholesterol, and fat, especially saturated fat, Moore says.

And while you may feel as though you could either take them or leave them, try to make vegetables the main dinner attraction more often. Let your sweet potatoes and salad fill up three-quarters of your plate and your chicken breast fill up one-quarter.

One area to keep an eye on is regularly making trips to fast-food restaurants for meaty meals. You're much better off cooking meat at home because you can control how much fat you're getting. Compare half a roasted chicken breast (7.6 grams of fat) to a chicken sandwich at Burger King (43 grams of fat). When you do eat fast food, choose a broiled chicken sandwich with a baked potato and a vegetable topping.

(continued)

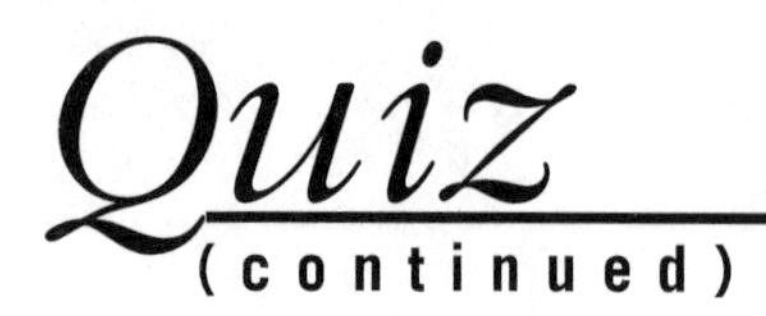

(continued)

Mostly *c*s

You have a burning need for carbohydrates, whether it's big crusty bread, pasta, or potatoes. If your cravings are really out of control, you may not be balancing your meals and snacks, Moore says. To lighten up on the carbs while still feeling satisfied, make sure that you're getting enough protein, such as 8 ounces of fat-free yogurt for breakfast, 2 to 3 ounces of tuna or turkey for lunch, and two or three golf-ball-size lean meatballs with pasta for dinner.

You also have a chance to turn your favorite food into a fat-fighting partner by choosing high-fiber foods, such as whole wheat bread, whole wheat pasta, and brown rice.

Cut way back on or eliminate high-fat cream sauces and deep-fried french fries. Instead, use tomato sauces on top of pasta, try chicken broth and garlic to season mashed potatoes, use low-fat Cheddar cheese and fat-free milk for macaroni and cheese, and drizzle a little olive oil over baked steak fries.

Mostly *d*s

Congratulations, you can't live without the foods that are ultra-healthy for you: fruits and vegetables. Keep letting them be the star of your meals, but make sure that you're preparing them in a healthy way. Simply steaming zucchini, broccoli, and corn saves on calories and helps retain the vegetables' nutrients, Moore says. In stir-fries, use cooking wines or broth instead of oil.

Balance your meals with brown rice, beans, and whole wheat bread and make sure that you get enough protein from lean meat sources. If you're a vegetarian, choose tofu, tempeh, and legumes.

The only thing that you really need to watch out for is that you don't prepare your vegetables swimming in butter, oil, cheese, or high-fat cream sauces.

Week Eight

Seeing a Difference

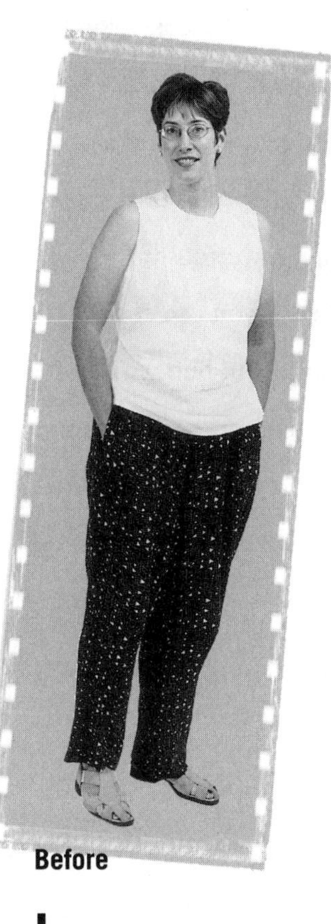

Before

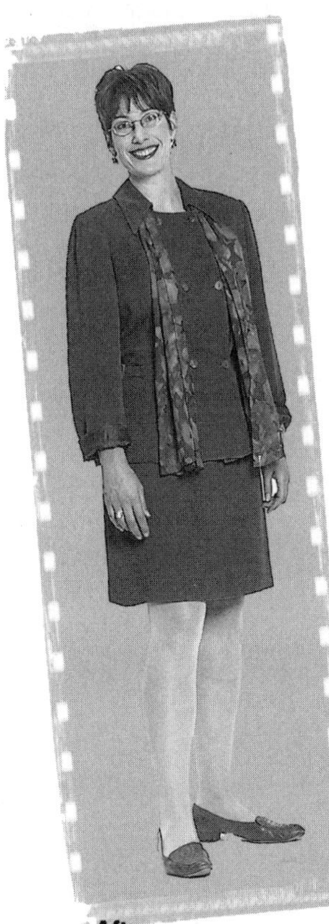

After

I PULLED ON A PAIR OF SHORTS, AND THEY PRACTICALLY FELL TO MY ANKLES. MAYBE THEY WERE MY HUSBAND'S? I CHECKED THE TAG. NOPE! THEY WERE MINE!

—Deb Gordon

Week Eight

For the past 7 weeks, you've worked on reducing overall body fat. By making gradual adjustments to your eating habits and exercising regularly, you've been getting thinner and looking younger. But if you're concerned that some stubborn trouble spots are resisting your efforts, you'll need to add some more powerful strategies to your arsenal.

In Week 8, you can choose from more than a dozen exercises to sculpt your stomach and butt, two of the most troublesome areas. You'll discover why drinking more water is one of the most effective weight-loss tools and how visualization can help you, too. Plus, now that you've shed some pounds, you may want to buy some core pieces for your new wardrobe. With these tips, you'll be able to pick out clothes that will make you feel comfortable and confident during these transition weeks.

Visualization Techniques That Work

IF YOU CAN THINK IT, YOU CAN DO IT.

SOUND TOO SIMPLISTIC?

IT'S NOT.

When you visualize an action, you use 80 percent of the neural pathways that are used in actually performing the action," says Howard J. Rankin, Ph.D., psychological advisor to the TOPS (Take Off Pounds Sensibly) Club and author of *Seven Steps to Wellness*. Just by picturing yourself thinner or envisioning yourself exercising and eating better, you are already 80 percent on your way there.

Take this classic visualization example: Imagine sucking on a lemon. Before you know it, your salivary glands kick in, as if an actual lemon were in your mouth. Your mind persuades your body that you taste a lemon, and it acts accordingly, says Emmett Miller, M.D., medical director of the Cancer Support and Education Center in Menlo Park, California; creator of the *Imagine Yourself Slim* relaxation/visualization audiotape; and author of *Deep Healing*.

Use this phenomenon to your advantage. Through visualization, your mind convinces your body that you are thinner, stronger, faster, and younger so that you act in a way that leads to being thinner, stronger, faster, and younger.

"When an image is created in a deep state of relaxation, it serves as a strong autosuggestion," Dr. Miller says. "There is a real tendency of the mind and the nervous system to do all those things that would bring about that image."

The Art of Weight-Loss Visualization

With visualization, you picture as reality the positive end result—what you want to achieve. It provides a clear, defined goal and the path to get there. So if you're not yet seeing the results you want in the mirror, take another look—this time with your imagination.

"People tend to focus on what they don't like and what they fail to do instead of getting a clear picture of what they want," Dr. Miller says.

There are three styles of visualization to help you with your weight-loss goals: visualization as motivation, visualization as a coping technique, and visualization as a stress reliever. No matter what style you use, keep in mind the three basic tenets of successful weight-loss visualization.

Wade into the deep end. To truly visualize for weight loss, it helps to be in a relaxed, calm, and thought-free state, especially at first. "Deep relaxation eliminates distracting thoughts. If not in a relaxed state, people have a tendency to think negative thoughts. But being relaxed allows the message to affect you more powerfully," Dr. Miller says.

Before doing a visualization exercise, try the following relaxation response. Find a comfortable, quiet place to sit. Close your eyes as you relax all your muscles, beginning with your feet and moving up toward your face, says Dr. Miller. Breathe in through your nose. Say the word *one*, or any word that relaxes you, with each exhale.

Think details, details, details. Don't just visualize yourself as slim. Picture the definition and the shape of your finely tuned muscles. Imagine the colors, textures, and patterns of a favorite outfit that you want to wear. The more realistic your vision, the more real it will be, Dr. Miller says.

Experience your vision, right down to your senses. This is not a game where you pretend to be someone else. When you visualize, you should be able to *feel* what it is like to be a thinner, younger you. Smell, hear, touch, and taste your vision. "The more senses that you can bring into it, the better," Dr. Miller says.

Picture This: A Thinner, Motivated You

An Olympic skier closes her eyes and sees herself maneuver and master the course. She pictures each turn, each hill, each bump in the mountain. By the time she actually skis, she has completed her run a thousand times in her mind. Then, the fun part: She visualizes herself up on that podium accepting a gold medal and hearing the National Anthem play as she enjoys the spoils of her success.

You too can use visualization just as elite athletes do. By seeing yourself as thinner, you ingrain in your mind the idea of what you want—and the actions that you have to take to get there. "By picturing yourself with a slim body, you'll find that your appetite will decrease, your desire to exercise will increase. You'll start doing the things that will bring about your image," Dr. Miller says.

Also, your image serves as motivation. You will see and feel what it's like to be a thinner, younger you. Tasting that success—even if it is through a mental image—encourages you to keep at it, even during the tough times. "The brain likes it when you show it a goal," he adds.

For support and motivation, you should visualize once or twice a day, Dr. Miller says. It takes 10 to 15 minutes each time as a beginner. As you progress, you'll be able to use these visualization techniques in 5 minutes whenever you need to.

Before you begin, find a picture—perhaps an old picture of yourself or one from a magazine—that represents what you want to look like. Pick a realistic one. "It's good to have a picture of the body you want," he says.

To start, go into a state of deep relaxation, then use the following as a visualization guide. If you have trouble using the technique during a state of deep relaxation, make an audiotape to guide you through or buy a guided-imagery tape, Dr. Miller suggests.

Your body. Picture how you want your body to look. Notice the definition of your muscles. Also focus on particular body parts—your thinner waist, your toned chin, your shapelier and firmer legs.

Your clothes. Visualize yourself in a specific outfit, one that you have always wanted to wear. See yourself in this outfit in your thinner, lighter, but also stronger body. Feel the fabric against your skin and how the clothes hug your body. Imagine every detail: the color, style, cut, and pattern.

Your look. What does the new you look like? Picture your new haircut, new makeup, new accessories. See yourself shopping for new clothes, picking out styles that you might not have worn before.

Your actions. What do you want to do with this new body? See yourself walking farther and faster or taking up new activities like jogging, biking, or waterskiing.

Your reactions. Hear the compliments people will shower on you: "You look fabulous!" "You've lost weight!" "How did you do it?" See their faces as they admire your new look. See your face as you beam with delight.

See Past the Roadblocks

Just as elite athletes visualize their paths to success and envision their victories, they also picture the obstacles that pop up. They think about what may block their way and then they visualize how they will overcome it.

You can use visualization in the same way for weight loss. Picture something that would normally lead you astray, then see yourself rise above that problem.

Basically, visualization acts as a fire drill, Dr. Miller says. "Now everybody knows the exits. You are much more ready to handle it when it happens to you. The correct response has been programmed in beforehand."

To use visualization as a coping or problem-solving technique, go into deep relaxation. Then think about the situation step by step, visualizing the most minute details. Make it as real as possible, which will increase the chance that when faced with the predicament, you'll react just as you had imagined, Dr. Miller says.

You may have your own personal circumstances that you want to visualize, but there are some that almost all people trying to lose weight want to overcome. Here are Dr. Miller's suggestions to see your way clear of temptation.

The buffet. Picture yourself walking up to the buffet table. Imagine what you take: a skinless piece of chicken breast; a side of broccoli; a whole wheat roll; a salad of lettuce, tomatoes, onions, and peppers covered in a light vinaigrette; and perhaps some strawberries for dessert. Watch yourself put the spoon down as you take small, reasonable portions. Pass over the candied yams, the cream sauce, the desserts. Walk away from the buffet as soon as you have what you want. Imagine how satisfied and happy you are with your food choices and how good it feels to push your plate away. Savor feeling full but not stuffed.

The saboteur. A friend offers you chocolate chip cookies. You say, "No, thank you." But she persists and tests your will by saying, "This one time won't hurt you," or "Oh, come on, don't ruin the fun." Look her straight in the eye and say, "I am in the process of choosing my food carefully, and I would appreciate your support on this by not offering, suggesting, or giving me food." Smile because you know that you successfully defeated a temptation. And imagine how good you feel physically, because you didn't eat the cookies, and emotionally, because you didn't give in to someone else's demands.

The fast eater. Imagine sitting down at the table. Take a good, long look at your plate. Savor the colors: the golden yellow of the corn, the deep green of the asparagus, the bright red of the tomato. Study each grain of rice, noticing the shape and texture. Smell the aroma, taking a minute to enjoy each food's distinct bouquet.

Finally, take your fork and pick up a small amount of food. As you bring it closer to your face, smell the food again. Put it in your mouth but don't chew. Let the food sit on your tongue for a moment. Then begin to chew, and roll the food around your mouth and tongue, touching all the different tastebuds. Chew the food at least 25 times, enjoying every second of flavor. After you swallow, take another moment to enjoy what you just ate before you take another bite. Take a sip of water. Begin the process again.

The exercise skipper. See yourself putting on your sneakers, anticipating your daily walk as a time of relaxation and fun. Picture your surroundings as you walk and imagine how the brisk air feels on your face. You grow stronger and leaner with each step. Visualize your lungs taking in the air and breathing it out without effort. Imagine how far you can walk and how good you feel afterward.

Take a Mental Vacation

Study after study has shown that stress is the number one reason that people fail to keep off weight. Faced with stress, your body often wants to reject all that is good for weight loss, so you wind up making bad food choices and skipping exercise.

But with visualization, you can short-circuit that response without endangering your progress. "When you use imagery, you develop a sense of mastery and control over your own circumstances," says Stephan Bodian, former editor of *Yoga Journal* and author of *Meditation for Dummies*. Stress-release visualization triggers your body to respond as if it were on vacation—tension slips away, breathing becomes slow and relaxed, and your mind lets go of all distractions.

Try one or all of the following visualization techniques to ease tension and reduce stress.

■ Imagine taking a warm shower, Bodian says. As the water falls around you, feel it wash away all your worries, problems, and concerns.

■ Imagine warm honey melting from the top of your head, Bodian says. It slowly covers your body, flowing down until it completely envelops you. Allow the warm, thick liquid to absorb all your tension and stress.

■ Picture yourself at your favorite getaway: a beach, the woods, the mountains. Imagine every aspect of the experience, says Kolleen Biel, program manager at the New Albany Health and Wellness Center in New Albany, Ohio. For example, if your dream spot is the beach, imagine seagulls flying overhead, smell the salt in the air, hear the gentle crashing of the waves, feel your toes sink into the cool sand beneath your feet.

■ Think of something that you love to do: gardening, doing needlepoint, reading a book, watching your favorite TV show, sitting in a beloved overstuffed chair, Biel says.

■ While under stress, take a second and say, "My mind is clear and relaxed. My muscles are loose and relaxed." Just the power of suggestion relieves stress and tension, Biel says.

A Taut Tummy

BELLY BULGES ARE AMERICA'S NUMBER ONE PROBLEM SPOT. ACCORDING TO A *PREVENTION/NBC TODAY WEEKEND EDITION* SURVEY, 52 PERCENT OF AMERICANS WANT TO TRIM THEIR MIDSECTIONS. AMONG WOMEN ALONE, MORE THAN 65 PERCENT TARGET THEIR TUMMIES AS THEIR MOST TROUBLING ZONES.

Why all the fuss over abs? Simply because that's where our fat goes. Though women tend to carry weight below their waists in the classic "pear" shape when they're younger, at menopause and beyond they start storing it in their abdominal areas, as men do. There, it causes all sorts of problems. It wrecks the waistline and makes pants tighter. It increases the risk for heart disease, puts extra stress on the back, and makes women look and feel older than they should.

"Abdominal fat can really weigh you down, both physically and mentally," says John Yetter, M.D., medical director at SSM Rehab Sports Medicine in St. Louis. "It's not only unhealthy for your heart and your lower back. For many people, it's the first wake-up call that they're falling out of shape. You can ignore a little weight gain here and there. But once you can't zip your pants anymore, you know you have to do something."

Of course, the reverse is also true, he adds. "When folks shed a few inches off their middles and can tuck in their shirts again, they get some spring back in their steps."

Slimming the Midsection

Though belly fat is tenacious, with just a little extra effort you can whittle your waistline down to size, says exercise physiologist Ann Marie Miller, fitness director of the New York Sports Clubs in Manhattan. "It sometimes takes a little longer to trim your abdominal region because that's where you carry your excess fat. So if you're a little overweight, you have to be a little more patient to see results."

The recipe for strong, flat abs is a mixture of daily calorie-burning activities and specific toning exercises that build tight, solid muscles. "You can easily strengthen this area with a few simple exercises," says Miller. But to really develop a flat, defined midsection, you also need to increase your daily aerobic activities. This will allow you to remove extra padding so those muscles show through.

In fact, if you do regular aerobic activity, you'll be less likely to store fat in your midsection to begin with. Researchers in Atlanta found that women who exercised, especially by walking or doing aerobics, were less likely to put weight on their waistlines than women who didn't. Women who exercised vigorously for 30 minutes a day had the best gains—17 percent less belly fat than those who exercised less. So you'll want to do at least ½ hour of aerobic activity about 5 days a week, along with the strength-training exercises described below.

Building the Abs

The abdominals are four muscles in your midsection. The most obvious one is the rectus abdominus, which runs from your rib cage to your pubic bone. It's separated into sections, which are responsible for the washboard appearance when the muscle is nicely defined. Even though the rectus abdominus is just one muscle, it's possible to work the upper and lower halves separately with specific exercises.

Other abdominal muscles are the internal and external obliques, which run from your ribs to your hips and along the front and sides of your torso. The fourth and deepest abdominal muscle is the transverse abdominus. It runs horizontally, like tree rings, across your torso. To slim your waist and flatten your stomach, you need to work all four muscles.

For the best results, you'll want to train your abs two or three times a week. "Start with two sets of 8 to 12 repetitions for each exercise. Then work up to three sets of 10 to 15 repetitions," says Miller. Always work the mus-

Get Off the Floor

Crunches are great for toning the abdominal muscles. But you don't have to spend all your time on the floor to get a flat tummy. Any aerobic exercise that requires the use of your upper and lower body will help build strong abdominals and obliques. Some of the best include:

- Rowing
- Tennis
- Cross-country skiing
- Cardio kickboxing
- Racquetball

cles slowly and with control: Count 3 seconds as you lift up, pause for a second, then count 3 seconds as you lower.

Here are the best exercises to target the entire abdominal area, says Miller. Try them all, then pick the three that work best for you. Be sure to include exercises that target your upper and lower abs (working these muscles automatically works the transverse abdominus) as well as your obliques.

Classic Crunches

"Everyone recommends crunches, and with good reason. The basic crunch is one of the easiest and most effective ways to work your abs," says Miller. "The trick to making them work is keeping proper form and doing them in a slow, controlled manner."

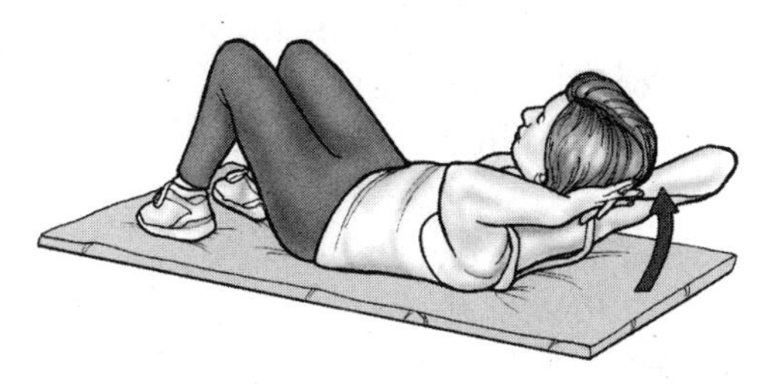

Lie on your back on a mat or carpeted floor, with your feet flat on the floor and your knees bent. Clasp your hands loosely behind your head with your elbows out to the sides. Tilt your pelvis slightly to flatten your back against the floor. Slowly curl your shoulders about 30 degrees off the floor. Don't pull up on your neck. Hold for a second, then lower. Repeat.

Muscles worked: Upper abs

Good Technique—It Works!

The abdominal crunch and all of its variations are the best ways to tone out-of-shape abs. But it's easy to do these exercises incorrectly, which can lead to a sore neck and poor results. Here are a few tips on form from the American Council on Exercise.

- Don't pull on your neck during the movement. Keep your chin a fist's distance from your chest.
- Clasp your hands behind your head. If you find this too difficult when you first begin, start with your arms across your chest.
- Don't "throw" or jerk your body to complete the movement. Keep it slow and controlled.
- Maintain pressure on the abdominals by imagining that your navel is pressing against the floor. This will help keep your back flat.
- Always exhale as you contract and inhale as you release.

Twisting Crunches

To target the obliques, you just need to add a twist to the basic crunch, says Amy Goldwater, a certified fitness specialist and fitness advisor to the TOPS (Take Off Pounds Sensibly) Club in Milwaukee.

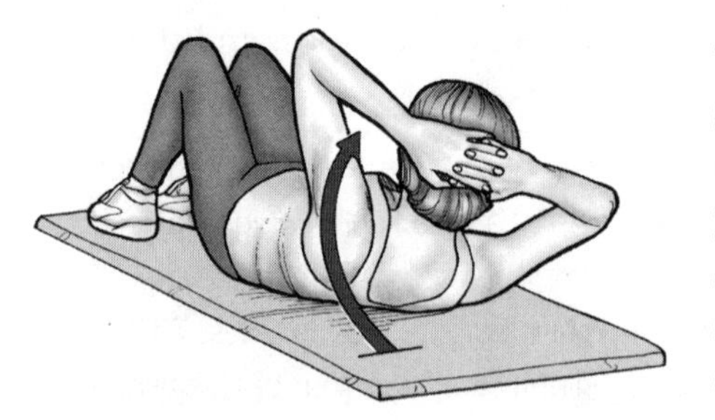

Lie on your back with your feet flat on the floor and your knees bent about 90 degrees. Clasp your hands lightly behind your head with your elbows out to the sides. Tilt your pelvis slightly to flatten your back against the floor. Slowly raise your head and shoulders off the floor, rotating your left shoulder toward your right knee as you come up. Hold for a second, then lower to start. Repeat the motion on the other side.

Muscles worked: Obliques

Chair Crunches

"To really isolate your abs during your crunches, put your feet up on a chair," suggests Goldwater. This minimizes the use of your hip muscles, so your abs have to work harder to complete the exercise.

Lie on your back with your feet up on a chair so your knees are bent about 90 degrees. Clasp your hands lightly behind your head and keep your elbows out to the sides. Tilt your pelvis slightly to flatten your back against the floor. Press your heels into the chair and slowly raise your head and shoulders off the floor about 30 degrees. Hold, then slowly lower. Repeat.

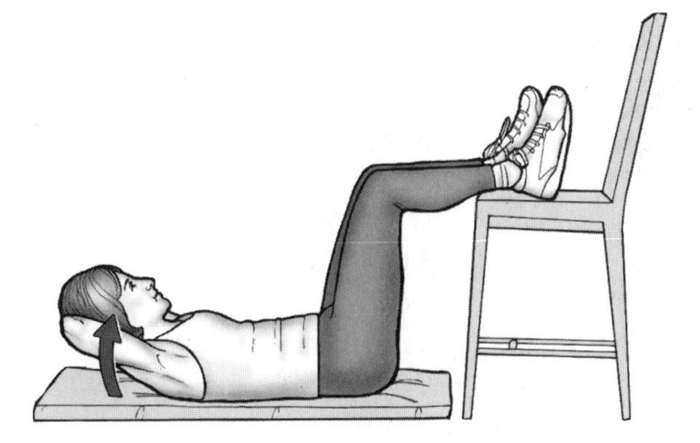

Muscles worked: Upper abs

Single-Leg-Raise Crunches

This crunch variation requires lifting one leg at the same time that you lift your shoulders. It's important to concentrate on keeping good form, so you're using your abs and not your hips or other muscles to complete the exercise.

Lie on your back with your feet flat on the floor and your knees bent about 90 degrees. Clasp your hands lightly behind your head, with your elbows out to the sides. Tilt your pelvis slightly to flatten your back against the floor. Contract your upper and lower abs and simultaneously raise your left knee and your head and shoulders, bringing your elbows toward the knee. Hold, then slowly lower. Repeat, alternating with your right leg.

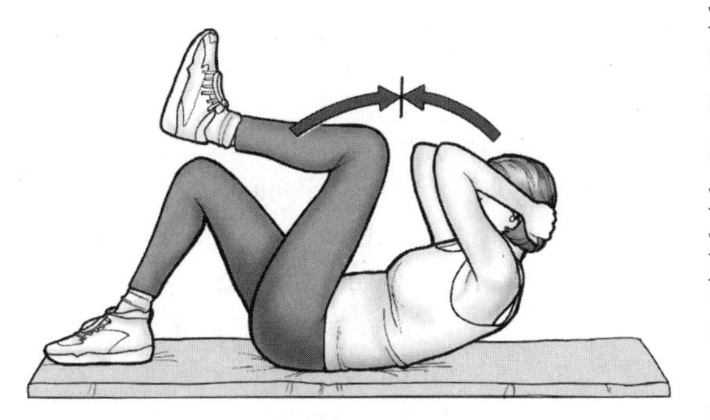

Muscles worked: Upper and lower abs

Knees-Up Crunches

"You can make regular crunches harder by lifting your legs," says Miller. "Just be sure to keep your back flat on the floor throughout the exercise."

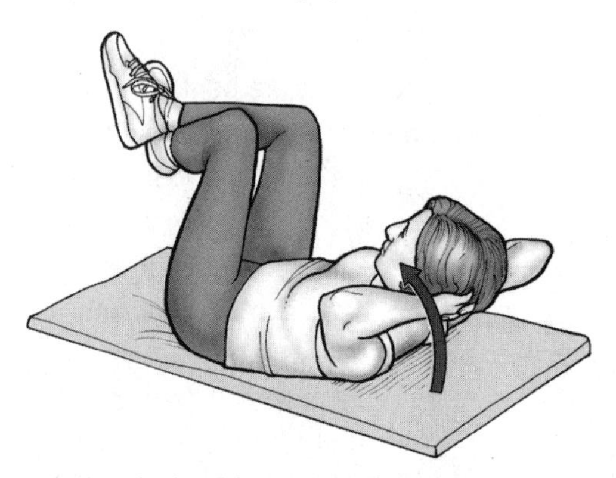

Lie on your back with your hands clasped lightly behind your head and your elbows out to the sides. Raise your legs so your thighs are perpendicular to your body and your calves are parallel to the floor. Cross your ankles and keep your knees open. Keep your back pressed against the floor. Fold your pelvis and rib cage together as you simultaneously lift your head, shoulders, and tailbone slowly. Hold, then lower. Repeat.

Note: You can make this an oblique exercise by alternately rotating one shoulder toward your opposite knee, as with the twisting crunch.

Muscles worked: Upper abs (obliques, if you add twists)

Pelvic Tilts

"With pelvic tilts, you don't look like you're doing much, but they really work your abdominals. As a bonus, they work your pelvic floor muscles, which can help prevent the urinary incontinence problems that sometimes occur as women get older," says certified fitness instructor Kelly Bridgman, wellness director for the Peggy and Philip B. Crosby Wellness Center of the YMCA in Winter Park, Florida.

Lie on your back, with your feet flat on the floor and your knees bent. Clasp your hands lightly behind your head, with your elbows out to the sides. Tighten your abs and slowly lift your pelvis as you curl it toward your rib cage. Simultaneously, press your lower back against the floor. Hold for a second, then slowly lower. Repeat.

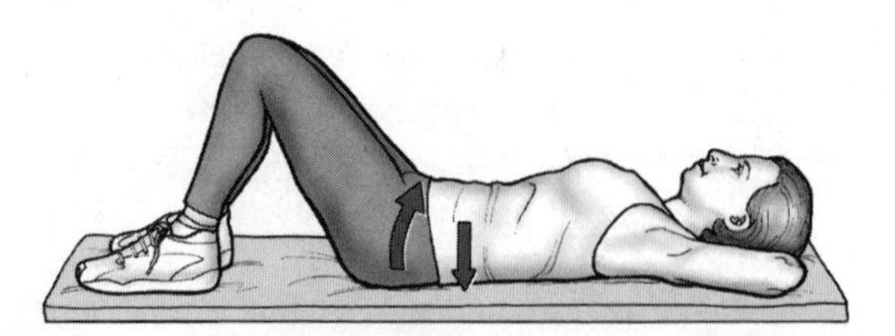

Muscles worked: Lower abs

Reverse Curls

"One of the best exercises for targeting the lower portion of your abdominals is the reverse curl, in which you concentrate on using your abs to raise your hips, instead of your shoulders, off the floor," says Bridgman.

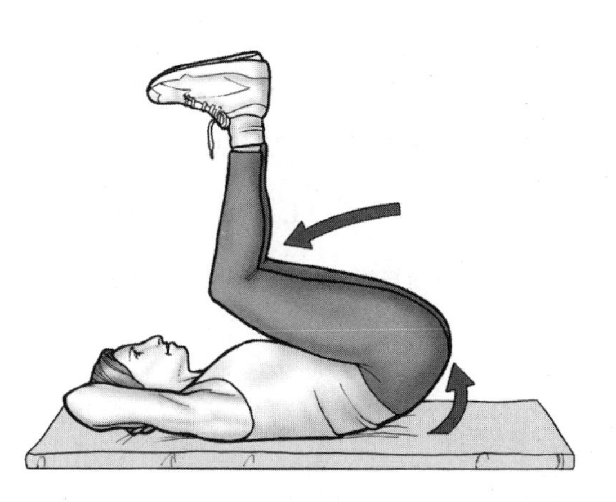

Lie flat on your back with your hands clasped lightly behind your head and your elbows out to the sides. Raise your legs so that your thighs are perpendicular to your body, with your calves parallel to the floor. Tilt your pelvis slightly to flatten your back against the floor. In a slow, controlled manner, raise your hips toward your rib cage, so your knees drop toward your forehead. Hold for a second, then slowly lower. Repeat.

Muscles worked: Lower abs

Ball Curls

Stability balls, those big inflated balls that you can sit and stretch on, are super for strengthening your abs. "When you do regular abdominal curls on a ball, you get more out of the exercise because your back is extended farther and your abs need to work harder to lift your torso. Plus, you're higher off the ground, so you're working more against gravity," says Bridgman.

Start by sitting on the ball, feet shoulder-width apart and flat on the floor. Keeping your weight centered and balanced, slowly walk your feet forward and lean back until the ball is positioned under your lower back. Clasp your hands lightly behind your head and hold your elbows out to the sides, just as you would for a regular crunch. Slowly curl your head and shoulders up slightly. Hold, then slowly lower. Repeat.

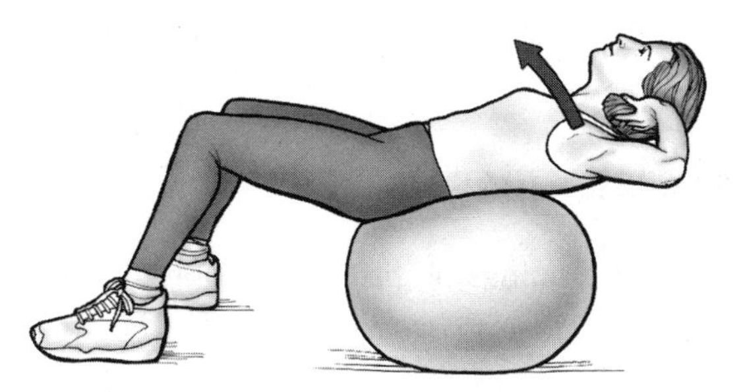

Muscles worked: Upper abs

A Tight Butt

MIGHTY APHRODITE, OR VENUS, AS SHE WAS KNOWN IN ROME, HAD SUCH A BEAUTIFUL BEHIND THAT SOME PEOPLE REFERRED TO HER AS VENUS *CALLIPIGE*—GREEK FOR "HAVING BEAUTIFUL BUTTOCKS." IT'S A SAFE BET THAT THE GODDESS OF LOVE AND BEAUTY DIDN'T SPEND TOO MUCH TIME SITTING ON THAT LOVELY DERRIERE.

We have a real problem with sitting in this country," says Majid Ali, a certified fitness instructor in Los Angeles. "We sit behind desks. We sit behind steering wheels. We sit in front of computers and televisions. Then we wonder why our backsides aren't as firm as they used to be. They've simply adapted to all that sitting."

The softening and sagging that most folks blame on aging has more to do with how we use our behinds, says Ali. "Sure, gravity has some effect on our bodies over time. But the simple fact is that the butt is a muscle—a big muscle—and if we don't use it to climb, walk, work, and play, as it was designed for, it will lose its tone and start to droop. If you want to have the high, round tushie you had when you were younger, you have to get off it and get moving."

It's a Woman Thing

It's only fair to warn you that even though toning and firming your butt isn't hard to do with the right exercises, shedding excess fat from the rear region

Tush Toning to Go!

No matter how much you work your tush muscles, they'll never show unless you also burn off some of the extra weight. Here are some fun aerobic exercises that really burn calories while giving your bottom an extra workout.

- Bicycling
- Inline skating
- Ice-skating
- Stairclimbing
- Trail walking
- Cross-country skiing
- Step aerobics
- Cardio kickboxing
- Snowshoeing
- Rowing machine

can take a little longer. Before menopause, most women naturally store fat in their hips, butt, and thighs. This fat can be stubborn, and it's often the last to go. But you can make a visible difference by regularly doing some kind of fat-burning activity, like fitness walking or strength training that targets these areas.

"It's important to set realistic goals when you're trying to trim trouble spots," says fitness instructor Kelly Bridgman of the Peggy and Philip B. Crosby Wellness Center. "You can't pick and choose where you lose weight first. And often the lower body is the last to go for women. But be patient and stick with it. And don't forget to give yourself credit for all the other improvements you make along the way."

Shape and Contour

We tend to think of the butt in terms of one big muscle. And in some ways, it is. The gluteus maximus is the bulkiest muscle in the body, and it makes up the roundest, fullest part of the butt. But its neighbors are the gluteus medius and the gluteus minimus. Collectively, these muscles form the gluteals.

A few muscles aren't technically part of the butt but do play a supporting role. These are the hamstrings, which run just below the butt down the backs of the thighs, and the lumbar muscles, which sit just above the butt. Toning these muscles along with the glutes themselves will help give you firm, shapely curves.

There are plenty of exercises that work more than one of these muscle groups at the same time. For the best all-around toning, be sure that the exercises you choose collectively hit the gluteals, hamstrings, and lower-back region.

You'll get the best results by doing glute workouts two or three times a week, says exercise physiologist Ann Marie Miller of the New York Sports Clubs. "Start with two sets of 8 to 12 repetitions, and work up to three sets of 10 to 15 repetitions for each exercise." Always do the exercises slowly and with control.

Here are the best exercises for toning the glutes and surrounding muscles, says Ali. Try them all, then pick the three that work best for you (being sure to include exercises that target all areas of the butt).

Kickbacks

"These work better than most exercises to develop really strong glutes," says Ali.

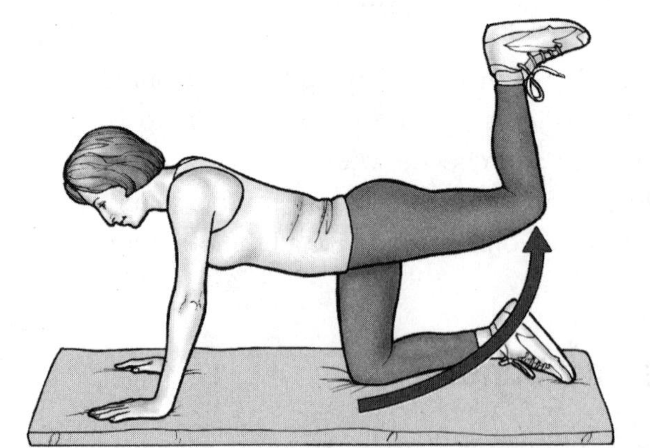

Get down on all fours. Extend your arms in front of you with your palms on the floor, your back straight, and your head in line with your back.

Keeping your back straight and your leg bent, slowly lift your left foot toward the ceiling until your thigh is parallel to the floor. Hold for a second, then return to the starting position. Complete a full set, then repeat with your right leg.

Muscles worked: Hamstrings (back of thighs) and gluteals

Way-Back Squats

"Regular squats are good for working your butt muscles, but if you really want to target them, hold on to the back of a sturdy chair and keep your butt way back," says fitness specialist Amy Goldwater of the TOPS (Take Off Pounds Sensibly) Club.

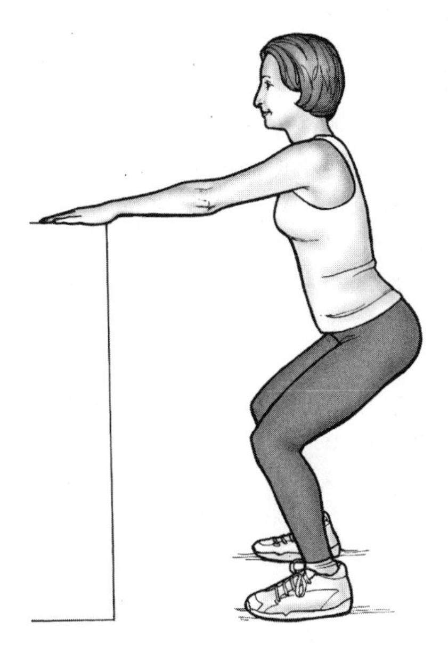

Hold on to a counter or the back of a heavy piece of furniture with both hands. Stand with your feet about hip-width apart.

Bend your knees and sit back, keeping your back and arms straight, until your thighs are almost parallel to the floor. Press your heels into the floor and stand halfway up. Lower again, then repeat.

Muscles worked: Gluteus maximus and quadriceps (front of thighs)

Resisted Side Steps

"You need a resistance band to do these exercises, but they work those outside gluteal muscles like nothing else. I guarantee your butt will be screaming!" says certified personal trainer Jana Angelakis, founder of PEx Personalized Exercise in New York City.

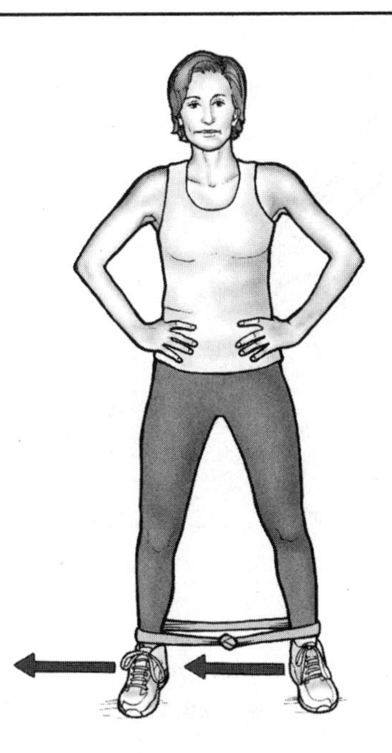

Stand with your legs about hip-width apart. Loosely tie an exercise band around both ankles.

Take 20 large side steps to the right with your knees slightly bent. Then take 20 large side steps to the left. Be sure you lead with your heel, not your toes.

Muscles worked: Gluteus medius and minimus

Romanian Deadlifts

This exercise is great for your butt, lower back, and hamstrings, says Ali. "Just perform it carefully since it puts stress on your lower back."

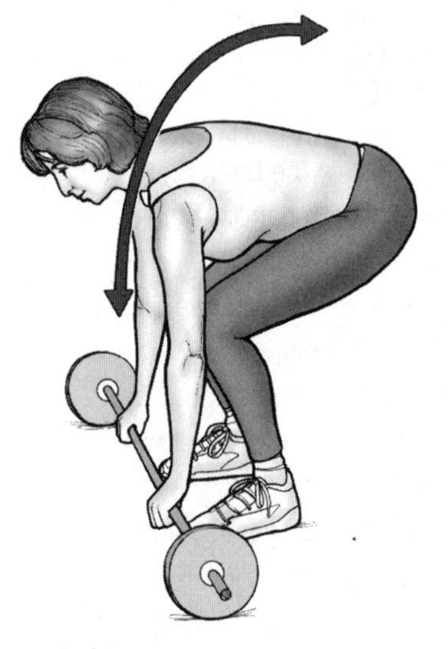

Hold a light barbell in front of you. Bend your knees slightly so that your hands hang at about midthigh. Your palms should face toward you; your hands, wider than shoulder-width apart.

Keeping your back flat and bending your knees slightly, bend forward at your hips and lower the weight toward the floor as far as you comfortably can (your knees will naturally bend). Slowly rise back to the starting position, keeping your back flat and your knees slightly bent throughout the movement. Repeat.

Muscles worked: Gluteus maximus, lower-back muscles, hamstrings (back of thighs), and quadriceps (front of thighs)

Bridges

"Bridges are easy, no-weight exercises that you can do anywhere," says Bridgman. "And they really target your glutes."

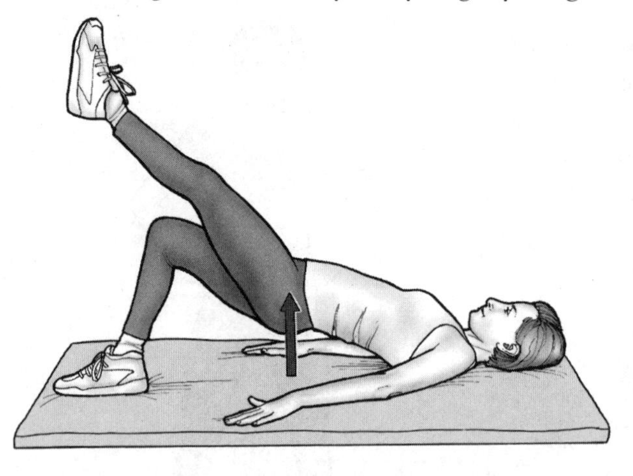

Lie faceup with your feet flat on the floor and your heels 12 inches from your butt. Hold your arms at your sides, palms down. While shifting your weight onto your right heel, raise your left leg straight up, with your foot flexed and your knee slightly bent.

Contract your buttocks while lifting your pelvis toward the ceiling. Raise your pelvis until your body is in a straight line from your bent knee to your shoulders. Don't arch your back. Hold for a second, then lower. Complete a full set, then repeat with your other leg.

Muscles worked: Gluteals and hamstrings (back of thighs)

Standing Hip Extensions

"Another very simple exercise that targets all the key muscles in your butt area is the standing hip extension," says Miller. "You can do it with ankle weights or while wearing heavy shoes if that's what you have. But it works best if you use a resistance band."

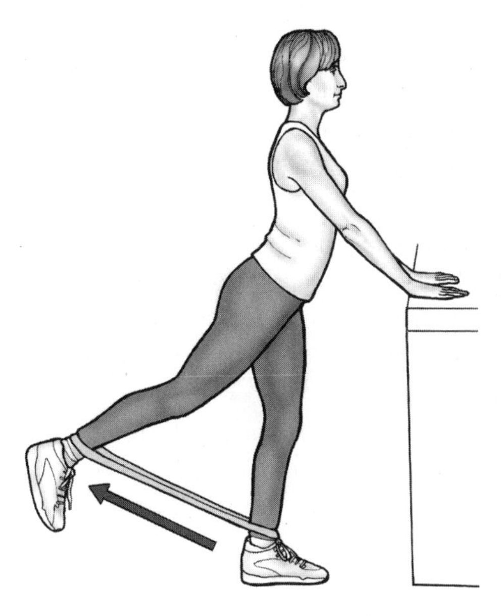

Stand facing a sturdy table or counter, with your hands resting lightly on it for support. Lean forward slightly, keeping your back straight and your knees slightly bent for balance. Using ankle weights or an exercise band tied loosely around your ankles, press your right leg back until your shin is about parallel to the floor. Hold, then slowly return to start. Complete a full set, then repeat with your left leg.

Muscles worked: Gluteals and hamstrings (back of thighs)

Grand Pliés

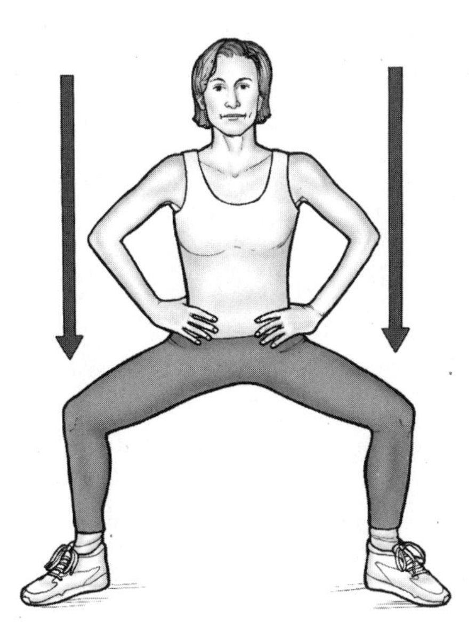

"Grand pliés take a wider-than-hip stance, so you isolate the glutes as you lower and raise your body weight," says Angelakis.

Stand with your feet wider than your hips, with your toes pointing slightly outward and your hands on your hips.

Bend your knees and lower your torso until your thighs are parallel to the floor. Do not bend your knees more than 90 degrees (they should not go beyond your toes). Pause, raise, and repeat.

Muscles worked: Gluteus medius and minimus

Leg Curls

"Leg curls give you firm, rounded hamstrings," says Goldwater. "This helps give the lower butt area a nice, toned appearance."

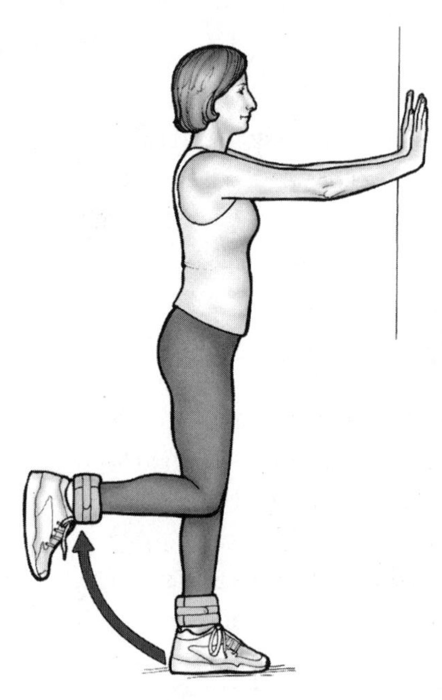

Wear either heavy shoes or ankle weights for resistance. Stand about an arm's length from a wall, holding on to it for balance. Keep your back straight and your head facing the wall.

Slowly bend your right knee, raising your right heel toward your butt, until your shin is parallel to the floor. Hold, then lower. Finish one complete set, then repeat with your left leg.

Muscles worked: Hamstrings (back of thighs)

Drink More Water

WHEN WEIGHT-LOSS SPECIALIST DONALD ROBERTSON, M.D., WANTS TO CONVINCE A PATIENT WHO DOUBTS THE FAT-BURNING POWERS OF PLAIN OLD *EAU DE TAP,* HE SAYS THIS: GIVE IT A WEEK, AND YOU WILL LOSE WEIGHT.

Hear echoes of a once-popular jingle for a quick weight-loss shake? Don't worry. Yes, you can get fast results with water. After 1 week of upping their water consumption to 3 quarts a day, Dr. Robertson's patients often lose up to 5 pounds. But unlike commercial quick fixes, water isn't a gimmick but rather an essential element of weight loss.

"Although most of us take it for granted, water is quite possibly the single most important catalyst in losing weight and keeping it off," says Dr. Robertson, medical director of the Southwest Bariatric Nutrition Center in Scottsdale, Arizona.

Our bodies are between one-half and four-fifths water, depending on the amount of lean body mass. That means that if you weigh 150 pounds, you're probably toting around close to 100 pounds of it.

In the course of a day, the average couch potato loses 2 to 3 quarts of water, depending on the climate, says Dr. Robertson. Your goal is to replace that lost fluid by drinking 8 to 10 glasses (8 ounces each) of water per day. Bump that amount up when you're physically active, when it's hot outside, or when you're traveling by plane. For every extra calorie you burn, you'll need an additional milliliter of water, or about 1 cup for every 240 calories you burn. And if you're overweight, your body's metabolic needs are greater, so have one additional glass for every 25 pounds of extra weight.

Here's how water can help you get thin and stay young.

Get Thin

Besides having zero calories, what makes water the number one weight-loss drink? For one thing, water naturally suppresses your appetite by filling your stomach up so that you eat less. It also helps your body metabolize stored fat and clear your system of wastes, Dr. Robertson says.

Here's why: Your kidneys depend on water to do their job of filtering waste products from your body. In a water shortage, they need a backup, so they turn to your liver for help. Your liver is responsible for mobilizing stored fat for energy. But if the liver has to do some of the kidneys' work, it can't operate at full throttle.

As a result, the liver metabolizes less fat. That means more fat remains in your body, resulting in less weight loss, says Dr. Robertson.

Even slight dehydration, especially the kind caused by taking diuretics, can cause a 2 to 3 percent decrease in your resting metabolic rate, says Wayne Askew, Ph.D., director of the division of foods and nutrition at the University of Utah in Salt Lake City. Since your resting metabolic rate—the number of calories burned when you're doing nothing—accounts for most of the calories you burn daily, even a small drop in it may have a significant long-term effect.

The bottom line is that when your body gets the water it needs to function optimally:

- Your body burns more fat.
- Fluid retention is alleviated.
- You feel less hungry.

Get Young

Meeting your daily water quota could make you feel more energetic and more alert than a kid on caffeine, according to Susan Kleiner, R.D., Ph.D., affiliate assistant professor of nutrition at the University of Washington in Seattle and coauthor of *Power Eating*.

The World's Simplest Weight-Loss Secret

It's so easy and effortless that it doesn't seem possible. But it's true: Drinking ice water can help you burn more calories.

Here's why: Ice water is absorbed faster than room-temperature water, says Dr. Donald Robertson of the Southwest Bariatric Nutrition Center. When you drink water that's 40°F or colder, your body has to raise the water's temperature to your body's temperature. In the process, it burns slightly less than 1 calorie per ounce of water. So if you down eight glasses of cold water a day, you'll burn about 62 calories. That adds up to 430 calories a week, or about 6½ pounds' worth of calories in a year.

Water is the most abundant compound in the human body, filling virtually every space in your cells and the space in between them. Every organ and bodily function depends on it. But when you don't drink enough, your cells start drying out. To quench their thirst, they start sucking fluid out of the bloodstream, leaving your blood sludgy, like olive oil left in the refrigerator. As a result, your heart has to pump harder to push the blood through, which can tire you out.

You don't have to lose much fluid to become mildly dehydrated. Just a 1 to 2 percent loss in body weight can affect your performance. Not getting your daily dose of this neglected but essential nutrient also increases your risk for developing everything from the common cold to certain types of cancer.

To tell if you're getting enough fluid to keep you in tip-top shape, check the color of your urine. It should be the color of straw, Dr. Kleiner says. If it's dark yellow or has an odor, you need to drink more water.

Go for the Goal

So how tough can it be to drink the right amount of water? Well, since so many of us don't do it, it's obviously tougher than it looks. Here's how to make it easy.

Make a water plan. Put together a schedule that reminds you to drink, suggests Dr. Kleiner. By the time you feel thirsty, your body has already lost 2 percent of its fluid, so it's important to drink before you're thirsty.

"You need to have a water plan, just like you have a food plan," she says. Drink a couple of cups when you first get up and throughout the day. Skip it in the evening so you don't have to get up at night.

Be sure to have water with every meal. Keep a pitcher of cold water in the fridge and another on your desk at work so that you're less tempted to drink coffee. "Since the thirst mechanism isn't a good one for maintaining hydration, I like to use visual cues, something kept right in view that's going to remind me," she adds.

Measure it out. Fill a bottle or pitcher with your daily water allotment and keep it on your desk at work or on the kitchen table at home. "Your goal is reached when the pitcher is empty," says Elizabeth Somer, R.D., a registered dietitian and author of *Age-Proof Your Body*.

Perk it up. Some folks just don't like the taste of water, especially what comes out of the tap. Try adding a twist of lemon or lime, mixing in a little fruit juice, or getting one of those filtration systems that not only improves the taste but also takes out contaminants. Or you can buy bottled water. "The point is, find water that you like," says Dr. Kleiner.

Quench your hunger. "Many people don't recognize the difference between thirst and hunger," says Dr. Kleiner. When her patients wake up in the middle of the night hungry, she suggests that they drink a glass of water first and wait 10 minutes to see if they're still hungry. Before the time's up, they're back catching their Zzzs.

Drink two glasses of water before every meal. Besides keeping you hydrated, Dr. Robertson says that drinking two glasses of water can make you feel less hungry, possibly reducing your food intake and aiding weight loss.

A Wardrobe in Transition

IT MAY BE AS OLD AS THE QUESTION OF THE CHICKEN AND THE EGG. WHICH COMES FIRST: SLIMMING DOWN OR BUYING A NEW WARDROBE? MANY WOMEN CHOOSE TO LOSE WEIGHT BEFORE BUYING CLOTHES, BUT THEY MAY BE SLOWING THEIR PROGRESS BY PUTTING THEIR LIVES ON HOLD.

Since you've journeyed into this program and shed some pounds, now may be a good time to pick up some new clothes—even if you still want to lose more weight. They'll make you look as though you're on your way to a svelte figure, and they'll help keep you pointed toward your goal.

"Feeling great about the way you look supports weight loss," says Diana Kilgour, an independent wardrobe and image consultant in Vancouver, Canada. Every woman, no matter how much she weighs, should have something to wear in which she feels comfortable and confident.

If you can't remember the last time you bought a flattering outfit, it's time to go shopping. If you know what to expect from your weight loss and can add some core pieces to your closet, you'll be on your way to finding that new wardrobe.

Watch your waist. Generally, we go down a dress size every time we lose 10 to 15 pounds. But where we lose the inches is what makes a difference in our wardrobes.

If the first 5 to 7 pounds come off your waistline, you could be dropping

Audit Your Closet

As you walk through a department store or peruse different designer boutiques, notice how clothes of coordinating fabrics and colors are usually placed on the same racks. That makes it easier for you to put outfits together—and spend your money on them. Yet getting the clothes in your own closet in sync can be difficult. The answer may be to reorganize your closet.

"Most people follow the 80/20 rule," says image consultant Georgette Braadt. "They wear 20 percent of their clothes 80 percent of the time. They have a lot in their closets, but they have nothing to wear."

If that sounds familiar, give away the clothes you don't wear and create space for your thinner and younger wardrobe. "You can't create a new picture without an empty canvas," she says.

Organize what you have left into capsule units, or sets of clothes with colors and fabrics that go together. Each capsule unit should be developed using two neutral colors combined with one or two accent colors that complement your skin tone.

Someone with a cool skin tone might build a capsule unit using a black jacket and pants coordinated with a red top, a white top, and a red/black/white print scarf. Someone with a warm skin tone might build around an olive jacket and skirt, adding an olive or brown tweed jacket with complementary brown pants and a beige sweater.

You can continue to expand each capsule unit or start new ones with new colors. Make sure that the fabrics and colors are complementary. Remember that the purpose of a capsule unit is to create flexibility in your wardrobe.

Once you meet your weight-loss goal, expand your wardrobe and create two or three more capsules.

a size in your jeans or skirts yet need the same shirts and jackets until you lose another 15 to 20 pounds or your shoulder size changes, Kilgour says.

Stick with simple styles. If you buy simple clothes that fit now, you can alter them more easily after you've lost weight. That means avoiding jackets with a lot of seams and staying away from pants with pockets, pleats, and belt loops, Kilgour says. The more complicated the style, the harder it will be to alter.

Instead, buy straight skirts and simple jackets. They can be taken in at least one size after you lose more weight. But because you'll never be able to take in a pair of pants a whole size, don't buy too many new pairs until you've reached your goal.

Also, avoid dresses that are anything but simple. If the tailor has to take out zippers and pockets to alter your clothes, the work will be too expensive to justify the alteration, Kilgour says.

Button up as you slim down. Buy a blazer that fits a little snugly at first and wear it loose and open, suggests Jan Larkey, author of *Flatter Your Figure.*

Once you lose inches in your stomach and hips, button it up. If you lose

Living Proof
PANEL

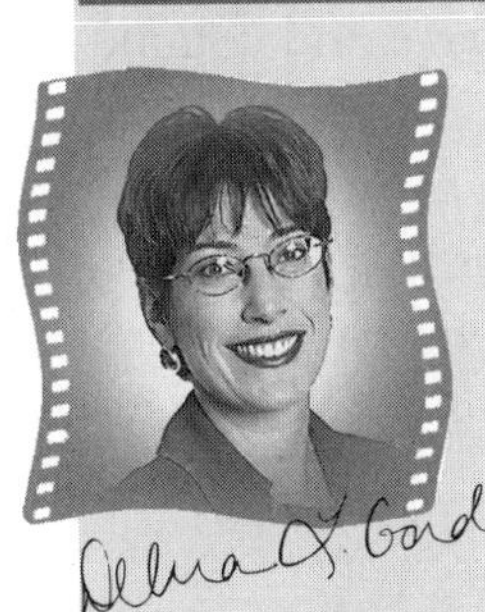

Tuck It In

Three sons in 9 years, and my body jiggled in places where bodies just aren't supposed to jiggle. Just as I'd given up on the idea of an uninterrupted night of sleep, so too did I relinquish those quaint notions of tucking my shirt into my pants, wearing dresses that nipped in at the waist, or encircling my waist with a belt.

But it took just 2 months of high-fiber foods, nightly walks with my neighbor, and a few fewer glasses of wine with dinner before the unbelievable happened. Not only did I tuck a shirt into a pair of jeans, eschew my normal overshirt, and buckle on a belt, I wore it out in public!

I've made this mistake before, mind you, only to find myself truly disgusted when I caught sight of my hips and stomach in the mirror later in the day.

Not this day. I didn't look ultraslim, but I also didn't look half bad.

Then came the night I pulled on a pair of shorts, and they practically fell to my ankles. Maybe they were my husband's? I checked the tag. Nope. They were mine!

My next step is a shopping spree—in a smaller size.

even more weight, you can always wear the jacket a little on the loose side, says Debbie Ann Gioello, professor of fashion design at the Fashion Institute of Technology in New York City and author of *Figure Types and Size Ranges* and *Understanding Fabrics*.

Mix and match to double your outfits—and fun. What if you could double your wardrobe by buying just six new pieces of clothes? That's what happens when you buy a capsule, a set of clothes made up of complementary fabrics and colors that provide wardrobe flexibility.

Here's how to do it: buy two skirts, one pair of pants, two blouses, and a blazer, suggests Gioello. As long as the clothes are solid colors that complement each other, you can mix and match the items and have enough to wear for almost 2 weeks. And solids could be accented with floral or geometric scarves and accessories to extend your wardrobe even further.

"If you mix and match just one unit, you don't need a lot of clothing during this transitional time," says Georgette Braadt, an image and communications consultant in Allentown, Pennsylvania.

Once you've reached your weight-loss goal, add more capsules in your new size. Along the way, reward yourself with new items as you achieve smaller goals. Before you know it, dressing thinner and younger will be a breeze.

Week Nine

Makeover Magic

Before

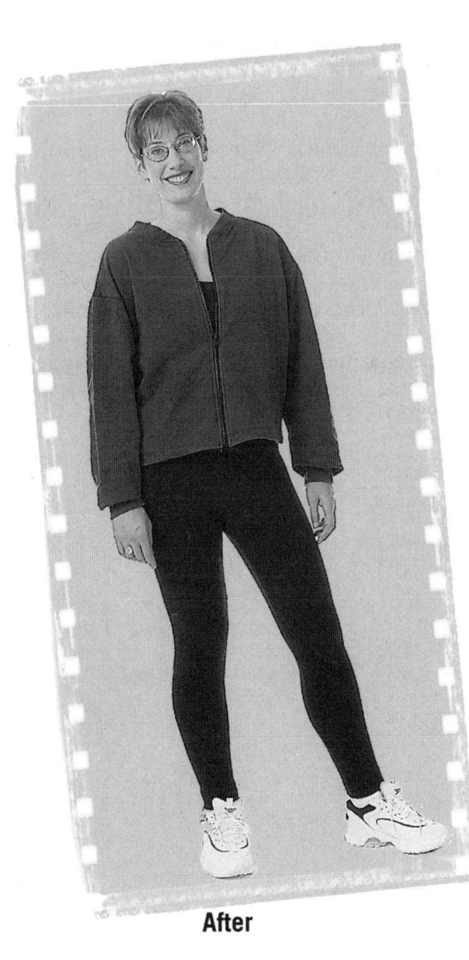

After

NOW MY REFRIGERATOR IS BURSTING WITH COLOR—FROM DARK GREEN ROMAINE LETTUCE TO ORANGE SQUASH, RED TOMATOES, AND YELLOW PEPPERS.

—Deb Gordon

Week Nine

As you've heard throughout The *Prevention* Get Thin, Get Young Plan, making small changes to your lifestyle will lead to a healthier set of habits that are easy to stick with. During each of the past 8 weeks, you added one goal from the eating plan to your daily strategy. Now that you've learned them all, how do you put it all together and grocery shop for your new, healthier lifestyle?

This week, you'll give your refrigerator a makeover so that it supports your thinner and younger eating habits, and you'll get some tips for navigating the supermarket aisles to steer clear of high-fat traps. As for exercise, you can choose from more than a dozen exercises to firm up flabby arms and tone your thighs—minor makeovers that will reveal a sculpted, stronger, younger-looking you.

Thinner Thighs

THE AMERICAN COUNCIL ON EXERCISE GETS ABOUT 400 CALLS A WEEK FROM FOLKS WHO WANT TO MAKE THEIR BODIES LOOK BETTER. MOST OF THE CALLERS ARE WOMEN. MOST OF THEM ARE WORRIED ABOUT THEIR THIGHS.

"How can I get rid of my fat thighs?" is probably the one question that trainers hear most, says exercise physiologist and certified personal trainer Ann Marie Miller, fitness director of the New York Sports Clubs in Manhattan. Because of the way in which women store fat, it's an entirely reasonable question.

Before menopause, estrogen causes women to store fat in their hips and thighs to accommodate childbearing. Nature wants women to maintain this extra energy source. As a result, thigh fat tends to be more stubborn than fat elsewhere in the body, and it's less responsive to changes in diet and exercise.

"You have to reduce your overall body fat through a combination of diet and aerobic exercise," says Miller. Plus, you have to do some strength training that targets areas where you want to build beautiful muscle tone—muscle that will show once the fat is gone. "You really can't do one without the other," she adds. "Doing a thousand leg lifts won't burn the fat from your thighs. It'll only give you tired legs."

It takes effort to tone your thighs, but the payoff is a leaner, younger look. You'll feel younger as well. "Having heavy legs can weigh you down and make it difficult to even walk," says Miller. "Losing that weight puts a lot more spring in your step."

Eight Great Thigh-Toning Exercises

To get really great thighs, you need to combine aerobic workouts with strength-training exercises. But in today's busy world, it's sometimes hard to find time for both. When you're crunched for time, try doing aerobic workouts that pull double-duty as thigh toners. Here are eight great choices.

1. Hill walking
2. Bicycling
3. Recumbent cycling
4. Step aerobics
5. Stairclimbing
6. Power walking
7. Inline skating
8. Racquetball

Work All the Angles

When you start working to tone your legs, it's important to remember that the area that is typically referred to as the thigh is made up of four different muscle groups: the quadriceps (front of thighs), the hamstrings (back of thighs), the abductors (outer thighs), and the adductors (inner thighs). You want to choose exercises that collectively work all of these muscle groups.

Miller recommends training your legs two or three times a week to get the best results. Start by doing two sets of 8 to 12 repetitions of each exercise. After a while, work up to doing three sets of 10 to 15 repetitions for each exercise. Do each exercise in a slow, controlled manner. The weight (when used) should be heavy enough so that the last four repetitions are fairly hard.

Here are the best exercises to target and tone your thighs, says Majid Ali, a certified fitness instructor in Los Angeles. Try them all, then pick the three that work best for you (being sure to include exercises that target all areas of the thigh). You can use either medicine balls or dumbbells for the weighted exercises.

Side Lunges

"Side lunges are great for strengthening the outer thighs, a spot a lot of women want to firm up," says Amy Goldwater, a certified fitness specialist and fitness advisor to the TOPS (Take Off Pounds Sensibly) Club in Milwaukee.

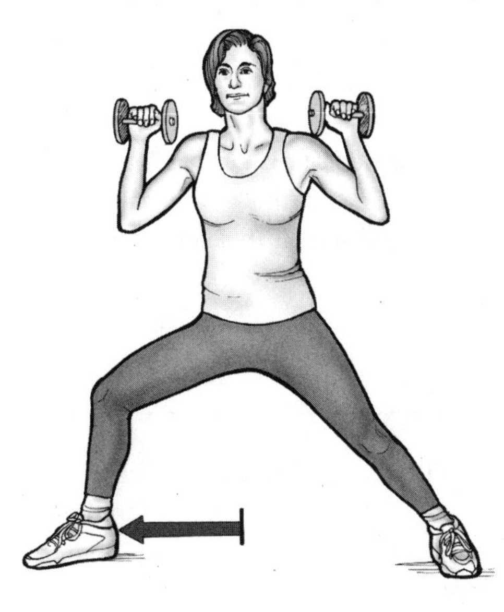

Stand with your feet about shoulder-width apart and your toes pointing out slightly. Holding a weight in each hand, raise your arms so that your hands are at shoulder level. Keeping your back straight and your abs tight, step to your right, landing heel to toe. Press your hips down until your right thigh is parallel to the floor and your left leg is extended. Your right toe should point to the side, while your left toe points forward. Hold for a second. Then slowly push back with your right leg and return to start. Complete a full set with your right leg, then do a set with your left.

Muscles worked: Adductors (inner thighs), abductors (outer thighs), hamstrings (back of thighs), and gluteals (buttocks)

Back Lunges

"Back lunges are great for working your hamstrings and quadriceps," says Miller. "And they're good for adding variety into your routine."

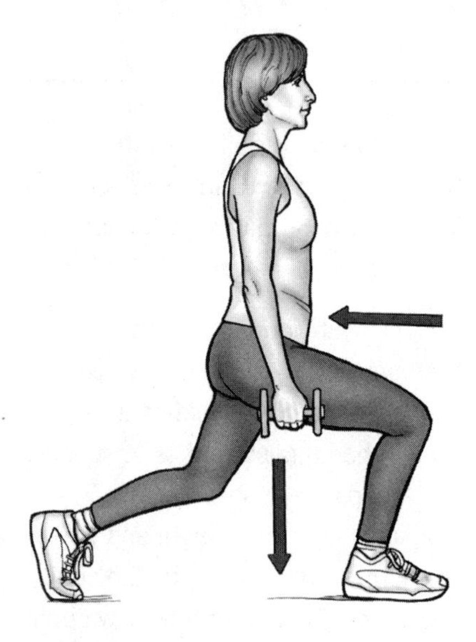

Stand with your feet hip-width apart. Hold a weight in each hand, with your arms down by your sides. Take a giant step backward with your left leg. Plant your left foot and slowly lower your left knee to the floor. Your right thigh should be parallel to the floor. Be careful not to let your right knee move forward beyond your toes. Then push off with your left foot and return to start. Repeat with your right leg.

Muscles worked: Hamstrings (back of thighs), quadriceps (front of thighs), hip muscles, and gluteals (buttocks)

Stepups

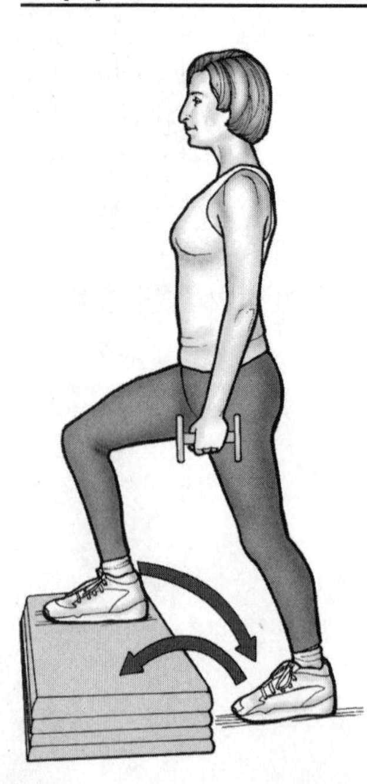

This exercise is harder than it looks. It's good not only for strengthening and toning leg muscles but also for improving coordination during everyday activities, says Ali.

Stand about a foot in front of a step or a sturdy box that is 12 to 18 inches high. Hold a weight in each hand, with your arms down by your sides. (If you're using medicine balls, you can hold just one ball in front of you at chest level.) Keeping your upper body straight, step forward with your right foot and place it on the step. Next, bring your left foot next to the right. Step back to where you started with your right foot and follow with your left. Repeat, starting with your left foot.

Muscles worked: Hamstrings (back of thighs), quadriceps (front of thighs), adductors (inner thighs), hip muscles, and gluteals (buttocks)

Seated Leg Lifts

"It's easy to work your legs with this simple home exercise," says certified fitness instructor Kelly Bridgman, wellness director for the Peggy and Philip B. Crosby Wellness Center of the YMCA in Winter Park, Florida. "You can do these unweighted to start. Then work up to doing them with ankle weights for added resistance."

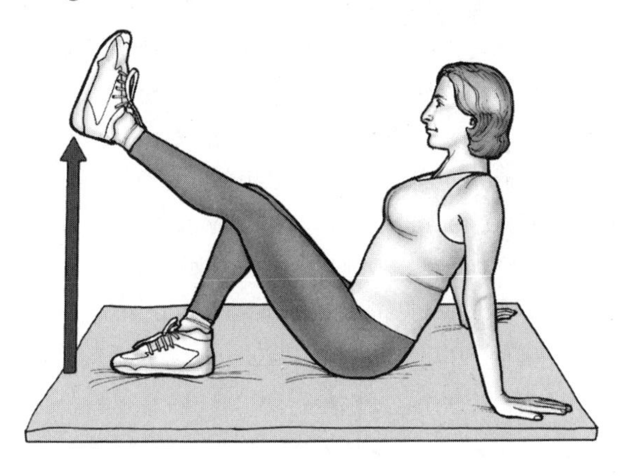

Sit on the floor with your legs extended in front of you and your hands on the floor behind you, supporting your trunk. Bend your right leg so your right heel is about 12 inches from your body. Keep your left leg extended, with your foot flexed. With your left knee slightly bent and your foot still flexed, slowly lift your left leg until your knee reaches the height of the knee of your bent leg. Then slowly lower the leg to the starting position. Complete a set with your left leg, then do a set with your right.

Muscles worked: Quadriceps (front of thighs)

Wall Squats

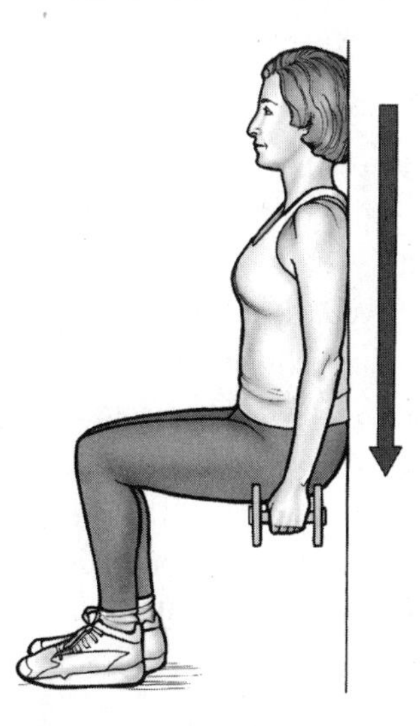

"Squats are great all-around exercises for your lower body, but especially for your quadriceps and hamstrings," says Bridgman. To really target the muscles in your thighs, try doing them against a wall.

Stand with your back against a wall. Your feet should be about shoulder-width apart, slightly out from the wall. Hold weights either down by your sides or up at your shoulders. Keeping your back straight and abs tight, slowly slide down, as though you're sitting, until your thighs are parallel to the floor. Don't let your knees move forward beyond your toes. Slowly return to start. Repeat.

Muscles worked: Quadriceps (front of thighs), hamstrings (back of thighs), and gluteals (buttocks)

Straight-Leg Lifts

This is an excellent exercise for strengthening and toning the muscles in your outer thigh, says certified personal trainer Jana Angelakis, founder of PEx Personalized Exercise in New York City. "After you can comfortably do several sets of 15 repetitions, you can use an exercise band tied around your legs above the knee for extra resistance."

Lie on on your left side, with your legs together and the bottom leg slightly bent. Bend your left elbow and rest your head comfortably on your arm. Place your right hand on the floor in front of you for balance. Keeping your top leg slightly bent, slowly raise it as far as it will comfortably go. Your foot can be pointed or flexed. There should be no swinging or momentum. Hold, then lower. Complete a set, then roll over and do a set with your other leg. When the exercise becomes too easy, loop an exercise band around your ankles for extra resistance.

Muscles worked: Abductors (outer thighs) and gluteals (buttocks)

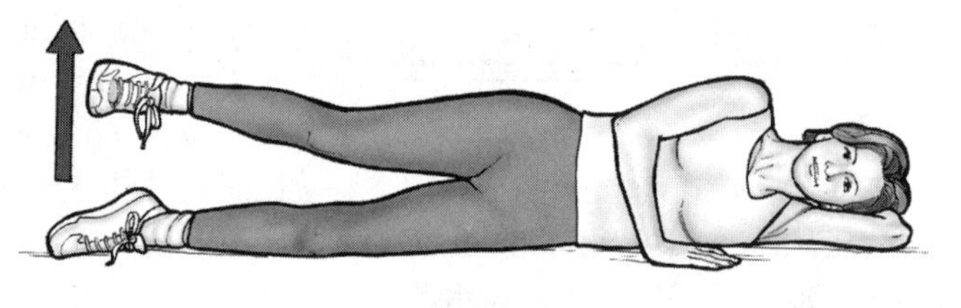

Plié Squats

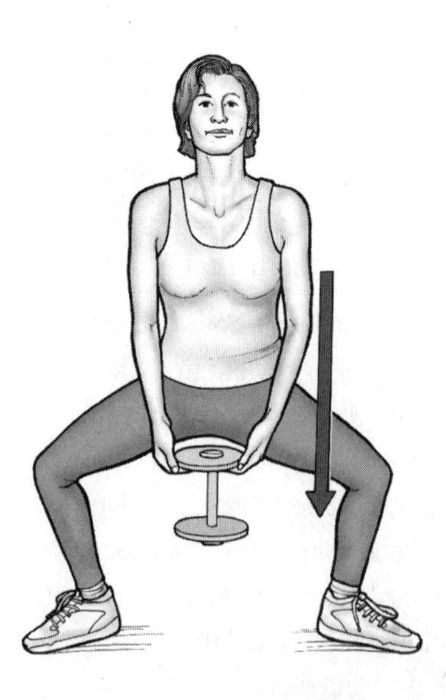

This exercise works inner thigh muscles that can be hard to target with other exercises, says Ali.

Stand with your legs more than shoulder-width apart, with your toes pointing out. Hold a weight with both hands, with your arms extended down in front of you. Keeping your back straight and your abs tight, squat until your thighs are parallel to the floor. Keeping your feet flat on the floor, slowly rise back up to start. Repeat.

Muscles worked: Adductors (inner thighs), quadriceps (front of thighs), and gluteals (buttocks)

Walking Lunges

"Walking lunges are one of the best exercises for your thighs," says Ali. "They raise your heart rate, so they provide some cardiovascular benefits, and they strengthen muscles that we use to sit, stand, and climb stairs, so they're very functional."

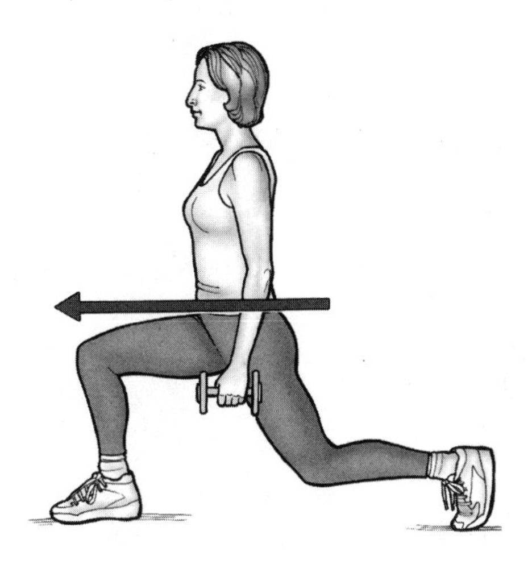

Stand with your feet hip-width apart. Hold a weight in each hand, with your arms down at your sides. Take a giant step forward with your right leg, landing heel to toe. Lower your right thigh until it is parallel to the floor; your left knee should be close to touching the ground. Hold for a second. Then, pulling forward and up with your right leg, bring your left leg forward and raise your body into a standing position. Repeat with your left leg. Keep alternating as you walk across the room.

Muscles worked: Hamstrings (back of thighs), quadriceps (front of thighs), hip muscles, gluteals (buttocks), and calf muscles

GOAL

Firm Arms

BELLY, BUTT, AND THIGHS. ASK MOST WOMEN WHICH BODY PARTS THEY WANT TO SLIM AND SCULPT, AND THOSE ARE THE ONES THEY'RE LIKELY TO NAME. UNDERSTANDABLY SO, SINCE WOMEN TEND TO COLLECT FAT IN THOSE TROUBLE SPOTS.

But if you spend all your time and energy on your lower half, you're overlooking one body part that responds quickly to just a few exercises and can make you look slimmer and sleeker in just a matter of weeks.

"The upper arm is a spot where women tend to store fat, which is what gives many women that jiggly appearance," says fitness specialist Amy Goldwater of the TOPS (Take Off Pounds Sensibly) Club. "But proportionately, since your arms have less fat than your legs, they respond more quickly to exercise, and you see results sooner. Seeing shapely arms in the mirror is a big confidence boost for a lot of women. It makes them look sleeker and stronger."

And, in case you're wondering, lifting weights will not give you manly arms, says weight-training researcher Wayne Westcott, Ph.D., training consultant for the American Senior Fitness Association in New Smyrna Beach, Florida. "Women simply do not have the hormones for developing big muscles. You'd have to spend hours in the gym every day to put on the kind of bulk that you see on female bodybuilders."

What you will get, he says, are firm, toned arms that look fabulous in short sleeves.

Six Things Strong Arms Help You Do Better

Looking good in short sleeves is nice, but don't think of your arms as just fashion accessories. Keeping them strong pays off in hundreds of ways every day. For example, you'll be able to:

1. Open stubborn jar lids
2. Stock your high kitchen shelves
3. Get up out of low couches or chairs
4. Hug loved ones
5. Carry shopping bags
6. Lift and hold children and grandchildren

Muscles Out of Balance

It seems surprising that your arms would be hot spots for fat to hang out. After all, women use their arms so often—for hefting children, shopping bags, and attaché cases. But most of those motions involve the biceps, or the muscles in the front of the arms, but barely use the triceps, the trouble spot in the back.

"Unless you lift weights or play sports like tennis, which use those muscles a lot, your triceps can stay underdeveloped and jiggly even if you're active," says Goldwater.

To get the best results, try doing two or three arm-intensive exercises two or three times a week, says exercise physiologist Ann Marie Miller of the New York Sports Clubs. "Work up to two sets of each exercise, completing 8 to 12 repetitions of each," she says. Be sure to do your arm exercises in a slow, controlled manner. The weight (when used) should be heavy enough so that the last four repetitions are fairly hard.

Here are the best exercises for developing strong, shapely biceps and triceps, says Dr. Westcott. Try them all, then pick the two or three that work best for you. Do them faithfully, and you'll see results in just 2 to 4 weeks. You can use medicine balls or dumbbells for the weighted exercises.

Shoulder Presses

Shoulder presses will do more than tone your triceps. They will also give you round, shapely shoulders. "Because they strengthen your shoulders and upper back, presses also improve your posture," says Goldwater.

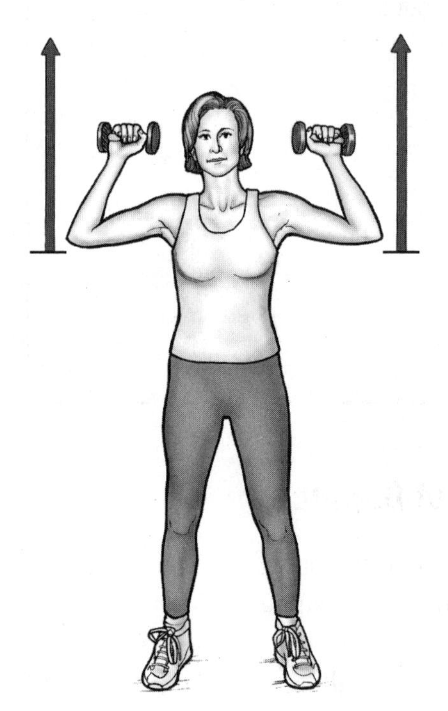

Stand with your knees slightly bent and your feet shoulder-width apart. Hold the weights at shoulder height. Slowly press the weights up until your arms are fully extended. Don't lock your elbows or arch your back. Hold for a second, then lower to the starting position. Repeat. If this exercise is difficult, you may try it seated instead of standing.

Muscles worked: Shoulder muscles, triceps (back of upper arms), and upper-back and neck muscles

Alternating Biceps Curls

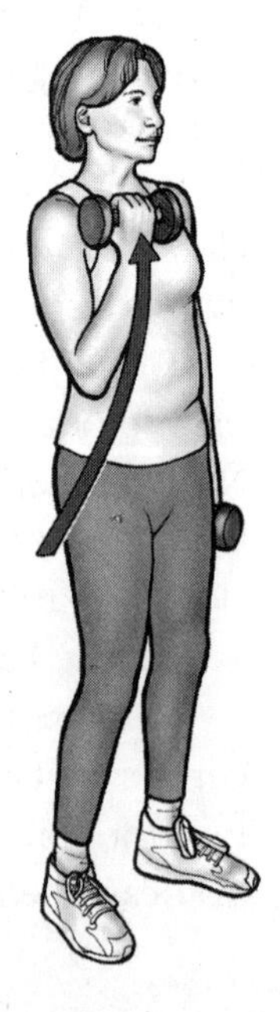

"Nothing gives you nice, curvy biceps like biceps curls," says Goldwater.

Start by standing with your feet shoulder-width apart and holding the weights down at your sides, palms facing in. Slowly curl the right weight up toward your collarbone. As you lift the weight, rotate your palm so that your pinkie ends up close to your body and your palm is facing slightly outward. Return to start and repeat with the left hand. "Adding the hand twist as you lift will give you nicer definition in your arms."

Muscles worked: Biceps (front of upper arms)

Adjustable Pushups

The pushup has gotten a bad rap as a punishing, military-like exercise. But nothing could be further from the truth. There are countless variations of pushups that everyone can do. "And the best thing is that pushups give you the biggest bang for your buck," says Miller. "You need no equipment to do them, and they develop your shoulders, chest, and triceps."

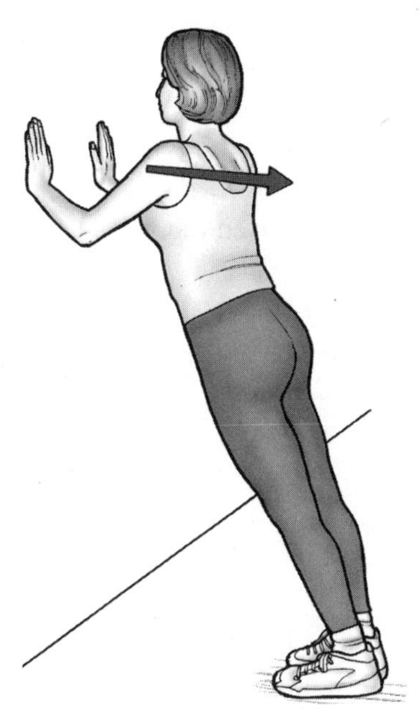

If you're just starting out, try doing pushups against a wall, recommends Dr. Westcott. Stand about an arm's length from a wall, with your feet together. Place your hands on the wall at chest height, about 6 inches apart. Keeping your body straight, bend your elbows so that they stay close to your body and point down (rather than out), then lower your chest toward the wall. Press up and return to start. Repeat. When these become easy, do them by pushing off a sturdy table instead of a wall. Then progress to doing them on the floor.

For floor pushups, place your hands shoulder-width apart. You can begin by doing pushups on your knees, keeping your back flat as you lower and raise your body. Then challenge yourself by trying them on your toes. You don't have to touch your chest to the floor. Just lower yourself until your shoulders are even with your elbows.

Muscles worked: Shoulder and chest muscles and triceps (back of upper arm)

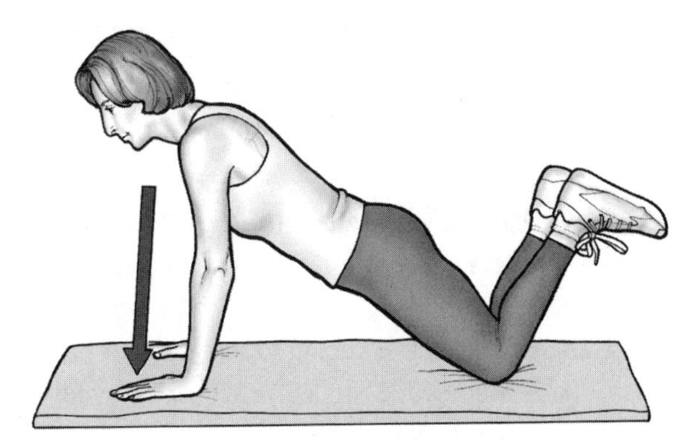

Wrist Curls

Sometimes women's wrists and forearms aren't strong enough to get the most out of their biceps and triceps exercises, says fitness instructor Majid Ali. If you feel as though your forearms fatigue before you get a chance to tire your upper arms, try adding these wrist curls to your routine.

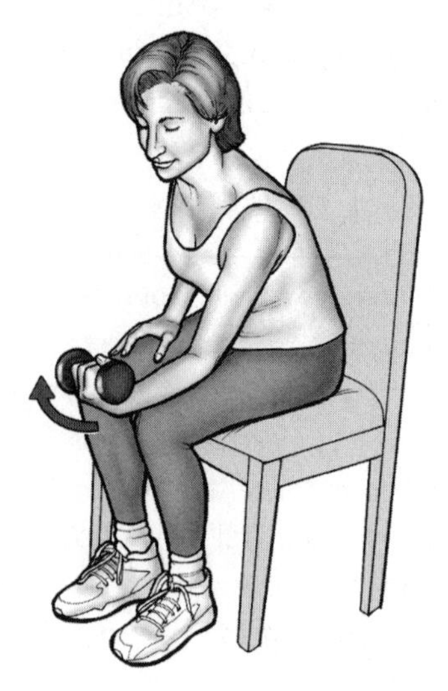

Sit in a chair and hold a weight in your left hand, with your palm up. Rest your right hand on your right thigh. Lean your left forearm on your left thigh, with the back of your wrist just slightly over your knee. Let the left wrist bend back naturally with the weight. Using your wrist, curl the weight up as far as it will go. Hold, then return to start. Complete a full set with your left hand, then do a set with your right.

Muscles worked: Forearm muscles

Overhead Extensions

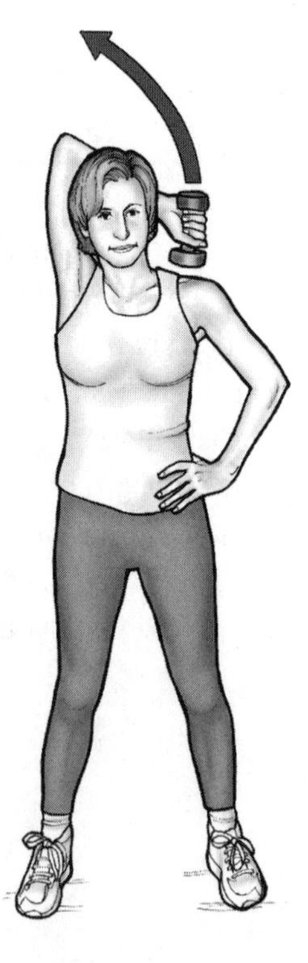

This exercise completely targets the triceps, says Miller.

Hold a weight in your right hand. Slowly raise it straight over your head, keeping your arm close to your ear. Bend your right arm at the elbow and lower the weight behind your head, as though you were going to scratch your back. Then raise it back overhead. Complete a full set with your right arm, then do a set with your left.

Muscles worked: Triceps (back of upper arms)

Triceps Kickbacks

Another exercise that isolates and tones the triceps is the kickback, says Ali. "It's a little tough, but it works!"

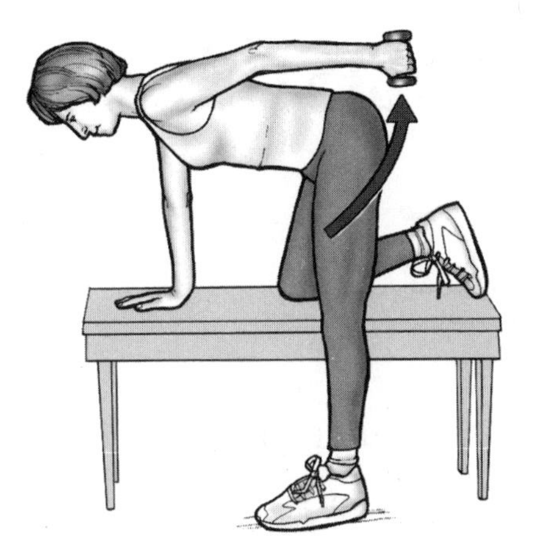

Hold a weight in your left hand. Bend over and support yourself by putting your right hand and right knee on a chair or bench. Keep your left foot on the floor and your back straight and parallel to the floor. Your left arm should be bent, with your elbow pointed toward the ceiling and the weight hanging close to your thigh. Straighten your left arm behind your body, so your entire arm is parallel to the floor. Then bend your arm back to the starting position. Complete a full set, then repeat on the opposite side.

Muscles worked: Triceps (back of upper arms)

Lying Triceps Extensions

Like overhead extensions, lying triceps extensions really focus on that underdeveloped area on the back of your arms, says Bridgman.

Lying on a carpeted floor or a mat, hold a weight in each hand, with your palms facing each other. (If you're using medicine balls, you can hold just one ball in both hands.) Hold your arms straight up, then angle them back so that they are tilted about 30 degrees toward your head. Bending your elbows, slowly lower the weights to either side of your head. Keeping your upper arms stable, slowly raise the weights again. Repeat.

Muscles worked: Triceps (back of upper arms)

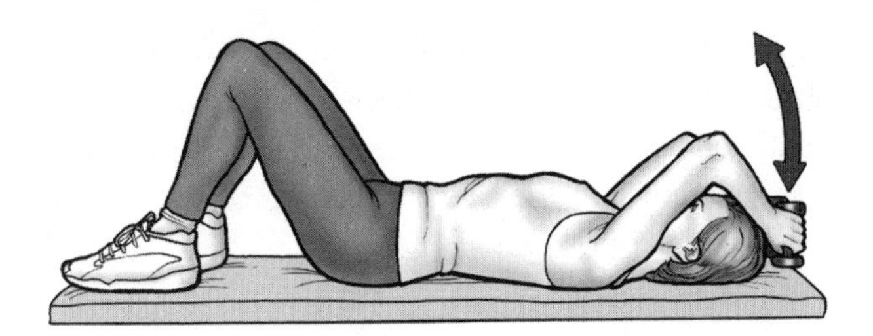

Supermarket Secrets of Slim and Satisfied Shoppers

YOGURT AND GREEN ONION. CHEDDAR AND HERBS. HONEY AND DIJON MUSTARD. THESE ARE JUST A FEW OF THE FLAVORS THAT POTATO CHIPS COME IN THESE DAYS.

Remember when your choices were pretty much barbecue and plain? Supermarket selections are booming nowadays, and not just with chips. Today, grocery stores may stock as many as 30,000 items—that's 10 times the amount of food on store shelves in the 1950s.

"The freedom of buying whatever you want, as much as you want, with no one looking over your shoulder can be challenging," says Mary Anne Cohen, director of the New York Center for Eating Disorders in Brooklyn and author of *French Toast for Breakfast*.

It's not surprising that you often have a tough time sticking to your healthy eating plan when you're that overwhelmed with tempting options. But in a very real sense, weight-loss success begins in the supermarket.

Here are some suggestions to make sure that grocery shopping enhances your new lifestyle instead of sabotaging it.

Keep your visits to a minimum. The more chances you give yourself to buy bags of cookies or chips, the better the chances are that you'll do it. The solution is to shop only once a week, says Linda Antinoro, R.D., senior nutritionist at the nutrition consultation service at Brigham and Women's Hospital in Boston.

Take a stroll. If you do have to pick up a few more groceries later in the week and there's a store in your immediate area, walk there. You'll get some exercise, and you'll be a lot less likely to buy 5 gallons of ice cream if you have to carry it home, Antinoro says.

Stick to the same store. Want to really minimize impulse buying? Experts say that you should shop at the same store every week. When you know your way around, you're less likely to grab candy from a sales rack, Antinoro says.

Cut out the crowds. Since you're less likely to fill your cart with chocolate when you have stress under control, it's probably not a good idea to shop during afternoons and evenings, especially on Thursdays, Fridays, and Saturdays—which are the busiest times. Make note of when your favorite store is least hectic, and visit then.

Snag a snack. You've heard it before, and you're going to hear it again: Eat something before you go shopping. Going to the store on an empty stomach makes all those foods look more enticing, Cohen says. At the very least, eat fruit or a piece of toast before your trip.

Check your list. Since a grocery list is your road map to healthy eating, be sure to keep it in front of you so that you don't get lost in the bakery section. You'll stay focused and, once again, minimize impulse buying. You may even cut your shopping time in half, Antinoro says.

If you have trouble remembering your list, keep it with your money or coupons, suggests Wendy Davis, R.D., a registered dietitian at Mercy Medical Center in Baltimore.

Get a good workout. If you think that a trip to the supermarket is exhausting, you're not too far from the truth—it can be a good workout. After pushing a cart around for 45 minutes and standing in line for another 15, you've burned 213 calories, about 3 calories shy of using a stairclimber for 30 minutes.

And, since the typical supermarket is more than 40,000 square feet in size, you'll make the most of your workout by walking up and down every aisle if you have spare time.

Tour the rim. Though you can walk anywhere you want in the store, the

Supermarket Shopping: By the Numbers

Want to know how your shopping habits relate to the rest of the country? Take a look.

- Most folks go grocery shopping twice a week, spending 8.8 percent of their weekly income.
- The busiest day to shop is Saturday, followed by Thursday and Friday.
- Women spend an average of $33 a week on themselves at the grocery store, while men spend $38.
- The average family spends $87 on groceries each week.
- People with children age 17 or younger buy more of the following than households without children: bagged salads, frozen main and side dishes, precut and seasoned meat or poultry, sandwiches or pizza to go, precooked meat and main dishes, rotisserie or fried chicken, and hot foods.
- Fifty-six percent of families with kids say that they plan meals at least fairly often, while 41 percent of them use leftovers.
- Fifty-four percent of married women do the shopping, while only 9 percent of married men pick up the groceries.
- Thirty-seven percent of married couples share the grocery shopping equally.

majority of your actual shopping should be done along the perimeter of the supermarket. That's where you'll usually find more unprocessed foods like fruits, vegetables, whole grain bread, dairy, fish, poultry, and lean meat, Antinoro says.

Cookies, crackers, and countless other processed foods, which usually have more sodium, fat, and preservatives, tend to be in the inner aisles.

Keep it convenient. Because cooking at home can help cut down on calories, buy precut onions, romaine lettuce, and baby greens to make dinner easier and faster, Davis suggests. If you're looking for a crunchy snack, try carrot chips—carrots cut to look like crinkle-cut chips for dipping.

Borrow from the bar. Choosing lettuce, tomatoes, broccoli, and chickpeas from the salad bar is one of the easiest way to get the ingredients for tonight's salad without having to prepare them yourself. But because you don't know how fresh they are, eat them soon, Davis says. They might not last as long as your other produce.

Buy lean. When you pass the meat counter, reach for flank steak, tenderloin, or top round. For pork, choose loin, tenderloin, or loin chops. And for chicken, stick to lower-fat white meat instead of dark, Davis says.

Beware of bargains. If some healthy food that's not on your list is on sale, should you stock up? That depends on what it is, Antinoro says. If crackers are on sale and you take home a month's supply, you might end up overeating. But if there's a sale on frozen carrots or some other ultra-healthy food, then by all means buy it.

Dodge bogus health claims. If you want to look past a food's low-fat promises, then flip the package over and read the nutrition label—you may end up with a healthier diet. A study by the American Dietetic Association found that people who read food labels get a healthier 30 percent of their calories from fat, while those who don't peruse the labels average 35 percent.

When you read a label, look for at least three items: the serving size, the number of calories, and the number of grams of fat, Davis says. If you only notice that your cheese-and-cracker sandwiches have 80 calories and 5 grams of fat, you'll be blissfully unaware that a serving is only six crackers. After just two handfuls, you've probably eaten about 160 calories and 10 grams of fat.

To keep your fat intake down, try not to buy food that has more than 5 grams of fat for a reasonable serving size or 20 grams of fat per meal, Davis suggests.

Ponder prepared products. Since stores are required to list only the ingredients on ready-to-eat food, such as rotisserie chicken, you'll have to do some detective work to find out if it's low in fat.

Check to see if the chicken is white meat instead of dark and if the skin was taken off, Davis says. Then ask the chef how the chicken was seasoned. Ask similar questions about other prepared food.

Enter "forbidden" territory. Remember, there are no bad foods. And avoiding a "bad" aisle in the grocery store, such as the potato chip section, almost guarantees that you'll end up bingeing on that food later, Cohen warns. Because forbidden fruit is always the sweetest, go ahead and wander down the aisle—and if you want some potato chips, simply buy an individual-size bag of them.

Rule out temptation. If taking your kids to the store usually means that you take home more tempting food than you planned, set some ground rules beforehand, says Jyl Steinback, a personal trainer in Scottsdale, Arizona, and author of *The Fat-Free Living Cookbook* series. She has a hard-and-fast rule: She'll buy only one thing that's not on the list, provided it's healthy. This way, she avoids having an abundance of enticing snacks in the house.

Insist on "kiddie" portions. If your kids are bugging you to buy a bag of chips, why not? Just as you'd buy yourself an individual size, do the same for your kids, Cohen suggests. You'll satisfy them as well as help them tune in to when they've had enough.

Ask for a manager. If you want a healthy food that your store doesn't carry, simply ask the manager to stock it, and you'll probably get your wish, Steinback says. When she can't find a particular food she likes, such as a fat-free salad dressing, she asks the manager of her local store to order it, and it shows up on store shelves within a month.

Build a pyramid in your cart. Before you go to the checkout counter, make sure that the food you're taking home matches the dietary guidelines of the USDA Food Guide Pyramid, suggests Dominique Adair, R.D., a registered dietitian in New York City.

Your cart should be full of whole grains, such as whole wheat bread and pasta, fiber-rich cereal, and brown rice; fruits and vegetables; some milk, yogurt, cheese, meat, fish, and eggs; and, if any, only a few items full of fats and sugar.

The Ultimate Refrigerator Makeover

TO SOME PEOPLE, A REFRIGERATOR MAKEOVER MEANS REMOVING THEIR 3-YEAR-OLD'S ARTWORK FROM THE DOOR AND TOSSING OUT OLD FOOD THAT'S SPROUTED A PICASSO PAINTING'S WORTH OF COLORS.

But if you want your refrigerator to support your thinner and younger eating habits for the rest of your life, give it an additional makeover: Toss out unwholesome goodies and keep its shelves stocked with healthy fare.

"When we open the refrigerator and we see pie, we eat pie," says Melanie Polk, R.D., director of nutrition education at the American Institute for Cancer Research in Washington, D.C.

Trading that pie and other high-fat goodies for healthier food will help you lose the weight that you want and keep it off. Here's how it's done.

Trash temptation. You wouldn't think twice about getting rid of leftovers with blue fur. You should take the same approach to more appealing items like cheese dip, slabs of bacon, fudge cake, and the other things that you know can pack on pounds. Simply put, you're more likely to overeat if you have high-fat stuff on hand, Polk says.

Focus on your favorite recipes. Now that you have some room, think about

The Adventurer's Makeover

Most folks wouldn't think to head to the produce aisle for adventure. But look beyond the oh-so-familiar bananas and broccoli, and you may find a new world of mysterious fruits and vegetables waiting for you.

Your tour guide for this trip, Katherine Tucker, Ph.D., associate professor of nutrition at Tufts University in Boston, will introduce you to 10 fat-fighting fruits and vegetables that you may never have considered buying.

Bok choy. If you like stir-fries, the next time you're cooking up onions, peppers, and mushrooms, add some bok choy to the mix, Dr. Tucker suggests. One cup of the shredded vegetable has only 20 calories and offers 2.7 grams of fiber, 73 percent of the Daily Value (DV) for vitamin C, 88 percent of vitamin A, and 16 percent of calcium.

Chayote squash. A cross between a zucchini and a pear with a citrus tang, chayote squash can be steamed, mashed, or sautéed in stock, she says. And since it has 4.5 grams of fiber and 38 calories per 1 cup, it's a perfect fat-fighting food.

Jicama. This high-fiber Mexican potato can be eaten raw or used in stir-fries, where its consistency resembles water chestnuts. One cup of jicama (pronounced HEE-ka-ma) has only 49 calories, 6.4 grams of fiber, and 43 percent of the DV for vitamin C.

Kumquat. If you really have a taste for the sour, try kumquats. They look like small oranges, but they have a sweet, edible skin and a very tart fruit. If eating them leaves you with a sour face, add them to preserves or marmalades for only 12 calories and 1.3 grams of fiber per fruit.

the healthy meals that you make often. Make sure that you keep your refrigerator—and pantry—stocked with the necessary ingredients, Polk suggests. If you like steamed vegetables over pasta, for example, keep some spaghetti, frozen broccoli, fresh tomatoes, chickpeas, garlic, olive oil, and Parmesan cheese on hand. That way, you'll never be more than a few minutes away from a healthy meal.

Remember your goals. Since you're going heavy on fruits and vegetables, you'll need to make sure that you have plenty of room for produce. That's because averaging 9 servings a day adds up to 63 servings for the whole week.

Leeks. These mild-tasting onions can be added to soups or quiches for only 16 calories per ½ cup. You can also cut them in half, marinate them in oil and vinegar, and then grill them, Dr. Tucker recommends.

Passion fruit. Scoop and eat the pulp and seeds of the native Brazilian passion fruit for a sweet and tart treat that has only 17 calories and nearly 2 grams of fiber. You can also eat it over frozen yogurt or use it for jam.

Persimmon. Once you learn that just one persimmon, with 118 calories per fruit, has a whopping 6 grams of fiber (20 percent of your 30-gram goal), its soft pulp will taste even sweeter. As a bonus, just one fruit will give you 73 percent of the DV for vitamin A. It's not ripe until it's very soft, so let it sit at room temperature for about a week after buying it. Then cut it open and spoon out the flesh.

Pomegranate. Lurking inside a pomegranate—105 calories per fruit—are hundreds of small, slightly tart seeds. Try adding them to a salad of mixed greens and red onion sprinkled with oil and vinegar, she suggests.

Star fruit. The star fruit looks like just what its name implies—a five-pointed star. And it's the right shape for snacks, fruit salads, and garnishes for chicken, pork, and fish. Simply slice and serve, Dr. Tucker says. For only 30 calories, you'll get 32 percent of the DV of vitamin C from this lemon-pineapple-plum-flavored delight.

Tomatillo. Attention tomato lovers: This south-of-the-border relative can be chopped for green salsa, guacamole, or salads, or cooked in Mexican sauces to pour over tamales or chicken, she says. For only 21 calories per ½ cup, it's a great addition to your diet.

Remember that one serving equals one medium-size piece of fruit, 1 cup of raw leafy vegetables, or ½ cup of fresh or cooked fruit or vegetables.

Add some color. The fashionably made-over refrigerator contains lots of color (even after you toss out that moldy mayonnaise).

That means stocking plenty of red apples and grapes, dark green spinach and lettuce, and bright orange carrots and apricots, says Katherine Tucker, Ph.D., associate professor of nutrition at Tufts University in Boston.

Put healthy food in its place. If you operate on the "seefood" diet (you eat everything you see), put a healthy bowl of washed grapes, apples, and oranges or a fresh green salad on the top shelf of your refrigerator. When you have all your produce tucked away in a bin, it's easy to forget that it's there, Polk says. Displaying fruits and veggies will help ensure that they are the first things you grab.

Hide the fat. If you simply must have marble fudge cake or some other fatty, tempting treat in your refrigerator, stash it in the back on the bottom shelf or in a drawer. Keeping it out of sight might just keep you from devouring the whole thing in a single sitting, Polk says.

Put Your Fridge on a Diet

Here's a list of some of the best foods to transform your fat-making fridge into a slim and sleek weight-loss partner.

Frozen Foods

Kick the Häagen-Dazs and frozen Snickers out of your freezer and replace them with these items.

- Fish fillets such as salmon or halibut
- Frozen fruit such as strawberries, blueberries, raspberries, and peaches
- Frozen vanilla yogurt
- Frozen vegetables such as corn, carrots, broccoli, Brussels sprouts, cut-up spinach, and blends of stir-fry and stew vegetables
- Ground turkey breast
- Lean red meat such as flank steak or ground round
- Low-fat frozen bean burritos
- Pizza crusts (preferably whole wheat)
- Skinless chicken
- Veggie burgers

Condiments

Since the door of the fridge is where you put the flavors that spice up your meals, choose the right condiments to keep your food tasty, yet low-fat.

- Barbecue sauce
- Butter-flavored sprinkles
- Chinese seasoning sauce
- Fat-free or light mayonnaise
- Garlic (fresh bulbs or a jar of minced garlic)
- Hot sauce
- Ketchup
- Lemon juice

Living Proof
PANEL

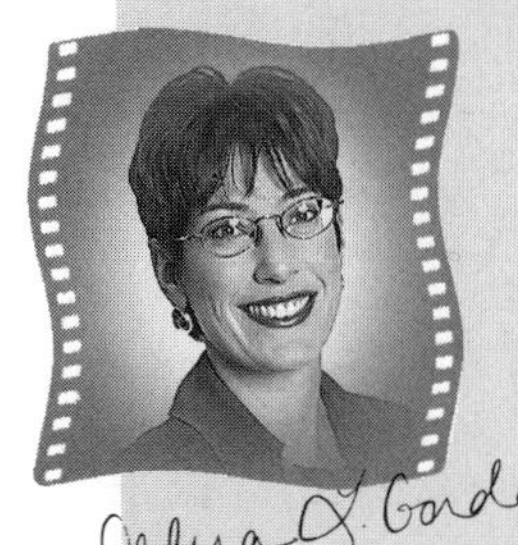

Great Food All the Time

I have always had good, healthy food in the house, but my kitchen lacked an important fat-fighting component: fiber. I knew that if I really wanted to make it easier to lose weight, I had to make some small but critical changes.

So I have made a conscious effort to buy more vegetables, and now my refrigerator is bursting with color—from dark green romaine lettuce to orange squash, red tomatoes, and yellow peppers. I make spaghetti squash, ratatouille, and vegetarian lasagna.

My cupboards are looking better, too. They're filled with whole wheat couscous and pasta. I cook exclusively with brown rice, and I eat Fiber One cereal instead of Cheerios.

I've also stocked up on chickpeas, white beans, black beans, and fat-free refried beans. I add chickpeas to all my salads and a can of white beans to spaghetti sauce.

Now I'm never at a loss for a high-fiber meal.

- Light salad dressing
- Low-fat bottled marinade (Indian, Chinese, Cajun, and others)
- Low-fat Parmesan cheese
- Mustard (if you're adventurous, try all the spicy and flavored types)
- Peppers (from a mild Anaheim to a fiery habanero, or something in between, like a jalapeño)
- Reduced-sodium soy sauce
- Salsa

Butter

Your butter dish can help make or break your healthy lifestyle. Since trans fatty acids have been linked to heart disease and other cardiovascular woes, stick with margarines that don't contain it.

If you do buy butter, use it sparingly. Each pound carries 3,252 calories.

Beverages

Soda—regular or diet—may be your beverage of choice, but it just doesn't stand up to these healthy drinks that you could stock on your shelves.

- Fat-free milk
- Orange juice or other fruit juices
- Soy or rice milk
- Vegetable juice such as V8
- Water in a gallon jug, either bought at the store or refilled from your tap

Dairy Products

Cream cheese, regular sour cream, and huge blocks of cheese aren't your companions on your journey to Weight-Loss Land. But that doesn't mean that you can't enjoy their slimmer counterparts.

- Fat-free vegetable dip
- Low-fat cheese slices
- Low-fat shredded cheese or blocks of cheese
- Low-fat sour cream
- Low-fat yogurt

Cold Cuts

If you have bologna, sausage, and beef hot dogs in your meat drawer, replace them with sliced turkey or lean ham.

Fruits

Unless you have a super-size fridge, you probably won't be stocking all of these at once, so choose a few of your favorites and rotate your selections each week.

- Apples
- Bananas
- Cantaloupe
- Grapefruit
- Grapes
- Honeydew
- Kiwifruit
- Oranges and tangerines
- Peaches and nectarines
- Pears
- Pineapples
- Plums
- Strawberries, blueberries, raspberries
- Watermelon

Vegetables

Again, you probably won't be able to fit all of these vegetables in your refrigerator, but choose different representatives from this list every week, depending on personal preference, what's in season, and what's on sale.

- Baby carrots
- Broccoli
- Cabbage
- Celery
- Corn on the cob
- Cucumbers
- Eggplant
- Green, red, and yellow peppers
- Kale
- Mushrooms
- Onions
- Romaine, Boston, or Bibb lettuce
- Scallions
- Spinach
- String beans
- Sweet potatoes
- Tomatoes
- White potatoes
- Yellow squash
- Zucchini

Week Ten

Accentuating the Positive

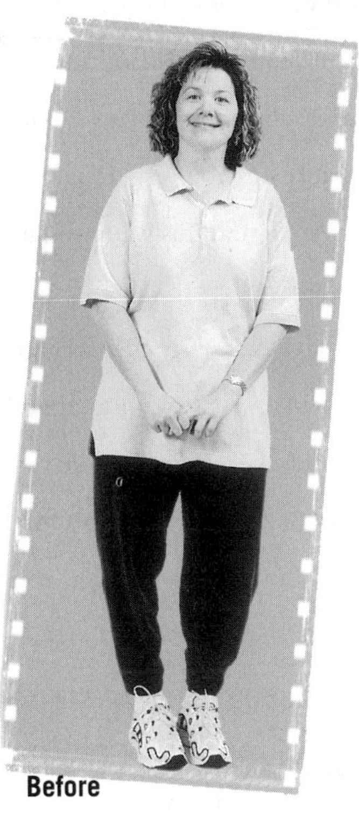

Before

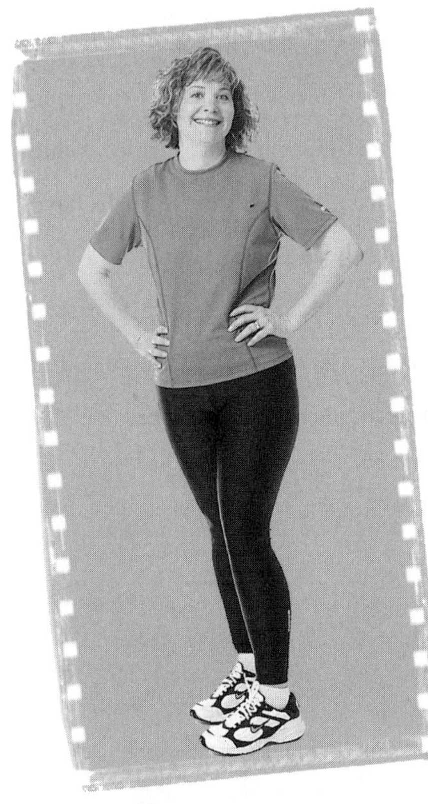

After

THE REAL CHANGE FOR ME HAS BEEN WITH MY SHIRTS. I NEVER USED TO WEAR SLEEVELESS SHIRTS. NOW I DO.

—Ana Reeser

Week Ten

You've worked your way through most of The *Prevention* Get Thin, Get Young Plan and are seeing some positive results from all your effort so far. You've discovered that you can lose weight without revamping your entire life all at once. You've gradually adopted many of the plan's strategies into your lifestyle, and this week you'll find a few more suggestions to accentuate your efforts.

Would you believe that something as easy as standing up straight will instantly make you look thinner and younger? It may even raise your spirits. You'll find exercises to improve your posture and strategies for building bone so that you'll stand tall for years to come. And even if you haven't reached your goal weight yet, you should be adding to your wardrobe. Because if your clothes are too loose, no one will notice your transformation. And to follow up your refrigerator makeover from last week, you'll learn the basics of restocking your pantry to support your new lifestyle.

Perfect Posture

EVERYONE WANTS QUICK WEIGHT LOSS. THAT'S WHY THOSE LOSE-5-POUNDS-IN-5-DAYS DIET SCAMS ARE SO DARN ENTICING, EVEN THOUGH WE KNOW BETTER. BUT EVEN IF YOU'RE TOO SMART TO BELIEVE THAT THOSE QUICK-LOSS GIMMICKS REALLY WORK, THAT DOESN'T MEAN YOU CAN'T LOOK 5 POUNDS LIGHTER IN JUST 5 DAYS—OR EVEN IN 5 SECONDS. ALL YOU HAVE TO DO IS STAND UP STRAIGHT.

Posture is one of the most overlooked—yet most important—aspects of our appearance," says Scott Krupkin, M.D., a physiatrist at the University Hospitals of Cleveland. "Hunching over when you stand or sit not only makes you appear heavier by shortening your waist and sinking your chest, it makes you feel heavier, both mentally and physically, as well. Your back aches, your neck aches, and you look and feel less happy, vigorous, and confident than someone who stands and sits up straight."

It's not that people don't know how to stand and sit straight, says Julio Kuperman, M.D., clinical associate professor of neurology at the University of Pennsylvania School of Medicine in Philadelphia and a longtime yoga instructor and yoga teacher trainer. It's just something we forget.

"Poor posture is a habit we develop over time, as we lean forward at desks and computers," Dr. Kuperman says. "Though it's occasionally okay

It's All in Your Head

Knowing that your posture needs improving is the bulk of the battle when it comes to standing stronger and slimmer, says Dr. Scott Krupkin of the University Hospitals of Cleveland. "Once you're conscious of your posture, you're more likely to improve it."

The trick is staying conscious of it. "You can correct someone's posture and watch it slip away about 5 minutes later," he adds. The following daily reminders can help.

- Hang a small mirror by your desk where you can't see your reflection until you slump forward into poor posture. When you see yourself, you'll straighten up.
- Stick brightly colored self-stick notes at the level your eyes should be if you're sitting up straight.
- Wear a rubber band loosely around your wrist for a few days. Every time you notice it, check your posture. It's an old trick, but it works. Eventually, you won't need the reminder to periodically check your posture.
- Check your posture every time a commercial comes on while you're watching television. This will help you avoid slumping while watching your favorite shows.
- Every time you stand, picture stacking your body parts atop one another like a tower. Your spinal vertebrae should all stack in a straight line. Your ears, shoulders, hips, knees, and ankles should all fall in line.

to lean forward when you need to, it becomes a habit, and we walk around with our shoulders hunched, our backs rounded, and our chins stuck forward all the time. This isn't the most efficient position for daily living, and we end up with muscular imbalances that cause fatigue and with aches and pains that leave us less energetic and productive in the long run."

Fortunately, poor posture is one bad habit that's easy to ditch. Just a few exercises will have you looking and feeling younger and thinner in no time. And that's a promise you can believe.

Sitting—And Standing—Pretty

Before you can work on developing good posture, you have to know what it is. "You can tell that your posture is efficient when your center of gravity is balanced down your body and you feel tall and relaxed," Dr. Kuperman says. You shouldn't feel as if your head is being pulled forward from hunching over or pulled back from slouching. Your back should feel straight, and your head should feel high. Can't find that posture-perfect spot? The following suggestions from Dr. Kuperman can help.

When You Sit

■ Keep your feet on the ground. Your chair should be positioned at a height where you can plant your feet firmly on the floor. The seat of your chair shouldn't be longer than your thighs, which can cause you to slump. And your knees should stay bent at about a 90-degree angle.

■ Push your butt back. Your rear end should be against the back of your chair, and your hips should be bent so that your lower back and thighs form at least a 90-degree angle. Your breastbone should be lifted, and you should feel a slight curve in your lower back. Avoid sticking out your rib cage, which can lead to muscle spasm and pain.

■ Lift your chin. You should lift your chin away from your breastbone without jutting it forward. Raise your computer monitor (or whatever you're looking at) to a level where you don't have to bend your chin into your chest to see it. Your chin should be up, and the back of your head should be in line with your back as much as possible.

When You Stand

■ Plant your heels. Your weight should settle back onto your heels when you stand, as if you had a big Godzilla tail or a long bride's train dragging behind you, Dr. Kuperman says.

■ Roll your shoulders back. You needn't feel like a cadet at a military academy, but your shoulders should fall back into their natural position, and your chest should be open and up. Again, avoid sticking out your rib cage.

Stronger and Straighter

The right exercises can help you out of a posture slump faster than you can say, "Attention!" The key is to strengthen the muscles that have weakened during years of underuse and to stretch and lengthen those that have shortened from being hunched together. Try performing the following exercises two or three times a week. (Yoga postures and stretches can be done daily.) For strength-training exercises, aim for one or two sets of 10 to 15 repetitions. Hold yoga poses and stretches for 20 to 30 seconds. Make sure that you are breathing calmly through your nose while doing them. If you can't breathe calmly, you need to back off by either holding the pose for less time or doing fewer repetitions.

Seated Twists

"Since you sit with your arms forward and your chest sunk in so many hours a day, it's important to open up your body and stretch those muscles so that they don't stay shortened all the time," says Dr. Kuperman. This seated stretch also relieves tension in your spine and hips.

Sit on the floor with your legs extended straight in front of you and your arms at your sides. Sit tall by lifting your ribs up from your pelvis. Then reach your left arm toward your feet while rotating your torso slightly and extending your right arm straight behind you. Hold for five full breaths, then repeat on the opposite side. Make sure that you are not leading with your chin or your shoulders.

Muscles worked: Chest and back muscles

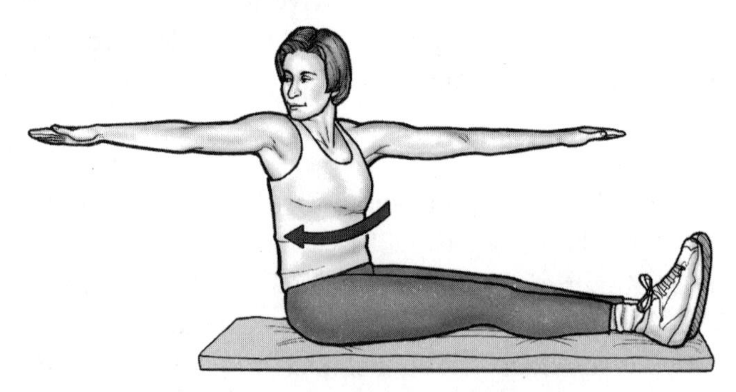

Mountain Pose

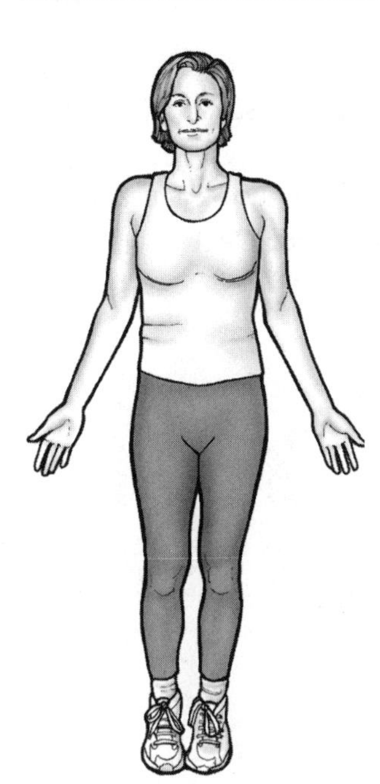

"Sometimes the hardest thing to do is simply standing straight on your own two feet, especially when you're prone to poor posture because you're imbalanced," says Dr. Kuperman. "This simple yoga pose restores that balance."

Stand straight up with your feet flat on the floor and close together so that the edges of your big toes touch. Standing with your knees gently locked and your thighs lightly tightened, breathe normally. Keeping your back straight, tighten your butt and stomach muscles. Then lift your rib cage and arch your back slightly while pulling back your shoulders. Hold your upper arms out and reach down. Hold the pose for 30 to 40 seconds. As you practice this pose, you will become more balanced and sway less as you stand.

Classic Crunches

Strong, tight abs are good for everything from zipping up your snuggest pants to standing taller and straighter. And the classic crunch is the best exercise for the job.

Lie on your back on a mat or carpeted floor, with your knees bent and your feet flat on the floor, about hip-width apart. Clasp your hands loosely behind your head, with your elbows facing out. Tilt your pelvis slightly to flatten your back against the floor. Slowly curl your shoulders about 30 degrees off the floor. Don't pull up on your neck. Hold for a second, then slowly lower. Repeat.

Muscles worked: Upper abs

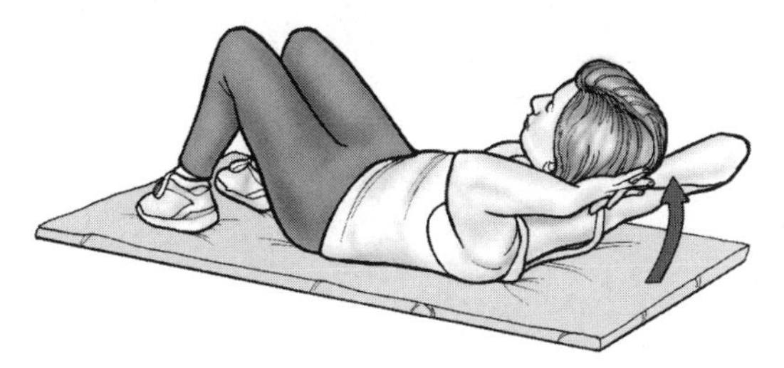

Arm-and-Leg Lifts

"Your lower-back muscles are what support your body and keep you upright, so they need to be strong for you to stand straight," says Dr. Krupkin.

Lie facedown on the floor with your arms extended over your head. Simultaneously raise your right arm and your left leg off the floor as far as is comfortable. Hold for 2 to 3 seconds. Lower and repeat with your opposite arm and leg.

Muscles worked: Lower-back muscles

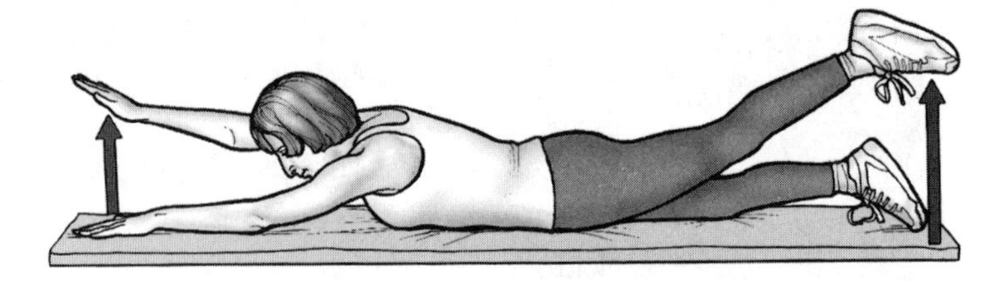

Horse Stance

"This is a popular posture for improving balance," says Dr. Kuperman. "It also helps strengthen balance-supporting muscles."

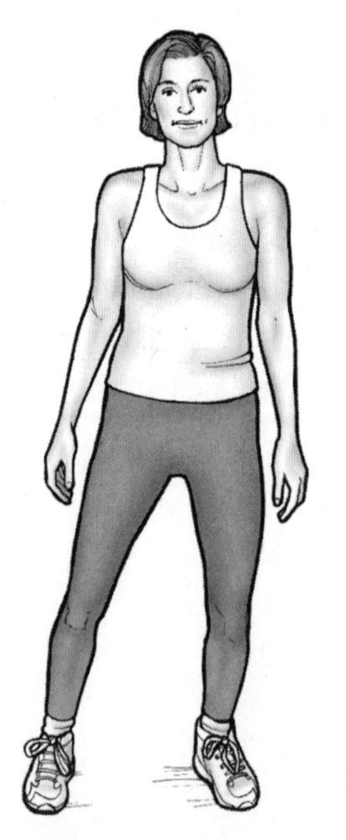

Stand with your feet 2 to 3 feet apart. Bend your knees so that they line up just over your toes (but not beyond). Settle your weight back onto your heels. Slowly shift your weight over to your left foot while still keeping your right foot fully planted on the floor and your spine straight. Then shift your weight to your right foot. Repeat slowly throughout the time you hold the pose.

Lying Pullovers

Any exercise that strengthens your shoulders and upper back will help improve your posture by helping you stand tall with your ribs high and shoulders back, says Dr. Krupkin. Here's one that hits your shoulders, back, chest, and triceps (back of upper arms) in one easy move.

Lie on your back on a bench (or on the floor) with your feet flat on the floor and your pelvis slightly tilted so that your back is pressed flat. Grasp a 5- to 10-pound weight with both hands and hold it above your chest. Keeping your arms straight, slowly lower the weight back over your head toward the floor. Stop when your arms are next to your ears. Hold, then return to start. Repeat.

Muscles worked: Shoulder, back, and chest muscles and triceps (back of upper arms)

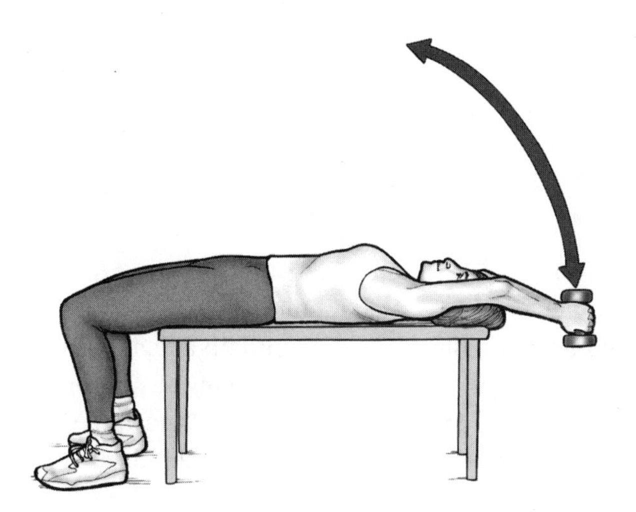

Building Stronger Bones

FOR KIDS, STANDING A FEW NOTCHES HIGHER ON THE DOOR FRAME IS A PROUD SIGN OF GROWING UP. FOR ADULTS, UNFORTUNATELY, THINGS SEEM TO GO IN REVERSE. MANY ADULT WOMEN, AND A FAIR SHARE OF MEN, FIND THEMSELVES SHRINKING WITH THE PASSING YEARS. IT'S A SIGN THAT THEIR BONES ARE GETTING OLDER—AND WEAKER.

Bones are living tissue, just like muscles. They can grow or shrink depending on how much or how little you use them. Every time you fitness walk, bound up a flight of stairs, hit a tennis ball, or lift weights, your body sends out chemical messengers calling for more bone to be added to your arms, hips, legs, and spine. The result over time is denser, stronger bones that help you stand taller, younger, and straighter.

On the flip side, if you put no more than minimal stress on your skeleton—say, by doing nothing more than walking around the house or office—your body gets the message that your bones don't need to be strong.

Unfortunately, you may not actually notice your bones getting weaker until your pants are suddenly too long or you begin to hunch. These are signs of osteoporosis, a skeletal disease in which the bones become so weak that they actually begin to compress. In some cases, they fracture or even crumble.

Exercise isn't the only key to keeping your bones young and strong. What you eat is equally important. Mostly, your body needs calcium. When you don't get enough in your diet, your body can't build new bone. Worse, it starts removing the calcium that it needs—to keep the heart beating regularly, for example—from the bone mass you do have, leaving weakened, porous bones behind.

"Your body is in a constant race between building bone and using bone. This race gets tougher as we get older because our bodies don't build bone as readily as when we're young and growing, and bone breaks down more rapidly. That's why we need to do everything we can to hold onto the bones we have and keep them strong," says Dickey Jones, M.D., cofounder of Orthopedic Specialists in Dallas. "You can't control everything as you age, but you can control whether or not your bones get weak and your shoulders hunch over."

Please Feed the Bones

Since calcium is crucial to building strong bones, you need to make sure that you get enough of this essential mineral, says Dr. Jones. Some people need to take calcium supplements, but you can get plenty of calcium from your diet as well.

Drink lots of milk. Bones are made mostly of calcium. Yet the average American woman gets only 550 to 600 milligrams of calcium a day. That's less than half of the 1,500 milligrams for people age 50 and older that the National Institutes of Health recommends. (The recommended amount for those under age 50 is 1,000 milligrams.)

The answer to this calcium deficit is to eat more dairy foods. "Dairy products are the best sources of calcium around," says Michele Trankina, Ph.D., professor at St. Mary's University of San Antonio in Texas and a nutrition consultant. "Foods like fat-free milk, low-fat cheese, and low-fat yogurt are superior for building bones because they're not only rich in calcium, most of them also contain vitamin D, which helps your body absorb calcium. Some leafy green vegetables such as spinach contain calcium, too, but they also contain binding fibers that make it hard for your body to absorb it."

How much dairy do you need to eat to get at least 1,000 milligrams of calcium a day? Just three glasses of calcium-fortified fat-free milk (at about 350 milligrams a glass) will do the trick. Other great sources are cheese (½

The Best Bone Test

We test our blood pressures to keep our hearts young and strong. We test our cholesterol levels to keep our arteries free and clear. But few of us ever test our bones to make sure that they're not aging quicker than we are.

There's a reason for this neglect. The gold-standard bone test for osteoporosis, called DEXA, involves using low-dose x-rays of the hips and spine. The cost ranges from $100 to $300, and many medical facilities don't offer it. But now there are "mini" bone tests, with names like accuDEXA, PIXI, and p-DEXA. They measure peripheral bones in the fingers, forearms, and heels. These are early screening tests that can detect thinning-bone problems, and they cost only about $35.

"I would encourage every woman, especially if she is at risk for developing osteoporosis or is menopausal, to have a bone-density test done. They definitely should get a full DEXA scan done when they begin menopause," says Theresa Galsworthy, R.N., of the Osteoporosis Center at the Hospital for Special Surgery. "We can do so much for this disease if we catch it early. Diet and exercise changes can make a huge difference. And we have some very effective medications such as the hormone estrogen or raloxifene (Evista) and nonhormonal medications such as alendronate (Fosamax) that can help suppress the breakdown of bone."

cup of part-skim ricotta provides 337 milligrams) and yogurt (1 cup packs 414 milligrams).

A bonus is that getting more calcium may actually make you *thinner* while it's making your bones younger. A 2-year study from Purdue University in West Lafayette, Indiana, found that women who got at least 1,000 milligrams of calcium a day, along with a diet of no more than 1,900 daily calories, had lower body fat and lost more weight (6 to 7 pounds) than women who ate less calcium. Lead researcher Dorothy Teegarden, Ph.D., believes that these positive results may have occurred because high levels of calcium suppress certain hormones that play a role in decreasing fat production and increasing fat breakdown. "Yet another good reason to drink your milk," she says.

Feed your skin some sun. Almost as important as calcium is vitamin D. Without enough of the "sunshine vitamin," you absorb very little bone-building calcium. If your primary source of calcium is dairy food, you needn't worry too much about vitamin D, since dairy foods are generally fortified with it, says Dr. Trankina. But if you get your calcium from other sources, such as fortified orange juice, you should be getting at least 400 IU of vitamin D daily. Salmon and other fatty fish are good sources of vitamin D, and so is the sun. Your body produces vitamin D when the sun strikes your skin, so you should spend about 15 minutes a day in the sunlight with your hands and face exposed.

Pile on the produce. Boston researchers found that men and women from the esteemed Framingham Heart Study who ate the most fruits and vegetables—especially potassium-rich foods like bananas and potatoes and magnesium-rich foods like spinach—during a 4-year study had greater bone density than those eating less of these foods.

Researchers believe that fruits and vegetables protect bones by acting as a buffer during the digestion process. Normal digestion produces acid in your body, and minerals like potassium and magnesium help neutralize that acid. If you don't get enough potassium and magnesium in your diet, your body still has to neutralize all that acid. It does this by pulling these minerals from your bones, leaving them weakened. So you have another great reason to eat 9 servings of fruits and vegetables every day, as nutritionists recommend.

Daily Insurance for Your Bone Bank

Before bottled teas, sodas, and juices started dominating dinner tables, many people used to drink milk with every meal, says Theresa Galsworthy, R.N., director of the Osteoporosis Center at the Hospital for Special Surgery in New York City. "Now that we've stopped that practice, it's hard for us to get all the calcium we need." Another problem is that our fast-food culture makes it difficult for us to get other nutrients that our bones need, such as vitamin D and magnesium.

Everyone should try to get their nutrients from fruits, vegetables, whole grains, and dairy foods, but calcium supplements can provide good insurance for your bones, says Dr. Trankina.

- Most over-the-counter calcium supplements are good, but your best bet is to use a supplement that contains either calcium citrate, calcium lactate, or calcium gluconate, says Dr. Trankina. "Calcium citrate is much more absorbable on an empty stomach than other compounds, like calcium carbonate."

Bone Robbers

You know that good lifestyle habits can help you store more calcium in your bones. Well, not-so-good lifestyle habits can rob your bones of this valuable mineral. Here's how to hold up the calcium thieves.

Kick the habit. Women who smoke lose bone twice as quickly as those who don't, says Dr. Dickey Jones of Orthopedic Specialists in Dallas. "There are many good medications that make quitting easier. Ask your doctor to help you out."

Can the carbonation. "Carbonated beverages, which are high in phosphorus, can cause excessive excretion of calcium and lead to a net loss of calcium from bones. Colas are particularly bad," says Theresa Galsworthy, R.N., of the Osteoporosis Center at the Hospital for Special Surgery. "Try drinking no more than two carbonated beverages a day."

Drink moderately. "Alcohol can interfere with the way the body activates vitamin D from the liver," says Galsworthy. "Without vitamin D, we can't absorb calcium." In general, limit yourself to one drink a day.

Eat less meat. Eating too much animal protein causes your body to excrete calcium, says Galsworthy. "Stick to 3 to 4 ounces of animal protein a day. That's a cut about the size of a deck of cards. And try to get more protein from vegetable sources like tofu and beans."

■ Figure out how much calcium you're getting in your diet, then supplement 500 to 1,000 milligrams to be sure that you're getting the recommended 1,000 to 1,500 milligrams a day. Avoid taking more than 500 milligrams at one time, however, because your body has a hard time absorbing more than that amount at once.

■ Though your body produces vitamin D from sunshine, and many dairy products are fortified with it, people synthesize and absorb less of this nutrient as they get older. Taking it in supplement form is probably a good idea. "You can get calcium supplements that include vitamin D," says Dr. Jones. "Or you can get it through a multivitamin. But it's important that you get it."

In a 3-year study of almost 400 men and women ages 65 and older, researchers at Tufts University in Boston found that those who took 500 milligrams of calcium and 700 IU of vitamin D daily had significantly less bone loss than those not taking the supplements. What's more, those not taking supplements experienced twice as many fractures as those taking extra calcium and vitamin D. The Daily Value for vitamin D is 400 IU.

■ Calcium and vitamin D aren't the only nutrients that help with the formation of bone. You also need magnesium, zinc, and copper, to name just a few. "You can cover your bases by taking a daily multivitamin to ensure that you get 100 percent of the Daily Value for all the essential nutrients," says Dr. Jones.

Building Strong Bones with Exercise

Like muscle tissue, bone operates on a use-it-or-lose-it policy. The more you challenge your bones, the stronger they get. The less you challenge them, the weaker they get. One 6-month study at the University of North Carolina in Chapel Hill compared two groups of women ages 40 to 50. Women in one group did resistance training, while those in the other group were sedentary. Researchers found that women who lifted weights 3 days a week gained 1 percent extra bone density in their spines. Those in the sedentary group actually lost bone during the same period.

To make the biggest impact on your bone health, experts recommend two kinds of exercise: weight-bearing and resistance-training. "Weight-bearing exercises are activities like jogging, walking, and dancing," explains Galsworthy. "These are important because your bones respond best when stressed against gravity, and therefore the impact of your weight against the ground stimulates bones to get stronger.

"But weight-bearing exercise isn't enough by itself. You also need some general resistance training, like lifting weights, to build muscle mass and strength," he adds. "This is especially important for the upper body, where women are at high risk for losing bone." The more muscle tissue you have, the more tension your muscles put on your bones. This stimulates your bones to grow stronger.

Since women are prone to losing bone strength in the hips, spine, legs, and wrists, cross-training is the best way to keep the entire skeleton strong, adds Galsworthy. "As little as three times a week of weight-bearing activity, combined with general strength training, can make a big difference—although, of course, if you can do more, that's even better."

Putting a Load on Your Feet

Any exercise is good, but to build stronger bones you need to subject them to more stress than they get during day-to-day activities, says Galsworthy. High-impact activities like jumping rope are ideal, but not everyone's joints appreciate that kind of jarring. Here are some good bone-building alternatives. Try doing one or more of these 3 days a week for 20 to 30 minutes per session.

Power walking. This involves walking briskly with short, strong steps, rolling heel to toe and keeping your arms bent and pumping by your sides. It puts enough stress on your legs, hips, and spine to maintain or build bone mass. But it won't jar your joints like running.

Treadmill jogging. Jogging on a treadmill can be easier on your joints than pounding the pavement, says Galsworthy. Regular vigorous activity like treadmill jogging may reduce a woman's bone loss after menopause by up to 50 percent.

Doing low-impact aerobics. This is easy on your joints but great for your bones since you're exerting more force on them than you usually do while walking. And all that stepping really tones your rear.

Rowing. Whether it's done on a machine or in a real kayak or canoe, rowing is an excellent spine strengthener. It will help your back stay straight and youthful. Women who are worried about getting a dowager's hump, that hunching upper back that may be caused by osteoporosis, can really benefit from including rowing in their routines.

Playing tennis. If you can't row, maybe you can swing. Playing tennis puts healthy stress on the spinal vertebrae. Plus, it builds super-strong bones in your swinging arm. "As a bonus, playing tennis or other sports regularly keeps your coordination and mind-body responses sharp," says Galsworthy.

Pushing Your Weight

Strong muscles yield strong bones. Here are some exercises that the American Council on Exercise recommends for building a strong skeleton from head to toe. For best results, do the following resistance exercises 3 days a week. Plan on doing one to three sets of each exercise, with 6 to 12 repetitions per set. For the weighted exercises, you can use either medicine balls or dumbbells.

Half Squats

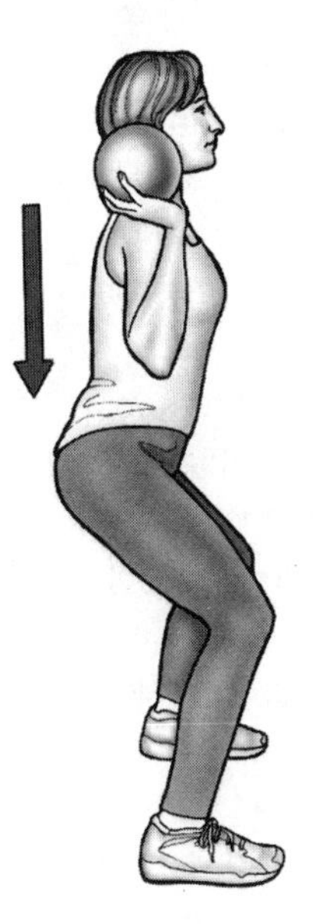

Stand with your back facing a chair (without armrests). Keep your feet flat on the floor and positioned slightly more than shoulder-width apart. Hold a weight in each hand at shoulder level, with your palms facing up. Keep your head in line with your upper body, facing forward.

Keeping your back straight, slowly bend at the knees and hips, as though you were sitting down. Don't let your knees extend beyond your toes. Stop just shy of sitting on the chair. Hold for a second, then return to the starting position. Repeat.

Muscles worked: Hip muscles, quadriceps (front of thighs), hamstrings (back of thighs), gluteals (buttocks), and lower-back muscles

Front Lunges

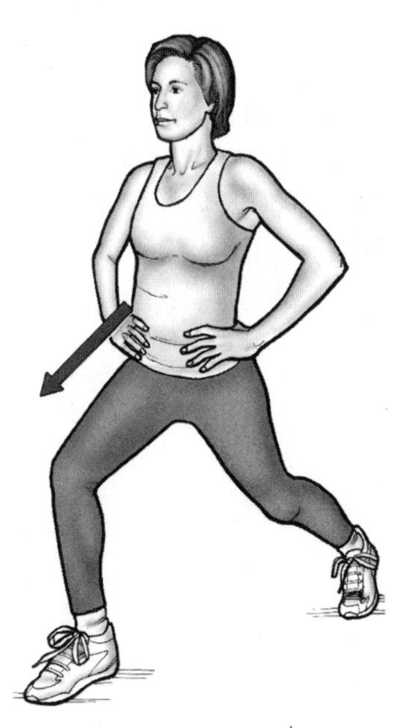

Stand with your feet shoulder-width apart. Take a large step forward with your right leg, dropping your left knee toward the floor. Be sure to keep your right knee in line over your ankle. Push back to the starting position, and repeat with the opposite leg.

Muscles worked: Quadriceps (front of thighs), gluteals (buttocks)

Side Lunges

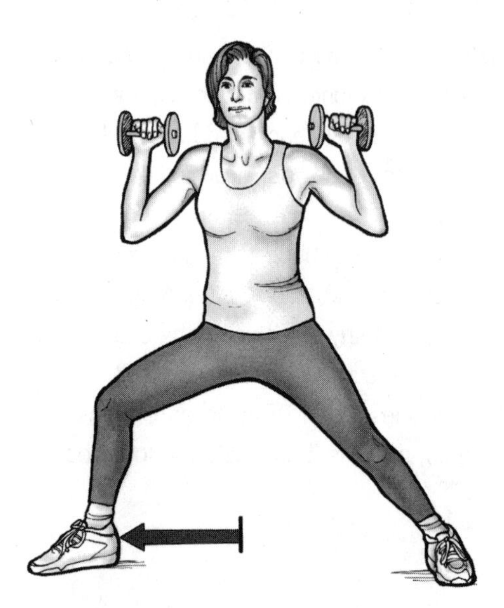

Stand with your feet about shoulder-width apart and your toes pointing out slightly. Holding a weight in each hand, raise your arms so that your hands are at shoulder level. Keeping your back straight and your abs tight, step to your right, landing heel to toe. Press your hips down until your right thigh is parallel to the floor and your left leg is extended. Your right toe should point to the side, while your left toe points forward. Hold for a second. Then slowly push back with your right leg and return to start. Complete a full set with your right leg, then do a set with your left.

Muscles worked: Adductors (inner thighs), abductors (outer thighs), hamstrings (back of thighs), and gluteals (buttocks)

Toe Raises/Heel Drops

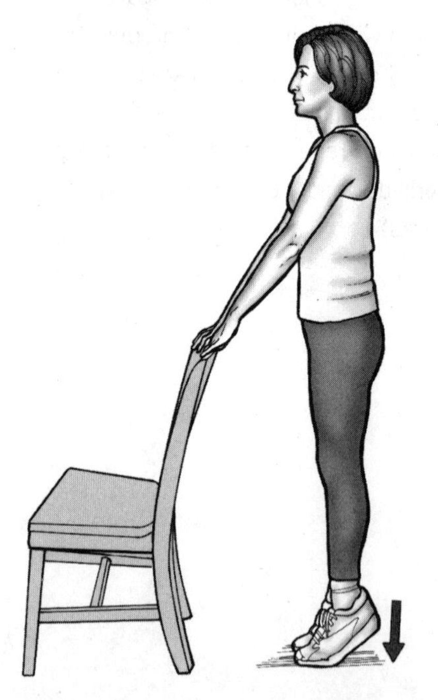

Rise up on your toes, drop back on your heels, then rock back. Repeat. You can hold the back of a chair for balance.

Muscles worked: Calf muscles

Pelvic Tilts

Lie on your back, with your feet flat on the floor and your knees bent. Clasp your hands lightly behind your head, with your elbows out to the sides. Tighten your abs and slowly lift your pelvis as you curl it toward your rib cage. Simultaneously, press your lower back against the floor. Hold for a second, then slowly lower. Repeat.

Muscles worked: Lower abs

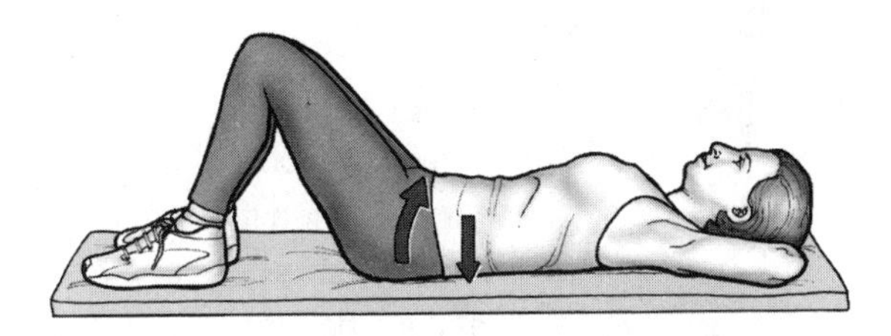

Biceps Curls

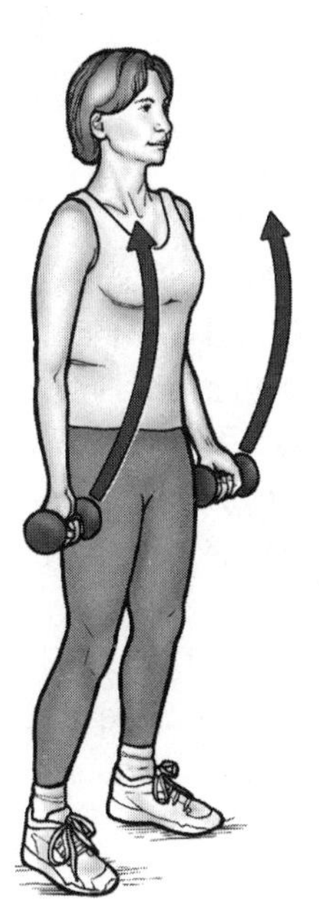

Stand with your knees slightly bent and your feet about shoulder-width apart. Hold a weight in each hand down at your sides, with your palms facing up. Keeping your elbows at your sides, slowly lift the weights up toward your collarbone. Don't arch your back. Hold for a second, then slowly lower to the starting position. Repeat.

Muscles worked: Biceps (front of upper arms)

Triceps Kickbacks

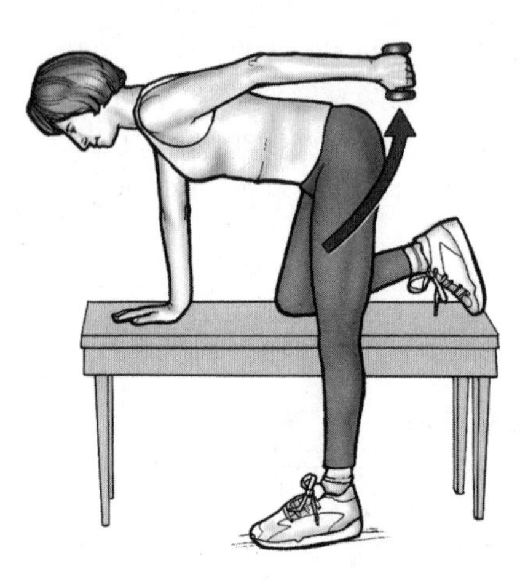

Hold a weight in your left hand. Bend over and support yourself by putting your right knee and right hand on a bench or chair. Keep your left foot on the floor and your back straight and parallel to the floor. Your left arm should be bent, with your elbow pointed toward the ceiling and the weight hanging close to your thigh. Straighten your left arm behind your body so that your entire arm is parallel to the floor. Then bend your arm back to the starting position. Complete a full set, then repeat on the opposite side.

Muscles worked: Triceps (back of upper arms)

Lateral Raises

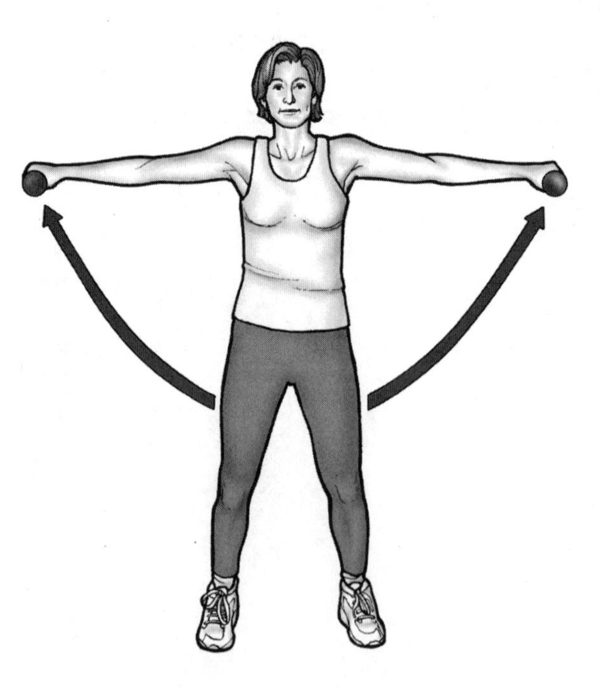

Stand with your knees slightly bent and your feet shoulder-width apart. Hold a weight in each hand down at your sides, with your palms facing in. Lift the weights out to the sides to slightly below shoulder height. Then slowly lower them again. Repeat.

Muscles worked: Shoulder muscles

Chest Presses

Lie on your back, with your knees bent and your feet flat on the floor and about hip-width apart. Hold a weight in each hand, with your arms extended up over your chest and your palms facing the ceiling. Your thumbs should face each other.

Bend your elbows and slowly lower the weights. Stop when they are about even with your shoulders. (If you're lying on the floor, your arms will be resting on the floor.) Slowly return to start. Repeat.

Muscles worked: Chest and shoulder muscles and triceps (back of upper arms)

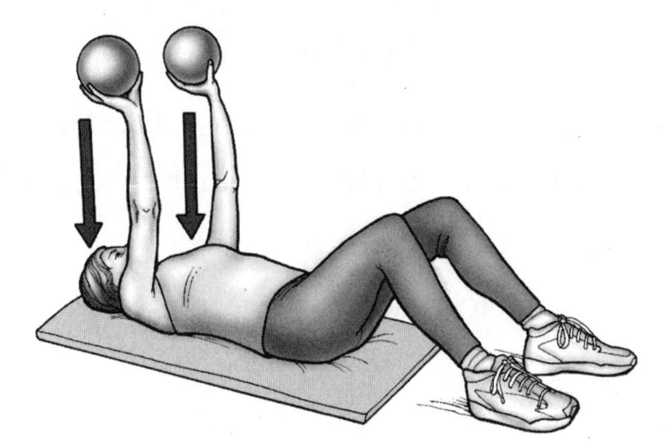

Lat Pulldowns

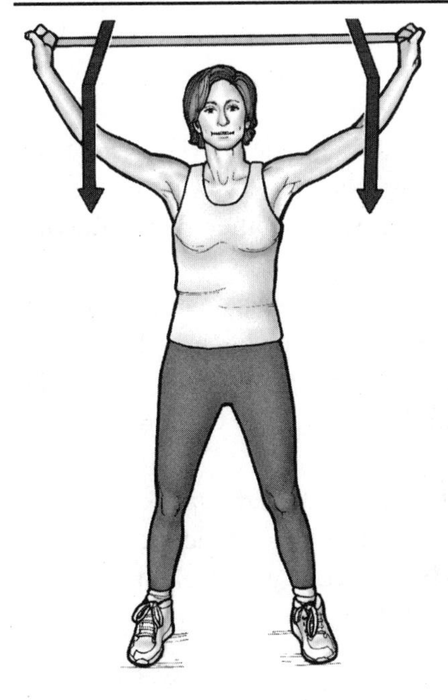

Grab an exercise band for this exercise. Stand with your feet shoulder-width apart. Hold one end of the exercise band in each hand, with your arms outstretched and positioned above and slightly in front of your head. Keeping your elbows straight but not locked, pull the band down in front to about chest level. Raise your arms back up, keeping your shoulders down. Repeat.

Muscles worked: Upper-, middle-, and lower-back muscles

The Perfect Pantry Makeover

YOUR REFRIGERATOR IS A MODEL OF WEIGHT-LOSS SUCCESS—BINS AND SHELVES BURSTING WITH COLORFUL PRODUCE, COMPARTMENTS NEATLY STOCKED WITH LOW-FAT DAIRY PRODUCTS, THE FREEZER PACKED WITH LEAN MEAT.

THAT'S GREAT. NOW, HOW'S YOUR PANTRY SHAPING UP?

In the good old days—days of creamy fillings, cheese-in-a-can, and licked fingers—your pantry was the perfect hiding place for snack cakes, fried corn chips, and other health-defying foods.

But if you want to stay fit and youthful, you must ensure that your pantry stays just as much of a healthy partner in your kitchen as your refrigerator, says Melanie Polk, R.D., director of nutrition education at the American Institute for Cancer Research in Washington, D.C. Here's how to do it.

Get motivated. Need some inspiration to clean out your cupboards? Hang a motivational image on the pantry door, such as a college picture of you in a bathing suit or a picture of someone who's at your goal weight, suggests

Laura Molseed, R.D., outpatient nutrition coordinator at the University of Pittsburgh Medical Center.

Clean it out. Since getting rid of temptation will help you enjoy healthy, disease-fighting foods more easily, it's time to do some serious housecleaning. That means giving away all those sweet treats, including candy and cookies, and making room for healthier alternatives, such as raisins, dried apricots, and cereals.

Raise your pantry's fat-fighting power. After you clean out your cupboard, restock it with plenty of filling, fat-trapping, high-fiber snacks.

For example, replace your crackers (less than 1 gram of fiber) with organic apple rings (4 grams of fiber); instead of Twizzlers (less than 1 gram of fiber), choose dried cranberries (4 grams of fiber); and trade in your cupcakes (1.8 grams of fiber) for rye wafers (5.7 grams of fiber).

Hide it high. If your family insists on keeping cookies and other goodies in the cupboard, designate a place for them—on a shelf that's up too high for you to see them or in a section that you don't usually open. If you can't see them, you're less likely to indulge, Polk says.

Have healthy food handy. Just as you keep a bowl of grapes front and center in the fridge, prominently display pretzels, whole wheat crackers, and high-fiber cereal in the front of your pantry for easy grabbing, Polk says.

Bag your snacks. Separate your pretzels, popcorn, and other snack foods into plastic sandwich bags. That way, you'll keep the portions of your snacks reasonable and have them ready to go with you to the office or on trips, Polk says.

Keep an emergency stash. Stockpile enough pasta, spaghetti sauce, and vegetable soup so that you won't have to resort to ordering take-out food during those weeks when you're running behind on your grocery shopping.

Behind Closed Doors

Here are the essentials that you need to maintain a pantry filled with satisfying, low-fat, and nutritious foods.

Staples

Always keep these staples on hand in your pantry.

- All-purpose flour
- Apple cider vinegar

- Baking powder
- Baking soda
- Bread crumbs
- Brown sugar
- Canola oil
- Cocoa (instead of chocolate chips)
- Cornmeal
- Cornstarch
- Extra-virgin olive oil
- Fat-free evaporated milk
- Green, black, or herbal tea (instead of hot chocolate)
- Herbs such as oregano, basil, thyme, parsley, and rosemary
- High-fiber cereal, such as bran flakes, shredded wheat, oatmeal, Grape-Nuts, or Kashi
- Low-calorie maple syrup
- Raisins or other dried fruit
- Red wine vinegar
- Spices such as chili powder, cinnamon, cumin, garlic powder, ginger, nutmeg, cloves, spice blends, salt, and pepper
- Wheat germ or flaxseed
- White sugar
- Whole grain bread
- Whole grain pancake and waffle mixes
- Whole grains, such as barley, bulgur, and quinoa
- Whole wheat flour
- Whole wheat pita bread

Canned Goods

Instead of foods like nacho cheese, cans of oil-soaked tuna, and fruit in heavy syrup, always think of healthier alternatives.

- Bamboo shoots
- Beans, such as pinto, kidney, navy, black, and chickpeas
- Canned fruit, such as pineapple, apricots, and peaches in juice
- Canned vegetables, such as corn, green beans, asparagus spears, beets, lima beans, peas, black-eyed peas, carrots, sliced mushrooms, greens, potatoes, and tomatoes
- Fat-free refried beans

- Low-fat spaghetti sauce
- Low-sodium chicken broth
- Natural peanut butter (best kept refrigerated)
- Reduced-sodium and low-fat soups, such as vegetable, minestrone, and lentil
- Roasted red peppers
- Tuna packed in water
- Water chestnuts

Snacks

Pack your pantry with this filling and flavorful fare.

- Baked tortilla chips
- Low-fat granola bars
- Popcorn
- Pretzels
- Sunflower seeds
- Walnuts and almonds
- Whole wheat crackers
- Whole wheat tortillas

Clothes That Accentuate Weight Loss

A CLIENT OF IMAGE CONSULTANT ANNA WILDERMUTH RECENTLY LOST 30 POUNDS. THE PROBLEM IS THAT YOU CAN'T TELL.

She wants to lose another 30 pounds, so the woman refuses to buy new clothes or have any of her old garments taken in until she has met her goal. Because her wardrobe hasn't undergone the same transformation as her body, no one has noticed that she is slimmer.

"You are putting on old clothes, and they probably feel loose—but not so loose that it makes a significant difference from the outside. When someone sees you in these old clothes, they aren't going to say, 'Oh, my gosh! You are losing weight, and you look great!'" says Wildermuth, owner of Personal Images in Elmhurst, Illinois. "You work so hard for this big change, but people won't notice until you make the little changes that will enhance it."

When you made the decision to lose weight, you took a monumental step toward looking and feeling great. After all that hard work and success, this is where you can really start to have fun. You get to create a whole new you.

Living Proof
PANEL

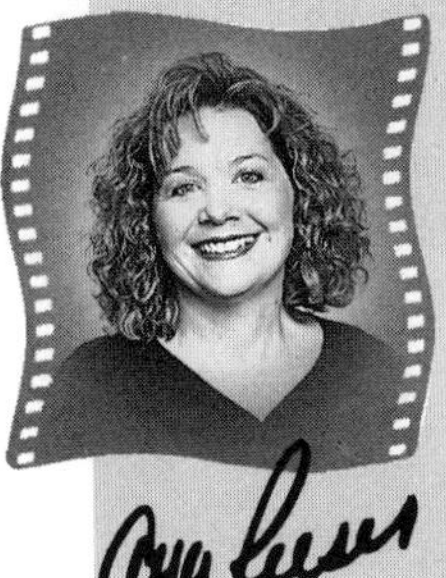

Wearing Clothes That Fit—And Flatter

I am more aware of what I wear now. Before, everything I wore was baggy, and I did everything that I could to hide my body. Now I don't mind wearing things that are tighter and form-fitting. In fact, when I go shopping, I actually look for things like that. Instead of an extra-extra-large T-shirt, I'll get a medium that actually fits me.

I'm also not as self-conscious as I used to be about my legs. I can, if I choose, wear midthigh-length shorts and skirts instead of knee-length ones.

The real change for me, though, has been with my shirts. I never used to wear sleeveless shirts. Now I do. I used to be very self-conscious about my upper arms because I thought they looked a bit flabby, so I covered them up.

But as I have participated in the program, lost weight, and done some resistance training, those muscles have firmed up, allowing me to show off my arms a bit.

"Losing weight makes you look younger and healthier. Play this up with an image that accentuates your new figure," says Princess Jenkins, an image consultant at Majestic Images International in New York City.

Why do you need a new image? Perhaps you don't even think about it, but you have probably developed a certain look, Jenkins says. Those old stonewashed jeans, your hair in the same ponytail that you've had for years, the blue eyeliner that's covered your eyelids for as long as you can remember. You continue to do it because it's easy, comfortable, and quick.

But over time, you "the person" disappears as "the look" takes over. Consciously or not, people don't even really notice you anymore. In their minds, the look *is* you.

So even after losing weight, if you don't shake up those mainstays of your image, friends and family won't be able to tell. "People are used to looking at you in this way," Jenkins says. "You have to help them see through all that. Everything about you is new, and now you need a new wardrobe and the look to show it off."

Dressing like a Star

Whether she wore playful capri pants or a sophisticated little black dress in *Breakfast at Tiffany's,* Audrey Hepburn always looked tall, slender, and elegant. Her secret was knowing how to dress in ways that complemented her small frame.

Hepburn wore clothes that were very simple, says Diana Kilgour, an independent wardrobe and image consultant in Vancouver, Canada. She didn't complicate her clothes with much detail at all.

Whether your shape tends toward the slight build of Hepburn, the natural athletic form of Loretta Swit, or the voluptuous curves of Oprah Winfrey, now is the time to showcase those extra pounds you've burned off. Here's how to look as thin and as young as you feel in smaller sizes and flattering styles.

Find your best features. Hepburn looked good because she knew what to accentuate. If you've just recently lost weight, though, you're probably more familiar with hiding your body than flaunting it. You can emulate her classy, slim style by taking a look at your best features.

"People tend to dwell on their limitations," says Georgette Braadt, an image and communications consultant in Allentown, Pennsylvania. Many women know what they don't like about themselves, but they fail to see that they have beautiful skin or that they walk elegantly or that they have terrific legs.

Step back and take a look at your body in a positive way. If you need help, ask a friend for advice and take notice when you get compliments.

Show it off. Once you know what to flaunt, don't be shy. "If you have great legs, wear your skirts a little shorter," Braadt suggests.

Duplicate the colors and styles of the clothes you wear when you hear compliments. Find pictures in catalogs and magazines of women whose body shape and features are similar to yours, and picture yourself in the clothes they're wearing before you go shopping.

For a fresh opinion on your look, take a friend with you to the store. "Bring someone who will help you go beyond your comfort zone," Braadt says, so you'll try on different styles.

Wear thinner fabrics for a thinner you. Remember those big, cotton-polyester-blend T-shirts that hid the bumps and bulges of your stomach and hips? Throw them out. It's time to wear thinner, more clingy fabrics, says Debbie Ann Gioello, professor of fashion design at the Fashion Institute of Technology in New York City and author of *Figure Types and Size Ranges* and *Understanding Fabrics*.

To appear longer and leaner, try wearing pantsuits with long jackets.

Stick with knit fabrics that have nylon or acrylic blends, she says. Or wear clothes made of Lycra or spandex, such as leggings and clingy T-shirts, because they emphasize your new shape. Sheer fabrics such as chiffon worn over a tank top will also highlight your figure.

Do your best Hepburn. Take some tips from the star herself. She had a very long waist, and she wore things that made her look even taller, as if she were miles long, says Irene Mak, professor at Parsons School of Design in New York City and technical design manager at American Eagle Outfitters.

If you want to make yourself appear even longer and leaner, try wearing pantsuits with long jackets. Wear them with a 1½- to 2-inch heel, suggests Claudia Kaneb, wardrobe head at NBC's *Today* show. The entire ensemble will make you look taller and slimmer.

Show off your legs with capri pants. Here's another youthful style that you can steal right from Hepburn's closet. "Capri pants show the definition of your legs," Mak says. If you have heavier calves, choose a length that covers part of your upper calves. If you have thinner calves, choose a length that falls above your calves.

Jazz up the classics. Classic clothes are well-constructed with quality year-round fabrics such as cotton, linen, silk, and wool. "Although classic clothes are fundamental to a working wardrobe, unaccessorized they can appear boring," Braadt says. Building your wardrobe around basic pieces that coordinate in color, fabric, and silhouette helps create wardrobe flexibility while maximizing your investment.

Classics are styles that are not influenced by current trends, which means that you can wear them for years without committing a fashion faux pas. The bulk of your wardrobe should consist of classics, she says, such as trousers, skirts, cardigans, and blazers. Proper fit ensures that people notice your figure instead of your clothes.

Dress up to keep your weight down. Accentuating your weight loss might even help you stay slim. "I've heard a lot of women say that when they like their appearance, it's just easier to stay out of the fridge," Kilgour says.

So dress up. When you change the way you dress, you change the way you carry yourself and the way you move. Just as you walk differently in different shoes, you may behave differently in a new wardrobe.

Week Eleven

Homestretch Secrets

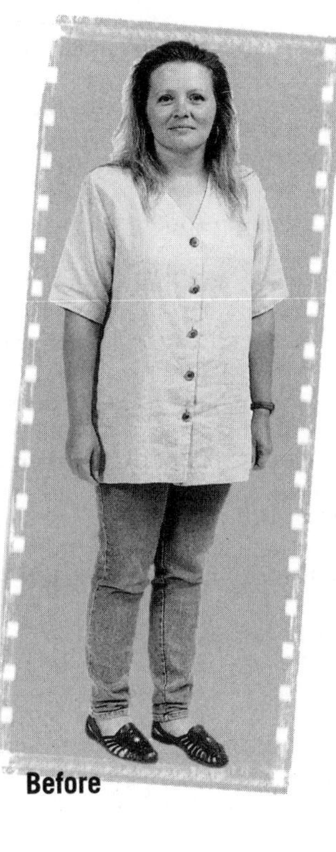

Before

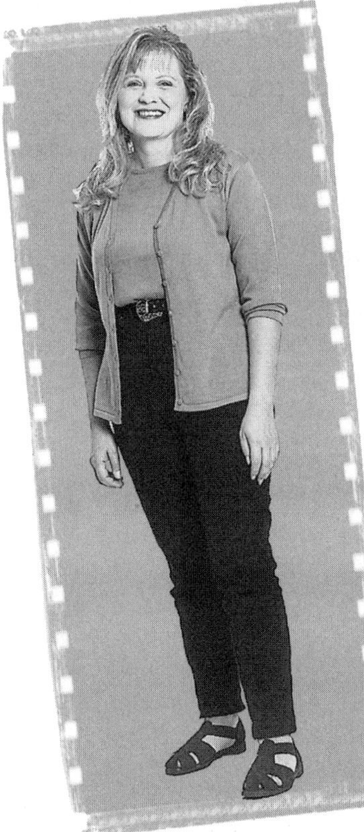

After

I WANTED TO BE HEALTHIER AND LOSE WEIGHT, SO I MADE A LIFESTYLE CHANGE, WHICH MEANT I HAD TO KICK MY QUARTER POUNDER HABIT.

—Pat Mast

Week Eleven

You're approaching the end of The *Prevention* Get Thin, Get Young Plan. You've made many small changes throughout the past few weeks that are becoming part of your healthier and slimmer lifestyle. And you've learned tips along the way to keep your motivation high. Now, it's time to add the finishing touches to the new you.

This week, you'll find plenty more advice. You've been experimenting with low-fat recipes for several weeks. But read the professional secrets to low-fat cooking, and you may discover some pointers to help you cook with ease and doctor your favorite recipes. Also, you'll learn how to make healthy choices at fast-food restaurants. Plus, with your new look come reactions—both positive and negative. Here's how to handle them and avoid sliding back into your old habits.

Bolster Your Bustline

WANT TO TAKE OFF 10 POUNDS AND 10 YEARS?

IT'S EASIER THAN YOU THINK.

ALL YOU NEED IS THE RIGHT BRA.

When a bra doesn't fit properly, it either allows breasts to sag too low or bunches them in so that they bulge out of the top and the sides. Both problems can add about 10 pounds and 10 years to a woman's appearance," says Berna Goldstein, vice president of merchandising for the Bali Company, a bra manufacturer in New York City. "And the problem is common. When we survey women, we find that 70 to 85 percent of women are wearing the wrong size or the wrong style bra for their figures."

Ill-fitting bras are especially common among larger-size women, the ones who can benefit most from the slimming effects of the right bustline support, Goldstein says. "You see many full-figured women who wear bras that let their breasts fall down to their waists. They look much older, heavier, and short-waisted than women who wear proper-fitting bras that put their breasts up where they belong."

Plus, wearing a bra that provides proper support, especially when you're exercising, can help reduce the stress to your ligaments and prevent your breasts from sagging in the first place.

Hands down, the biggest mistake that women make is buying bras that don't fit, Goldstein says. "Bras come in many different cuts and styles. Just as you can't wear every pair of size 12 pants you put on, you can't expect that every 36C bra will fit you the way that it should." Here are some helpful hints to get the best wear out of your underwear.

Measure up. A surprising number of women have never had their bra sizes measured, Goldstein says. "They just buy what they've always bought, which may or may not be the right size and style."

The best plan is to go to an undergarment specialty store and have a salesperson size you properly. You also can do it yourself, however. First, find your band size. Measure yourself under your breasts (underbust) to get your rib cage measurement and add 5 to this number. For example, if the measurement is 29, add 5, and your band size is 34. If the result is an odd number, say, 35, you could try either the size above or below, which in this example would be a 34 or a 36.

Next, determine your cup size. Start by measuring the circumference of your torso from your back, under your arms, and across your chest (over your breasts) at the fullest point of your bust (overbust). Next, subtract your band size from this measurement. Use the resulting number and the chart below to determine your cup size. This is a general guide, since sizes may vary depending on the brand.

Figuring Out Your Cup Size

DIFFERENCE BETWEEN OVERBUST AND BAND SIZE	CUP SIZE
Less than 1 inch	AA
1 inch	A
2 inches	B
3 inches	C
4 inches	D
More than 4 inches	DD or larger

Fill up without overfilling. When you put on a bra, each cup should completely contain each breast.

"If the cup wrinkles or sags anywhere, it's too big," says Goldstein. If you bulge over the top or the sides, you have the wrong size or the wrong style. "If the bra generally fits well and feels comfortable but you still have a little bulging, try a style with a fuller-cut cup to fit fuller shapes of the same size."

Lower the back. The lower the strap fits on your back, the more support you get. "Wearing a bra strap high on your back will allow your breasts to hang low and give you a frumpy appearance, not to mention making you very uncomfortable," says Goldstein. The lower edge of the band should run straight around your body. If the back rides up, the cups may be too small, the straps may be pulled too tight, or the bra's band is probably too big for you. The straps should be comfortable, without digging into your shoulders.

Dial in the straps. For the slimmest, youngest appearance, your bra should hold your nipples about 2½ inches below an imaginary line that connects the folds of your underarms. Adjust the straps so that your breasts fall to this point, while the back strap sits slightly lower than the front. "At no point should the straps dig into your shoulders," Goldstein says. "If that happens and the bra fits otherwise, try one with wider, more padded straps."

Test the band. The center of the bra should fall against your breastbone. The band should be snug all the way around, but you should be able to run your finger all the way around beneath it. "Larger women often make the mistake of buying a bra that is super-tight because they think that's what they need for support," says Goldstein. "What they end up with is a bra that digs into them all over and gives them very unflattering, heavy-looking lines as they spill out around it. Try larger, wider straps and bands instead of a tighter bra. It'll support you better and make you look slimmer, too."

Pick something pretty. When was the last time you bought a pretty bra? If you can't remember, it's high time, Goldstein says. "Women often stop buying themselves pretty underwear after they're married or if they've gained weight, which is a shame because pretty underwear makes you feel young and pretty."

Worried that pretty bras aren't functional? Don't be. "Bra technology has come a long way. Even the biggest, most supportive sizes come in beautiful colors, prints, and fabrics," she adds.

The Bounce-Free Workout

Before 1977, women who hoped to exercise bounce-free were left to their own devices. The first sports bra, in fact, was two jockstraps sewn together by a pair of resourceful athletes, now renowned as the mothers of the Jogbra.

But even after manufacturers started producing commercial exercise bras, large-breasted women were left out in the cold until the 1990s.

Today, there are sports bras available for women of all shapes and sizes. But they don't all work equally well for everyone. The American Council on Exercise reports that a large majority of women still experience breast dis-

Means of Support

Wearing a quality, supportive bra is rule number one for maintaining a youthful bustline. Rule number two is to build up the muscles beneath your breasts.

"To firm up your breast area, you need to build the pectoral muscles that lie directly beneath your breasts," says Amy Goldwater, a certified fitness specialist and fitness advisor to the TOPS (Take Off Pounds Sensibly) Club in Milwaukee. "When you pump up those muscles, you fill out that area and give your bustline a little lift."

Chest presses. Lie on your back, with your knees bent and your feet flat on the floor and about hip-width apart. Hold a weight in each hand, with your arms extended up over your chest and your palms facing the ceiling. Your thumbs should face each other.

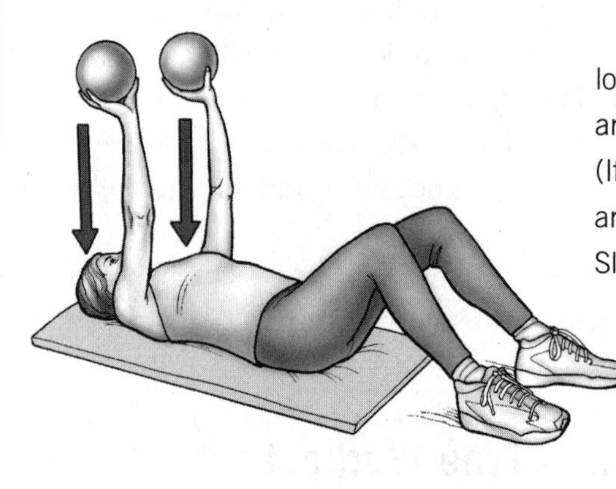

Bend your elbows and slowly lower the weights. Stop when they are about even with your shoulders. (If you're lying on the floor, your arms will be resting on the floor.) Slowly return to start. Repeat.

comfort when exercising. That not only makes exercising unpleasant, but too much bouncing is bad for your bustline.

"Many large-breasted women will wear two sports bras to prevent these problems," says Susan Verscheure, who has researched sports bras in the department of exercise and movement science at the University of Oregon in Eugene. "But with the right bra, most women can get the support they need with just one."

Here are some characteristics to look for.

Here are two exercises that she recommends. Do them two or three times a week, with at least 24 hours between exercise sessions. Be sure to do the exercises in a slow, controlled manner, counting 3 seconds as you lift, pausing a second, and counting 3 seconds as you lower. The weights should be heavy enough so that the last four repetitions are fairly hard.

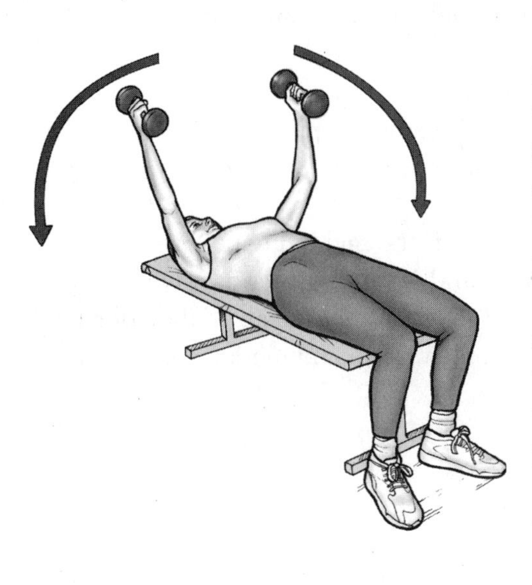

Chest flies. Lie on your back on a bench or the floor, with your knees bent and your feet flat on the floor. Holding a weight in each hand, extend your arms up over your chest, with your elbows slightly bent and your palms facing each other.

Bend your arms slightly to the sides at your elbows, creating a wingspan effect, and slowly lower the weights out to the sides until they are about level with your shoulders. Hold for a second, then raise the weights to the starting position. Repeat.

Encapsulation. There are essentially two styles of sports bra. For women with C-cup breasts or larger, encapsulation is the way to go, Verscheure says. An encapsulation (also called isolation) bra holds each breast separately in a supportive cup. The other style, a compression bra, pushes your breasts against your chest wall and holds them there.

"We found that one encapsulated bra worked better than two compression bras, and it was more comfortable," she adds.

Don't be fooled by their appearance when you shop for one. Many encapsulated bras have hooks and seamed cups like regular bras, so they don't look the way you might expect.

"They're not the kind of sports bras that most women would wear without a shirt over them," Verscheure says. But the added performance makes up for the lack of appearance.

A broad back. Sports bras come as T-backs and cross-backs (with straps that run toward the middle of the back) or as scoop backs (with straps that run straight over the shoulders).

T- or cross-backs pull the entire bust up, so they're good for controlling bouncing. But they can dig into the trapezius (upper-back) muscles of larger-breasted women. "The rule of thumb with T-back bras is the bigger the back panel, the better the comfort," says Missy Park, founder of Title IX, a women's athletic supply company in Berkeley, California. Or you can opt for a large scoop back, provided the shoulder straps are wide and supportive.

Thick bands. Any bra for larger-breasted women should have wider straps than the average sports bra, Park says. "Narrow straps will dig into your shoulders and be uncomfortable. Look instead for wide, padded straps going over the shoulders."

Stay-put power. Never buy a sports bra off the rack without trying it on, says Park. "Go into the dressing room and bounce up and down. Your breasts should pretty well stay put, with minimum bouncing. If they don't, take it off and try another one until you find a make and model that is comfortable and supportive."

Steps to Shapely Legs

When the flappers roared into the 1920s, waistlines dropped and hemlines rose, finally giving women the hard-fought permission to show some leg. Since then, women have been liberated with miniskirts, A-line dresses, short shorts, and, of course, the bikini. But there are still many women who would just as soon put them back under wraps.

In many cases, the cover-up isn't because their legs are out of shape. It's to hide bulging blue varicose veins or purplish webs of spider veins that can make even great legs look (and feel) not so great.

About 15 percent of adults have vein problems, says Luis Navarro, M.D., founder and director of the Vein Treatment Center in New York City. And those problems are much more common in women than they are in men.

Varicose veins were not likely something that you worried about on prom night, but they're not just an "old lady's ailment" either. They affect a surprising number of young women and more than half of women over the age of 40. Birth control pills and pregnancy can make you more susceptible to them. They're also hereditary.

And if you're overweight, you're more likely to have problems. "Carrying around excess weight puts more strain on your veins, especially around the pelvic area during pregnancy, where varicose veins often start," Dr. Navarro says.

Cultivate Curvy Calves

Shapely, strong calves are good for more than just turning heads. They also strengthen your "second heart," the system of muscles and vessels in your legs that pumps blood back up to your heart.

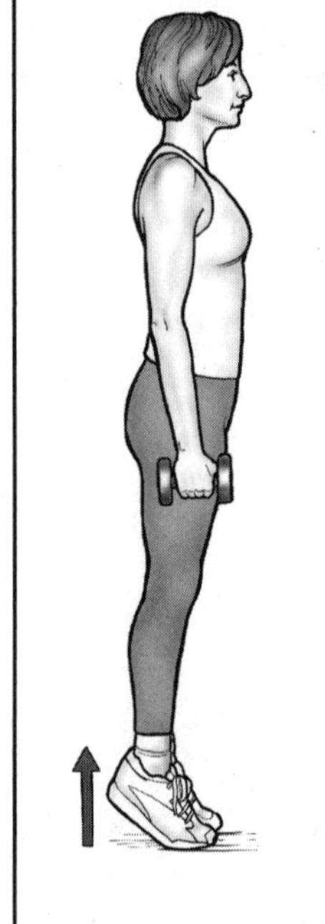

A strong second heart also helps keep your legs looking lovely by keeping spider veins and varicose veins at bay. Brisk walking and other aerobic exercise can help keep your calves toned, but it's also a good idea to exercise those muscles.

"Calf raises are probably the best exercises for these muscles," says Dr. Luis Navarro of the Vein Treatment Center. "They're quick and simple. And you have to do them only a couple times a week to benefit from them." Here's how.

Stand with your legs about hip-width apart and hold a weight (dumbbell or medicine ball) in each hand down by your sides. Slowly lift your heels off the ground, shifting your weight up on your toes, keeping your knees straight and your torso erect. Hold, then lower. Repeat 10 to 15 times.

Begin with just one set, and after 2 weeks increase to two sets of 10 to 15 repetitions, two times a week. This workout should be done only every other day.

Fortunately, with the right preventive measures—and the right treatments—you can keep your legs "bareably" lovely no matter what your age.

The Vein Culprits

Both spider veins and varicose veins are caused by a problem with circulation. There are valves inside your veins that keep your blood flowing back to your heart. When those valves fail to open and shut properly, blood pools inside your veins, causing them to stretch out and bulge.

When that happens in small veins or capillaries, you see a small weblike netting of red, blue, or purple spider veins pop up. When it happens in a larger vein, the result is a bluish, bulging varicose vein. These unsightly veins don't just make your legs look older than they are, they make them feel older, too, as they cause heaviness, night cramps, and, in the case of large varicose veins, uncomfortable throbbing and swelling.

"Genetics plays the biggest role in whether or not you're prone to these vein problems," says Dr. Navarro, "but lots of outside factors contribute to them."

Female hormones are a common cause, he says, because estrogen can weaken your vein walls, making them more prone to bulge. Pregnancy makes you especially susceptible because the added weight on your pelvic veins, additional circulating blood, and excess female hormones leave your veins at their most vulnerable.

While there's not much that you can do about your genes, hormones, or what happens when you're pregnant, there are other preventive measures that you can take to keep vein problems to a minimum. Here's what experts recommend.

Make your "second heart" strong. The system of veins, valves, and muscles in your feet and calves is called the second heart because it pushes blood from your legs back to your heart, Dr. Navarro says. "Like the heart in your chest, you need to keep your second heart strong through exercise for it to work properly. Just walking 20 to 30 minutes every day can help. But it's important that you get up and move whenever you can."

Move your feet. Even if your second heart is relatively strong, unless it has a chance to work, you're still at risk for developing vein problems. That's why both sitting and standing for long periods of time can increase your risk for varicose and spider veins, says Arielle Kauvar, M.D., associate director of the Laser and Skin Surgery Center of New York in Manhattan.

"When you're in a position where you just stand a lot or sit for very long periods of time, your calves don't have a chance to propel your blood back, and it's more likely to pool over time," she says. "Your best defense is taking a break and walking whenever you can."

But if you can't manage that, at least rock back and forth on your feet and flex and stretch your calf muscles at least once or twice an hour.

Eat your fill of fiber. Doctors have noticed that people who eat their daily fill of fiber (25 to 30 grams a day) are less prone to varicose veins, Dr. Navarro says. "We're not exactly sure of the connection, but it's likely related to constipation. People who don't eat enough fiber tend to be constipated.

When you strain to go to the bathroom, you put additional pressure on your veins."

A quick way to get half the fiber you need each day is to start your morning with ½ cup of a high-fiber cereal like Fiber One (14 grams).

Wear some support. Women who have a history of vein problems can benefit from wearing compression stockings, Dr. Kauvar says. Available at medical supply companies and some drugstores, these stockings fit tightly around your ankles and fit gradually looser as they rise up to the thighs.

Estrogen can weaken your vein walls, increasing your risk for vein problems.

"Because they're snug around your calf, they help prevent blood from pooling in those lower veins. And they press on your veins, so they help push the blood back up to your heart," she says.

Loosen your jeans. Clothes that fit snugly at your groin can put pressure on your leg veins, discouraging circulation back to your heart and encouraging veins to stretch and bulge. "Regular stockings can be a problem because they're tight at the thigh," says Dr. Navarro. The same is true for skin-tight jeans. Do your veins and your thighs a favor, and loosen up.

Kick your feet up. Gravity is not your friend in the fight against vein problems. Since your legs literally fight an uphill battle all day, do them a favor and prop them up when you lie down to rest, Dr. Navarro says. Put a pillow under your feet to elevate your legs 6 to 12 inches above your heart so blood can flow freely out of your legs with no strain on your veins. "It also feels wonderfully relaxing to kick your feet up after a long day," he says.

Uncross your legs. You may look pretty and ladylike, but crossing your legs won't keep them looking pretty in the long run. "Crossing your legs slows the upward flow of blood from your legs to your heart and increases pressure in your veins," Dr. Kauvar says. "When sitting at your job, try to sit up straight and keep both feet flat on the floor as much as possible."

Eschew extra estrogen. Estrogen can weaken your vein walls, making them more susceptible to stretching and bulging. So, if you're prone to varicose or spider veins, it's probably not a good idea to pour more estrogen into your system than you already have, says Dr. Navarro.

"Both hormone-replacement therapy and birth control pills can increase your risk for vein problems. If you can't avoid using hormones altogether, ask your doctor about low-dose contraceptives or hormone therapy," he suggests.

Strengthen with flavonoids. Bioflavonoids are substances in certain fruits, vegetables, and herbs that help strengthen capillary and vein walls. To get the most beneficial dose of these helpful compounds, Dr. Navarro suggests that people prone to vein trouble take flavonoid-rich herbal supplements such as butcher's broom and horse chestnut. You can find these in your local natural food store. Take as directed. Horse chestnut may interfere with the action of other drugs, especially blood thinners such as warfarin (Coumadin). It may also irritate the gastrointestinal tract. Horse chestnut should not be used during pregnancy.

A Vanishing Act

Even if you do everything right, you still may find yourself with a bulging vein or two down the line, especially if you have had multiple pregnancies, have used hormones for a long period of time, or have a strong family history of vein problems.

"If you have a strong genetic tendency for varicose veins, it's pretty tough to prevent them 100 percent," Dr. Kauvar says. "You can minimize them, but you may not be able to completely avoid them."

Fortunately, varicose veins are more easily treated than ever. And with a few fairly painless procedures, you can have your vein-free legs back again in a short amount of time. "The new chemical and laser treatments for eliminating veins are so refined, we can eliminate even very big blue varicose veins with just a few treatments," Dr. Kauvar says.

When you're looking to vanish veins, you have two avenues to choose from: sclerotherapy or laser surgery. Both work by eliminating the stretched-out vein and rerouting blood to healthy vessels. Which method your doctor chooses depends mostly on the size of the vein and your personal preference.

Sclerotherapy. This procedure involves injecting a chemical solution into your affected vein, causing it to become inflamed and eventually collapse. During the following weeks, your body breaks down and reabsorbs the defunct vein.

"We can use sclerotherapy for small spider veins to large varicose veins," says Dr. Kauvar. "The needles we use are very small and very fine, so they are not too uncomfortable. And, though the older solutions used to sting quite a bit and could be quite irritating to the skin, there are new solutions that are not painful and are much more gentle to the skin."

If the vein being treated is larger, you may need repeat treatments.

Laser surgery. Until recently, lasers could treat only smaller spider veins, Dr. Kauvar says. "But during the past 5 years, the laser technology has advanced so we can use them on even larger veins."

Lasers work by heating your vein with light energy that essentially "cooks" it. Your body then absorbs the unused vein during the next few weeks. As with sclerotherapy, if the vein is very large, repeat treatments may be necessary. But as laser technology improves, the number of repeat visits required for removal drops, Dr. Kauvar says. "With the latest techniques, spider veins and smaller varicose veins can be cleared in two to four treatment sessions."

With either therapy, you can usually resume normal daily activities immediately, though more strenuous exercise may have to wait a few days to a week.

Professional Secrets to Delicious Low-Fat Cooking

YOU'VE PLANNED A GREAT MEAL, BOUGHT THE FRESHEST INGREDIENTS, AND ARE READY TO COOK. WHETHER YOUR DISH IS A DELIGHT OR A DISASTER COULD DEPEND ON YOUR PREPARATION TECHNIQUE.

Even if you have been cooking for years and have always gotten compliments galore, you can learn from the experts when it comes to low-fat cooking. Here's how to avoid the five most common pitfalls.

Invest in Nonstick Pans

Instead of your regular pans, use nonstick cookware to create low-fat skillet and stovetop dishes as well as baked goodies. Most people have a tendency to add oil to a dish while it's cooking if the food starts to stick. And you can easily double the amount of fat in a recipe with a few injudicious splashes of oil.

"If nothing else, at least buy a nonstick 10-inch skillet, preferably with a lid," says Tom Ney, author of *The Health-Lover's Guide to Super Seafood* and director of *Prevention* magazine's Test Kitchen in Emmaus, Pennsylvania.

Such a pan will prove its versatility immediately. You'll be able to use it to water-sauté, which is browning meats without adding fat, and to create braised dishes, which are browned meats cooked with added liquids.

If you must use a regular skillet, first coat it thoroughly with a nonstick spray, says Barbara Gollman, R.D., a registered dietitian and author of *The Phytopia Cookbook*.

"You should do this even if you plan on adding a little oil or butter to the dish," she says. If sticking occurs, add some broth, juice, or plain water to the skillet. Use it to soften and scrape the browned bits from the bottom of the pan—they'll add flavor to the dish.

Go Low-Fat, Not Fat-Free

A little bit of fat adds enormously to a dish's flavor and texture, so if you're watching portion sizes and otherwise eating generally healthy, there's no reason not to have some fat in a dish, especially if it's a heart-healthy monounsaturated fat, says Gollman.

For some foods, there's a big difference between low-fat and fat-free. Low-fat cheeses and sour cream, for instance, melt and blend much better than their fat-free counterparts, which often contain sticky gums.

Low-fat cheeses handle even better if you fine-grate them straight from the refrigerator, while they're still chilled. They melt best when heated for a longer time at a lower temperature. Or, if you're using a microwave oven, keep the food on a lower setting, cover it with microwaveable plastic wrap or a microwaveable cover, make sure the food rotates, and stir frequently. Low-fat cheeses taste best when they are used in dishes that have added moisture—lasagna, for instance.

And while fat-free sour cream might be okay on top of a baked potato, the gums and thickeners found in such a product make it hard to incorporate smoothly into sauces or batters, Ney says. Low-fat is a better choice here. You can also use combinations of fat-free, low-fat, and full-fat to come up with your own tasty, healthy versions of dishes.

Even if you are cooking low-fat, it's not unreasonable to add up to 1 tablespoon of an oil to a dish that serves four to six, Gollman says. To get maximum flavor out of that spoonful, use extra-virgin olive oil or a flavorful walnut or sesame oil.

If you are baking, you can usually reduce the fat called for in a recipe by

The Perfect Low-Fat Cake

You *can* have your cake and lose weight, too. The same goes for your cookies and muffins. The secret is using the techniques that professional chefs use to trim the fat. Here's how they do it.

If the recipe is an old classic—Betty Crocker, pre-1990—chances are that it can tolerate trimming both fat and sugar by about one-quarter with no problems.

- Cut back on butter or shortening by replacing it with an equal amount of fruit puree: for white batters or doughs, use applesauce; for chocolate, use prune puree. With most recipes, you can replace up to half the fat with puree without noticing a difference.
- Replace up to half of the whole eggs in a recipe with egg whites, or use ¼ cup of silken tofu, put through a blender, per egg.
- For every ounce of melted unsweetened chocolate in a recipe, substitute 3 tablespoons of cocoa powder dissolved in 2 tablespoons of water and mixed with 1 tablespoon of prune puree.
- Cut back on the amount of saturated fat in a cake or muffin recipe by substituting canola oil for half of the butter or shortening. With cookies, it's probably better to just eliminate one-quarter of the butter or shortening.
- Instead of spreading on icing, dust a cake with powdered sugar or a mix of powdered sugar and cocoa. Or serve it topped with a few slices of fruit and a fat-free whipped topping.

about one-quarter, and replace about half of the amount of butter or margarine with canola oil to reduce total saturated fat or trans fatty acids.

Spice Up Your Life

It's an unfortunate fact of food: Fat brings out flavors, so using less fat requires that you add more flavor in other ways.

"Don't be timid about using more herbs and spices," Gollman says. Instead of ¼ or ½ teaspoon of a dried herb, try a full teaspoon or two for a recipe that serves four to six. Or use 1 tablespoon or more of fresh herbs, such as basil, rosemary, or dill, which are available year-round at most big supermarkets.

Add fresh herbs toward the end of the cooking time to keep their delicate flavors from fading from the heat. (For maximum flavor, you need to use three times as much fresh herb as you would dried.

Low-fat foods tend to dry out while they cook.

Think of flavors as layers, Gollman says. To your herb flavors, add another layer—sweet—by using fruit juice, dried fruits such as cranberries, flavored vinegar, or the colorful zest from orange, lemon, or lime peel. You could add apricot juice to a dish of chicken tenders, lime juice to broiled scallops, dried cherries to the ground beef going into a meat loaf, or a touch of cooking sherry to a vinaigrette, Gollman says. (Wines are often too dry to add the taste of sweetness to a dish, but grape juice works just fine.)

"Deep, complex flavors take time to develop in a dish," Ney says. Since time is one thing many of us don't have much of these days, you can buy additions to your dish that have already had the flavor cooked into them. Roasted red peppers, roasted garlic, broths, and tomato sauces all fit this bill.

You can also take advantage of blended seasonings, including teriyaki sauce, peanut sauce, pesto, chutneys, relish, green chili sauce, tarragon mustard, horseradish, and curry pastes, Ney says. Most products have recipe suggestions on the labels.

Toasting raw seeds and nuts before adding them to a dish will deepen their flavor, Ney suggests. Simply toss them into a medium-hot, dry frying pan and toast them until golden brown. (Just be sure to stir them frequently so they don't burn.) Experiment with raw sesame seeds, sunflower seeds, pine nuts, walnuts, almonds—whichever kinds of seeds and nuts you prefer.

And don't forget garlic. Use roasted garlic as a creamy, no-fat spread on toasted Italian bread, or add garlic early on to a dish for a mild flavor. To keep its flavor fresh and lively, put it through a garlic press and add to the dish shortly before it's done cooking.

Beware of Overcooking

Fat doesn't evaporate, but water does, which means that low-fat foods tend to dry out while they cook and are truly miserable to eat if they're overcooked even the least bit. So cooking times and temperatures are extra important. Plus, you may need to add ingredients that bind moisture, such as soluble fiber or egg whites, to a low-fat dish.

That old rule of thumb for cooking times for fish—10 minutes for every inch of thickness—was and still is bad advice, Gollman says. "If you are grilling or sautéing, 6 to 7 minutes is plenty of time." Baking may require slightly more time.

Poaching fish guarantees a moist finished product. You can add a bit of lemon or orange juice to the poaching fluid for flavor, and lemon juice helps cut down on the fish aroma.

Lean meats do better with moist, slow-cooking methods, such as braising or stewing. You will get better flavor if you brown the meat—chicken breasts, beef cubes, or pork tenderloins—before you add the liquid, such as broth, wine, or juice. Then cook at a simmer. Boiling toughens meats.

If you're broiling, marinate the meat first and brush on marinade as you broil to help retain moisture. You can also spray the meat with the same nonstick spray you use on pans, or use a mister to put a fine coat of olive oil on the meat, Gollman suggests.

Sear meats at a high temperature first when cooking, to seal juices inside the meat. Don't cut into the meat to see if it's done. Instead, insert an instant-read thermometer. The temperature should reach 160°F at the center of the cut. If you're cooking chicken breasts, leave the skin on for extra flavor and moisture and cook to 170°F. Remove the skin at the table.

If a meat comes out of the oven or off the grill slightly underdone, Gollman says, simply zap it for 30 seconds on high in the microwave oven. "It already has the flavor and the look," she says. "It just needs a little bit more cooking."

Low-fat baked goods, too, dry out quickly if they are overdone. Make sure that your oven temperature is correct—check it against another thermometer if you suspect it's off.

Learn the Label Lingo

It's not too hard to be fooled by ingredients that appear to be low-fat but really aren't. To figure out how much fat is in a hunk of Swiss cheese or a can of chicken soup, you look on the label and see how many grams of total fat you'll get per serving. When it comes to meat, especially ground meat, though, it's an entirely different, often elusive story.

Some major grocery store chains do put nutrition labels on their ground beef, but ground meat does not yet come under the labeling requirements of other foods, and the USDA hasn't decided how it should be labeled.

So meat that is labeled "80 percent lean" has 20 percent fat *by weight*—not percent of calories. That means per 3.5-ounce serving, it has 10 grams of fat, getting almost 70 percent of its calories from fat. Meat that is "90 percent lean" still gets 51 percent of its calories from fat. And extra-lean, at 5 grams of fat per serving, is hard to find.

Don't think that if you get ground chicken or turkey you are automatically getting a low-fat product, Gollman says.

"If the skin is ground along with the meat, it can be quite fatty," she says. In this case, it's best to buy ground skinless breasts of chicken or turkey. And when you're buying chicken or turkey sausage, franks, or other processed meats, check the label to be sure that there are real fat savings.

You can always buy meat and ask to have it trimmed and ground for you while you wait.

Enjoying Guilt-Free Fast Food

IF FINE DINING IS CAUSE FOR CELEBRATION, THEN WOLFING DOWN A BURGER AT A FAST-FOOD RESTAURANT IS OFTEN CAUSE FOR A GUILTY CONSCIENCE.

It doesn't have to be. At some point, almost all of us find ourselves queued up in the drive-thru lane or taking our kids in for the latest toy craze. Indeed, the average American now eats an average of four meals a week away from home.

The problem, as we all know, is that most of this stuff is high in fat and calories and very low in nutritional value. Some fast-food sandwiches pack a whopping 1,000 calories. But not all of it is unhealthy and fattening.

"There are a million bad choices and a few good ones," says Jayne Hurley, R.D., senior nutritionist at the Center for Science in the Public Interest in Washington, D.C. "As long as you know what those good choices are, you can walk out of the restaurant without blowing half a day's calories and fat on one sandwich."

Like everything else in weight loss, a little planning and preparation go a long way. While it's certainly not a good idea to eat french fries every day, if you make the right choices at the drive-thru window, your waistline won't suffer, says Jeanne Goldberg, R.D., Ph.D., director of the center on nutrition communication at Tufts University in Boston. Here's how.

Living Proof
PANEL

Getting Back to Usual

Pat Mast

My usual at McDonald's had always been a hamburger, a small order of french fries, and an iced tea. But when my sons got older and started ordering Quarter Pounders, large fries, and large sodas, I did the same. Suddenly, I realized that I was eating more in general, including having seconds at home. All those extra calories ended up on my waistline, and I gained 40 pounds in 5 years.

Finally, I decided to put an end to overeating. I wanted to be healthier and lose weight, so I made a lifestyle change, which meant I had to kick my Quarter Pounder habit.

It wasn't easy. It took awhile before I felt satisfied eating a hamburger and small fries again, but now I feel and look healthier—with a smaller waist.

Get an education. Learning just how much fat and calories are in some items might ruin your appetite for fast food. Among the more offensive are the following:

- Double Whopper with Cheese at Burger King—1,010 calories and 67 grams of fat
- Nachos Bellgrande at Taco Bell—770 calories and 39 grams of fat
- One slice of Stuffed Crust Pizza with pepperoni at Pizza Hut—438 calories and 19 grams of fat

For more bad—and some good—news, ask for a nutrition guide at the counter. You'll learn what to stay away from and what you can eat, like a Grilled Chicken Soft Taco at Taco Bell for 200 calories and a relatively slim 7 grams of fat.

Keep the guide in your car to plan ahead, suggests Tammy Baker, R.D., a registered dietitian in Cave Creek, Arizona, and a spokesperson for the American Dietetic Association. Or go online before you head out to the fast-food emporium. Many chain restaurants have their nutrition information on their Web sites.

Shop around. Food doesn't have to be from drive-thru windows to be fast. Scout out other eating choices to meet your nutrition needs, such as convenience stores and supermarkets, says Olivia Bennett Wood, R.D., associate professor of foods and nutrition at Purdue University in West Lafayette, Indiana.

Many stores offer fresh salads, fruit, deli foods, stir-fry vegetables, and even sushi. Exploring your options will help you get a variety of food to balance your diet.

Boost your nutrients. Wherever you go, make the most of your options. For example, two slices of tomato add only 5 calories to your sandwich and provide some vitamin C, lycopene, and potassium. Order extra lettuce and tomatoes; choose a lean type of meat, such as turkey, roast beef, or grilled chicken; and put it on whole wheat bread, suggests Baker. You've managed to get a meal full of protein and fiber with a minimum amount of fat.

Kick the value meals. Being able to get more food for less money may be good for your wallet, but it's sure to pack on the pounds. A small order of fries has 210 calories and 10 grams of fat, while a large order has 540 calories and 26 grams of fat. "They have value in terms of money, not necessarily in terms of nutrition," Wood says.

Living Proof PANEL

Yo Quiero Taco Bell

I can't give up my Taco Bell. Passing up candy and ice cream is a cinch, but when I crave a tostada, I get one. What I can do is cut down on how often I eat it. Now, instead of making fast food a weekly ritual, my husband, John, and I go to Taco Bell for lunch once a month, and we balance out the extra calories we're eating with a light dinner.

The same holds true for bigger-and-badder sandwiches, Hurley says. A McDonald's Quarter Pounder with Cheese has 530 calories and 30 grams of fat, while their hamburger has 270 calories and 9 grams of fat.

Avoid extra calories. A chicken sandwich is healthy, right? Not if there's 1½ tablespoons of mayonnaise on it. The mayo alone adds a whopping 160 calories and 17 grams of fat. If you really want the mayo, ask for a light version (40 calories and 4 grams of fat) and get it on the side so you can control how much of it you eat.

And while you're cutting out the fat, order a grilled chicken sandwich for only 9 grams of fat over a fried one, which has 16 grams of fat. Also, skip the cheese, which adds 90 calories and 8 grams of fat, and the bacon, which adds another 40 calories and 3 grams of fat.

Back off the bubbles. On top of your meal, a 22-ounce nondiet soda will add 280 calories. Ask for water or fat-free milk instead.

Kicking your high-fat fast-food habit won't be easy. But when you figure out a way of making it a healthy part of your diet, you can kiss your guilt goodbye.

Getting a Reaction— And How to Handle It

ONE DAY, TAMMY HANSEN WAS DRIVING DOWN THE STREET IN HER HOMETOWN OF ROCKFORD, MICHIGAN, WHEN A MAN STARTED HONKING AND WHISTLING AT HER.

HER FIRST THOUGHT: DID I LEAVE MY PURSE ON THE HOOD OF MY CAR AGAIN? THEN IT DAWNED ON THE 33-YEAR-OLD SCIENCE TEACHER: HE WAS HONKING AT *HER*.

It's not exactly the type of reaction she was hoping for after losing 61 pounds, but since this was attention she didn't get before she lost weight, she took it as a compliment.

Back at home, her husband's reaction took her by surprise, too. He tried to reward her weight loss with chocolate-covered raisins.

If you're someone who wants to keep your weight loss to yourself, forget about it. It's inevitable that people will react to the new you. The question is, how will you deal with it, says Howard J. Rankin, Ph.D., psychological advisor to the TOPS (Take Off Pounds Sensibly) Club and author of *Seven Steps to Wellness*.

Here's how to handle all that extra attention—wanted and unwanted.

Learn how to accept a compliment. While it's perfectly normal to feel over-

Living Proof
PANEL

Shoofly, Don't Bother Me

Instead of canceling dinner dates for fear that I'll overeat, I serve myself smaller portions when I'm at other people's houses. That way, I don't leave any food on my plate, and I don't hear comments about how much—or how little—I've eaten.

But when I refused dessert at my cousin's house—a slice of freshly made shoofly pie with blackstrap molasses—I had some explaining to do. Instead of crumbling under pressure and eating it, I told my hosts that I prefer fruit in place of dessert. I even persuaded them to take my daily 30-minute walk with me.

I'm excited about my lifestyle change, and it shows. Although people comment on the way I look, I'm complimented far more often on my positive attitude and energy, which keep me motivated.

whelmed by comments about your weight loss, the best thing to do is to acknowledge them. Simply say thank you.

If you feel particularly uncomfortable, end the conversation by saying something like "I feel a lot better." Or say, "I find I'm more energetic," suggests Joyce A. Hanna, associate director of the health improvement program at Stanford University and an exercise physiologist in Palo Alto, California. Then change the subject.

Ignore negative comments. While most of the comments you hear will be encouraging, you're bound to get at least one negative comment. If someone tells you, "I bet you won't keep the weight off," shrug it off, Dr. Rankin says. Keep your mind positive.

Share your weight-loss secrets. Another way to deflect negative comments is by confiding in your friends about how you lost weight. The next time someone gives you a hard time about indulging in dessert, let them know that your weight loss came from a lifestyle change, says Stephanie Noll, a clinical psychologist at Duke University Diet and Fitness Center in Durham, North Carolina. Tell them that you stayed on track with a food diary and that you found exercises you enjoy, so it's okay if you enjoy dessert once in a while.

Ease those insecurities. Ever notice how some family members and friends will do little things to undermine you when they're insecure? Whether it's your best girlfriend or your sweetheart, if they feel insecure about all the attention you're getting, they'll try to persuade you to have seconds at dinner or make you feel guilty about losing weight.

Since they're probably worried that your relationship with them will change, simply reassure them that you're the same person you were before you lost weight, Hanna suggests. Treat them just as you've always done, but put an end to forced food and guilt.

Living Proof
PANEL

Impressing Family and Friends

There wasn't much of a reaction from the people who see me every day because the weight loss was gradual and progressive. But when I visited my family and friends out in California who hadn't seen me in a while, the reaction was: "Wow!"

I was back to where I was before I had my son and before I gained all of my weight. It was nice that my weight loss was noticed. They all said that I looked great. Then, at Christmas, my husband's family reacted equally as well. They were asking me how I lost all of this weight. They were quite impressed.

My husband, John, likes it a lot. He thinks it's great for me because the compliments I get from others improve my mood and self-confidence. I think the whole program, and the reactions that I have gotten since going through it, have been great for us. It has helped make our strong bond even stronger.

Set boundaries. If you suspect that they're really trying to sabotage your healthy lifestyle, it's time to develop a script. The next time you're confronted with someone waving a scoop of rocky road ice cream, say, "That was a very nice thought, but I've chosen not to eat high-fat food."

"The interaction happens so quickly, chances are very high that you'll end up saying okay if you're not prepared," Dr. Rankin says. The more you have rehearsed, the more likely it is that you'll repeat your script in a stressful situation.

Make healthy compromises for friends. If you've noticed that your friends stopped inviting you to lunch at the greasy spoon because they know you want to stay away from high-fat fare, maybe you should suggest a healthy alternative. Invite them to a restaurant that serves healthy entrées.

Instead of making a date for the movies, ask a friend to go for a walk or a hike, suggests Robert Abelson, Ph.D., health and fitness instructor at BSBM Abelson Enterprises in Redondo Beach, California, who has lost more than 200 pounds.

Stay motivated. You'll be less likely to let other people's negative reactions affect your weight loss if you stay focused on your goals. Dr. Abelson keeps a picture of himself at his heavier size in his wallet to stay motivated.

Like Dr. Abelson, Hansen has stayed focused on her goal. Seven years later, she's still 61 pounds slimmer. Now, instead of getting chocolate from her husband, she gets a colorful bouquet of carnations—her favorite flower.

That's the kind of reaction to her weight loss that she appreciates.

Week Twelve

Making It Last

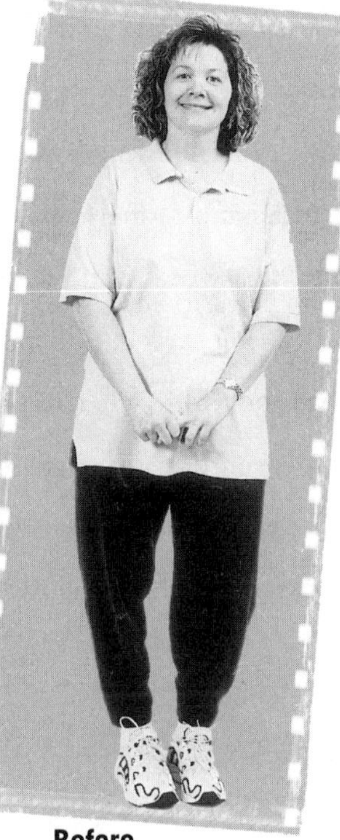

Before

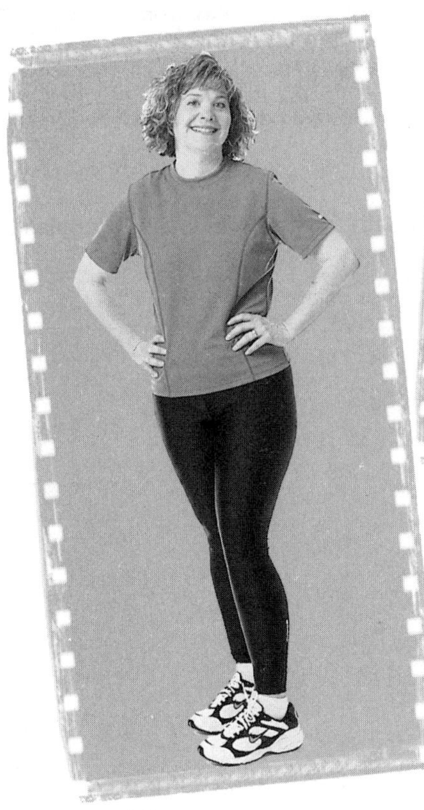

After

WE COULD SEE OURSELVES MAKING THESE CHANGES AND STICKING WITH THEM. THEY DIDN'T REQUIRE MAJOR ALTERATIONS IN OUR DAILY LIVES.

—Ana Reeser

Week Twelve

You've reached the final week of The *Prevention* Get Thin, Get Young Plan. But it's not really the end—it's the beginning of your slimmer, younger, and healthier lifestyle. This week's advice will help you stay on the straight and narrow, while allowing you to enjoy special occasions.

If you're like most Americans, you're eating, on average, four meals away from home each week. And you may think that you have very little say in what you're being served. But you'll be happy to learn that you're more in control than you realize when dining out. Festive occasions and holidays naturally tempt you to let your guard down. But with this week's strategies you'll steer clear of pitfalls. Plus, you'll learn how to set up an action plan to guard against gaining back the weight you've lost.

Slimming Strategies for Dining Out

GOING OUT TO EAT USED TO BE RESERVED FOR SPECIAL OCCASIONS. NOW, IT'S A WAY OF LIFE.

The average American eats four meals away from home each week. Dining out can mean anything from eating in the finest restaurant to wolfing down a burger in the car. Often, it's a matter of convenience or even necessity—a part of our busy lifestyles.

But let's face it. Anytime you don't have to cook can seem like cause for celebration. The problem is that your waistline can spread quickly if every meal out is a holiday from healthy eating. And from the looks of it, that's exactly what we're doing.

"The increase in obesity is directly correlated with the trend of eating away from home. It's almost perfectly correlated," says Paul Lachance, Ph.D., executive director of the Nutraceuticals Institute at Rutgers University in New Brunswick, New Jersey. "The more we eat out, the fatter we get."

That's because the more we eat out, the more calories we take in. A study of 129 women found that those who ate out the most—more than six times per week—consumed an average of 300 more calories per day than women who ate out less frequently.

The extra calories didn't add up to extra nutrition, either, notes Linda Eck Clemens, R.D., Ed.D., professor of clinical nutrition at the University of Memphis, who led the study. They came primarily from fat.

So the question is: How can you enjoy dining out and stay on track with your weight-loss goals? Even dietitians have a hard time estimating fat and calorie content when they're perusing an artfully worded menu.

Luckily, you can slash those excess calories and fat without being an expert.

Stay in Control

You don't need a scientific study to tell you that when you eat out, it's easy to eat too much. Just look at those colossal portions on your plate. What you really want to know is how to have a healthy, satisfying, and pleasurable meal without going into calorie overload.

Your first slimming strategies start at home. Before you head out the door, try these tricks to exercise a little appetite control.

Spoil your appetite. Mom was wrong. Sometimes it is a good idea to eat before meals. "You shouldn't go into a restaurant hungry any more than you should go to the grocery store hungry. Why? Because you're going to make bad decisions," says Don Mauer, author of *Lean and Lovin' It* and *The Guy's Guide to Great Eating*.

Weight-loss experts suggest eating a small amount of high-fiber food or protein before you leave for the restaurant. To dampen your hunger just a bit, snack on a piece of fruit, fat-free yogurt, a salad, air-popped popcorn, or a healthy drink.

Wear fitted clothing. Make an extra effort to avoid loose-fitting or stretchy clothing when you're going out to eat, says Julie Waltz Kembel, a behavioral counselor at Canyon Ranch spa in Tucson and author of *Winning the Weight and Wellness Game*.

It turns out that the oh-so-comfortable feel of elastic is as liberating for the lips as it is for the hips. So Kembel relies on a snug waistband to serve as a gentle reminder that she's had enough. "It helps boost your resolve to eat less," she says.

Hold off on the alcohol. Alcohol relaxes your control and stimulates your appetite. So have that glass of wine or beer with your meal, not before it,

Breakfast: A Reason to Stay Home

Eat breakfast out, and you can easily blow a day's worth of fat, not to mention 1,000 calories, by 10:00 A.M.

Sure, you know that eggs are high in cholesterol and bacon isn't a diet food. But who would have guessed that pancakes with butter or margarine and sausage has as much artery-clogging power as a McDonald's Quarter Pounder and an order of fries?

The bottom line is that if you're trying to start your day on the right foot, nutritionally speaking, don't go out for breakfast, says Dr. Linda Eck Clemens of the University of Memphis.

When researchers at the university compared the nutrient quality of meals at home with meals at restaurants, breakfast came up the big loser. People who ate breakfast out consumed more fat, more calories, and half the fat-fighting fiber that people who ate at home did.

Of course, it is possible to get a healthy breakfast when you eat out. Go for hot or cold cereal, fruit, juice, plain toast, an English muffin, a small bagel, or some fat-free yogurt.

Many restaurants offer egg substitutes. Combined with hash browns and plain toast, you have a pretty decent breakfast.

suggests Kembel. Instead of ordering a cocktail, ask your server to bring a pitcher of ice water to the table.

Mastering the Menu

Whether you're headed to a burger joint or splurging on five-star cuisine, when someone else is doing the cooking, your goal is to take control of the food you order by asking questions and making creative selections from the menu.

"Think of yourself as someone on a treasure hunt as you look for all the healthy options," says Gayle Reichler, R.D., a registered dietitian and consultant in New York City and author of *Active Wellness*.

Don't be wowed by fancy descriptions like "mouthwatering" and "luscious." Instead, review the menu by considering the food itself. Is it generally healthful? Or is it fatty? Mix and match from the entire menu. For instance, if you want to start your meal with some fresh fruit but it's listed under desserts, feel free to order it as an appetizer.

When you dine out, you're more in control than you think.

Let your server know that you want to eat a low-fat meal, and you're likely to get it. A survey by the National Restaurant Association found that more than 96 percent of restaurants will alter their preparation methods if requested.

"When you dine out, you're more in control than you think," says Reichler, a former pastry chef who now trains chefs on healthy food preparation. "You are the customer, and in the restaurant business, the customer is always right."

When you make the right decisions at this stage of the game, the rest of meal is easy—just wait for your food to arrive and enjoy it.

Crack the code. You're generally better off ordering meals that are baked, broiled, grilled, steamed, roasted, or boiled. Even so, don't assume that you know how a dish is prepared until you ask a few questions.

Chefs are in the business of creating great-tasting food, and one way they do that is by using fat to boost flavor.

"Restaurants are notorious for adding butter to food in order to make it tender and moist," says Reichler. When she surveyed 447 chefs, more than two-thirds correctly answered questions about nutrients and how cooking affects them.

But they fell short on questions about fat and cholesterol and were likely to neglect healthful cooking practices about one-third of the time.

Reichler tells her clients to grill the waiter about ingredients, not nutritional content (fat, carbohydrate, protein). Instead of just asking for a low-fat meal, refer to the specific type of fat that should be reduced—butter, oil, mayonnaise, or cream.

Downsize your dinner. Restaurants almost always serve double portions. Order appetizers, side dishes, or half-orders of high-calorie entrées.

"I look the waiter straight in the eye and say, 'I'll pay for the whole thing, but bring me half,'" says Kembel. You're saving a lot more than a few hundred calories. It means that you're in control of what you eat instead of leaving the decision to some stranger in the kitchen preparing the food.

"It develops a sense of competence and confidence," she adds.

Go halvsies. Ask restaurants to use only half of the normal portion for high-fat ingredients such as cheese, oil, béarnaise sauce, or gravy, says Mauer, who started using this trick to slim down one of his favorites—pizza. "You'll get the flavor with half the calories. No one has turned me down yet," he says.

To slim down Asian cuisine, top double the quantity of rice with half the entrée. Or mix equal parts of a steamed entrée with a regular stir-fried order, and you'll get the same amount of food and flavor with half the fat.

Get souped up. Have a bowl of soup first, and you'll fill up on fewer calories. "Calories are consumed more slowly because they are less concentrated," says James J. Kenney, R.D., Ph.D., a nutrition research specialist at the Pritikin Longevity Center in Santa Monica, California.

Researchers at Johns Hopkins University in Baltimore found that diners who began with tomato soup ate 25 percent fewer calories by meal's end than people who started with cheese and crackers.

And there's no need to stick with plain tomato soup. Minestrone, gazpacho, Manhattan clam chowder, consommé, or soups such as chicken with rice, vegetable, or bean will have the same effect.

Order extra vegetables. Whether they're dressing a sandwich or part of a stir-fry, ask for less meat and more of these low-calorie, high-fiber gems, says Melanie Polk, R.D., director of nutrition education at the American Institute for Cancer Research in Washington, D.C.

People who dine out tend to eat 25 percent fewer fruits and vegetables than people who eat at home. Maybe that's because it's not always easy to get a hefty serving of healthy fare on the typical American menu. Sometimes, it seems as if the closest thing to a vegetable on the menu is fried onion rings or fried zucchini sticks dipped in batter.

So don't be shy to ask to substitute a particular vegetable for those french fries or greasy onion rings. Many restaurants are happy to honor off-menu requests for healthy side dishes, such as steamed broccoli or fresh fruit, says Polk.

Master the art of dressing yourself. Salad dressings average 68 calories per tablespoon. By the time the kitchen staff has ladled it over your plate of healthy greens, you're way into the triple digits.

The solution is to order salad dressings and sauces on the side. Dip the tines of your fork into the dressing or sauce first and then spear your food.

"I'm amazed at how well this works," says Mauer. "Odds are I won't go through more than 2 teaspoons of dressing for a large salad."

Play around a little. Order foods with high "play value" such as steamed clams, crab claws, lobster in the shell, artichokes, relish trays, or fruit platters, says Kembel. The busier you keep your hands during a lengthy meal, the easier it will be to avoid eating extra food.

Add your own condiments. Order your sandwiches dry and then spread your bread with one of these flavorful, low-fat alternatives: honey mustard, chili or cocktail sauce, horseradish, chutney, cranberry sauce, ketchup, barbecue sauce, or jalapeño jelly.

"These items have some sugar and salt. Some of them may even have a little fat," says Kembel. "But when compared to butter, margarine, mayonnaise, or oil, any of them is a good choice."

When You Can't Resist

Does this mean that you should never order dessert? Or french fries? Or spareribs? Not at all. Sometimes, you just have to have your favorites without feeling like a nutrition criminal. Here are a few tips on how to indulge wisely.

Go big on the grease. If you really want something fried, choose large-size items: a breast of chicken instead of five or six chicken fingers, or seven or eight steak fries instead of 20 or more thin french fries. The smaller items have more total surface area, so they absorb more oil, making them higher in fat and calories, says Reichler.

Learn to share. Order one serving of a favorite high-fat food, such as fries or spareribs, and share it with everyone at the table, says Kembel.

Have a doughnut. Despite their fat-filled image, you can get fewer calories and less fat if you order a glazed yeast doughnut (170 calories, 9 grams of fat) with your coffee instead of almost any kind of muffin, including banana nut (360 calories, 15 grams of fat), chocolate chip (400 calories, 17 grams of fat), and bran (390 calories, 12 grams of fat).

Think small and satisfying for dessert. It may be easier than you think to skip the gooey treats—and about 80 percent of us do when we eat out. But if you really can't resist ending on a sweet note, Kembel suggests ordering two or three chocolate mints with your coffee or tea.

Declare a holiday twice a month. Letting yourself enjoy an occasional "free" meal is as much a part of slimming down as that high-fiber cereal stocked in your pantry.

"Anticipating something special is the spice of life for all of us," says Kembel. And there has to be a place for the occasional extravagance in your thinner, younger lifestyle.

Rather than depriving yourself of birthday cake or a romantic dinner on your anniversary, plan to indulge. Eat whatever you want in whatever quantity you want, but limit it to twice a month, says Kembel.

Think of this little piece of contrarian advice as a way to strike a balance between your desire to eat a healthy low-fat diet and your need to have a little fun.

Celebrating the Holidays

ROASTED TURKEY, MASHED POTATOES WITH THICK POOLS OF GRAVY, MOUNDS OF SNOWBALL COOKIES—AND, OF COURSE, THE UBIQUITOUS CHEESE BALLS. THAT'S A LOT OF FOOD. AND MOST OF IT ENDS UP ON OUR WAISTS.

The average American gains 5 to 7 pounds between Thanksgiving and the New Year," says Ross Andersen, Ph.D., assistant professor of medicine at Johns Hopkins University School of Medicine in Baltimore and one of the nation's leading researchers on lifestyle activity and weight loss.

Getting through the holidays—and enjoying your favorite foods—requires a plan all its own. You just need to develop a holiday eating strategy.

Of course, holiday treats between Thanksgiving and New Year's aren't the only temptations. There are boxes of chocolates and other sweets for Valentine's Day, Easter, and Halloween. Burgers, hot dogs, and barbecues abound at Memorial Day, the Fourth of July, and Labor Day.

Whether your challenge is eating a healthy Thanksgiving dinner or avoiding burgers at a Fourth of July cookout, you can still enjoy holiday traditions. Once you get through a holiday—and even a whole holiday season—without gaining weight, you'll feel empowered, Dr. Andersen says. Especially when you discover that it's still possible to have fun and enjoy important traditions.

Here are slimming strategies for the most common holiday scenarios.

Making Holiday Parties More Fun and Less Filling

Accepting an invitation to a holiday party doesn't have to mean accepting weight gain. Here's how to enjoy yourself without waving goodbye to weight loss.

Start new traditions. Who says a party has to include fruitcake and chicken wings? Do something different. Throw a house-decorating, wreath-making, or gift-wrapping party. Want to get out of the house? Invite friends and family to go caroling, sledding, or skiing, or to build snowmen, suggests Marsha Hudnall, R.D., director of nutrition programs at Green Mountain, a weight-loss program for women in Ludlow, Vermont. You can have fun while burning calories instead of consuming them.

Be choosy. If you're concerned about overeating at holiday parties, it might be a good idea to skip a few of them, Dr. Andersen suggests. Only attend the ones that are important to you.

If you do decide to go to more than one a week, set some ground rules, such as having dessert at only one party and punch at another, suggests Laura Molseed, R.D., outpatient nutrition coordinator at the University of Pittsburgh Medical Center.

Eat before you get there. Having a piece of fruit or yogurt before going to the party will help you cut back on trips to the buffet table, without interfering with your good time, Dr. Andersen says.

Keep some calories in your food "bank." By skipping extra calories early, you'll have room to enjoy the treats to come. Think of your body as a savings account, Molseed says. Passing on run-of-the-mill appetizers and bread means that you don't have to worry about having a piece of raisin pumpkin pie.

Choose appetizers wisely. Avoid the chicken wings and go for the shrimp on a skewer—it has only 10 calories and no fat. Other good choices are sushi for only 71 calories and 1 gram of fat, and chicken on a skewer for only 74 calories and 3 grams of fat, even with a dab of peanut sauce.

And, of course, if those goodies aren't on the party menu, you still can't go wrong if you pick strawberries, grapes, slices of melon, baby carrots, or broccoli florets, Molseed says. But skip the dip unless you know that it's low-fat.

Take your own. Here's how to be absolutely sure that you'll have something good and healthy to eat at a party: Make it yourself. Tell your host that you'll take a dish, says Joyce Nelsen, R.D., nutrition instructor at the Culinary Institute of America in Hyde Park, New York, such as a tray of thin-crust mini pizzas, each for 54 calories and 2 grams of fat.

Be fashionably late. If you tend to crumble under the pressure of cream puffs and piping hot meatballs, arrive an hour late. After all, the buffet table isn't quite as appetizing once it's been picked over a few times. Stray napkins and cold stuffed mushrooms may keep you away from the food, Nelsen says.

Cut your calories from wine in half by asking for a wine spritzer.

Keep your glass full. Of water, that is. Since 12 fluid ounces of light beer will run you about 99 calories, stick with water if you don't want to overload on calories. One and a half ounces of gin, rum, vodka, or whiskey contains about 100 calories, and 6 ounces of wine will cost you about 120 calories.

If you really want to drink, ask for a wine spritzer. By filling your glass half full of club soda, which has no calories, you'll cut your calories from wine in half. Or even try rotating between glasses of alcohol and water, and keep your drink maximum to two, Molseed suggests.

Stay in control. There's another reason to stay away from the alcohol. Because it tends to lower inhibitions, drinking could affect your eating plan. Alcohol lets your guard down, Dr. Andersen says, which could result in more splurging than you had planned.

Enjoying Your Holiday Meal

A few appetizers are nothing compared to the temptation of a table-long holiday feast, complete with your grandmother's stuffing, sweet cranberry sauce, and warm biscuits—not to mention the nudging of your relatives to fill your plate.

Set a goal. We are all familiar with all-you-can-eat holiday dinners, but they are obviously the wrong approach to weight loss, Dr. Andersen says.

"For many, the goal is to sit down and eat until you just can't eat one more piece of food," he says. "And then you rest and come back to the table an hour later for dessert." You could end up gaining 4 pounds over a 4-day weekend eating this way. This year, set a new goal: getting through the big dinner without overdosing on food.

Have a game plan. If you have a holiday meal coming up, plan your whole weekend so that you'll do as little damage as possible. Get up early on that holiday morning and take a long walk, Dr. Andersen says. And while it may seem obvious, eat a light breakfast and lunch before the big dinner, and follow that up with light meals and exercise for the rest of the weekend.

Envision your plate. Your visualization skills will really come in handy during the holidays. Imagine what your dinner plate is going to look like ahead of time, then don't eat anything else when you sit down to the real meal. Will you grab a drumstick or a slice of turkey breast? Will you have sweet potatoes or carrots with green beans? Will you have a piece of pumpkin or apple pie? How many glasses of wine will you drink? Take everything into account and commit to it on paper so you'll be more likely to stick to it, Dr. Andersen says.

Enjoy your favorite. When you think about what you're going to eat, make room for holiday favorites. Choose one food that you get the most pleasure from and include it on your list, Dr. Andersen suggests. If you've always loved the stuffing, choose it instead of something you have once a week, like mashed potatoes. This way, you won't leave the dinner table feeling as though you haven't enjoyed your meal or the festivities.

Leave plenty of room. Another way to keep from overeating—and to show some appreciation for your mother's china—is to make sure that you can still see the plate after you take your food, Dr. Andersen says. It's an easy way to control your portions without counting calories.

Avoid leftovers. You've enjoyed your feast and dodged extra calories, so don't let leftovers ruin your hard work. After all, who can resist a post-Thanksgiving turkey sandwich with a slice of pumpkin pie? Your solution: Refuse to take home leftovers, Nelsen says. If you're hosting the dinner, wrap food for your guests to take home. And if you still have leftovers, donate them to a soup kitchen.

Sweet Solutions

Just like greeting cards, candy in shiny colored wrappers has made its way into almost every holiday. Whether it's Valentine's Day, Easter, or Halloween, here's how to ignore the twinkle of wrapped calories.

Enjoy the rituals minus the sugar. Have fun on the holidays with a minimum of sugar. If your children are too young to eat all that Halloween candy—and you're afraid you'll pick up their slack—limit the amount of candy that they bring home. For example, if you have two kids, send them out trick-or-treating with only one bag, Nelsen suggests. You'll cut the amount of candy you have around the house in half.

Get rid of it. Here's a good rule to have: Whether it's leftover Halloween candy bars or half of a chocolate bunny, get it out of the house. Take it to work. "It will disappear in 10 minutes," Nelsen says. Or donate it to a food bank.

Pass up fat. If you must have candy in the house, make it fat-free. Two fruit-flavored Life Savers have only 20 calories, but one Snickers bar has 190 calories and 10 grams of fat.

Give and ask for nonedible gifts. If your heart is usually filled with chocolate on Valentine's Day, insist on doing something different—go hiking or take a walk at sunset, Hudnall suggests.

Surviving a Grilling

If you choose to eat the right food, summer holiday cookouts can be the healthiest holidays you have, especially if you remember to take advantage of low-fat grilling.

Grill better. Skip the typical hot dogs and burgers and find healthier alternatives. While a beef hot dog has 180 calories and 16 grams of fat, a light dog has only 100 calories and 7 grams of fat. And a 4-ounce hamburger has 328 calories and 24 grams of fat, while a frozen vegetarian burger has only 140 calories and 2 grams of fat.

If turkey dogs and veggie burgers don't tempt your palate, try a 4-ounce grilled chicken breast without the skin for 130 calories and only 3 grams of fat.

Stick with healthy salads. You know your homemade potato salad is high in fat, so take a green salad this year. Romaine lettuce, tomatoes, sweet peppers, mushrooms, carrots, and a tablespoon of oil-free blue cheese dressing has only 75 calories and 1 gram of fat.

If it's not a cookout without it, make your potato salad healthier by using less mayonnaise, Hudnall suggests.

Crunch well. Did you know that a 1-ounce serving of potato chips has 150 calories and 10 grams of fat? Crunch some crisp green, red, and yellow peppers instead. You'll not only save calories and fat, you'll get vitamins A and C.

Use your melon. A cookout is a great excuse to have the perfect dessert: a big slice of watermelon. It has only 50 calories per cup, plus vitamin A.

Run around. Burn some calories and stay away from the picnic basket with fun activities. Play badminton, volleyball, softball, or football. Throw a Frisbee, go for a walk, or have a water-balloon war, Hudnall suggests.

Refresh with water. After acing that volleyball serve, you'll need to quench your thirst. Have lots of cool water handy instead of soda, Hudnall suggests.

The Cellulite Solution

"BRITAIN'S DIANA DONS LONG COAT TO HIDE CELLULITE." THAT WAS THE HEADLINE SEEN 'ROUND THE WORLD IN 1996, WHEN BRITISH TABLOID PHOTOGRAPHERS ACTUALLY PHOTOGRAPHED SIGNS OF CELLULITE ON DIANA'S FAMOUS LEGS. THOUGH MOST FOLKS FOUND THE PHOTO OFFENSIVE, MANY ALSO FELT A TOUCH OF GUILTY RELIEF TO DISCOVER THAT EVEN PRINCESSES DON'T HAVE PERFECT LEGS.

That's the simple truth about cellulite. If you're a woman, you probably have some. If you don't, you probably will. "More than 85 percent of post-adolescent women develop at least a little cellulite somewhere on the lower body," says Jeffrey Sklar, M.D., assistant professor of dermatology at Columbia University and director of the Center for Aesthetic Dermatology in Woodbury, New York.

That doesn't mean that you have to spend the rest of your life in sarong skirts and long beach cover-ups, however. Though you may not be able to eliminate cellulite completely, there are steps you can take to minimize its appearance for younger, trimmer, and smoother legs.

Another Name for Fat

Ask some medical experts, and they'll tell you that cellulite doesn't even exist. It's not that they think you're imagining the dimply skin on the backs of your thighs. They just believe that those puckers and bulges are nothing more than ordinary fat. Cellulite, they say, is a term coined by the beauty industry in order to make this ordinary fat sound like a condition that women can "cure" with the right products or treatments.

Other doctors believe that these lumpy deposits are something more: They say that cellulite is an abnormality caused by a combination of poor circulation, swelling from inadequate lymph drainage, and the fat-storing actions of female hormones such as estrogen.

"The fact is, we don't completely know what causes the areas of dimply fat we call cellulite, why women get it, or how to eliminate it," says Dr. Sklar. "We do know that hormones play a role and that gaining weight contributes to it. So the real truth probably lies somewhere in between."

Though we don't like its appearance, the fat stored below the waist (where cellulite often appears) serves a useful purpose. Women naturally store fat in their lower bodies because the body calls upon these fat reserves to provide extra energy during pregnancy and breastfeeding. Though women have surplus fat there most of their lives, they don't start calling it cellulite until the dimples appear, most often in their late twenties and early thirties, says Alan Kling, M.D., clinical assistant professor at Mount Sinai Medical Center in New York City.

Previously smooth hips and thighs begin to bulge mostly because of a natural weakening of the skin, which allows fat to push to the surface, says Dr. Kling. You see this more on women than on men because of differences in connective tissue.

Everyone has strands of connective tissue that separate fat cells into compartments and that connect fat tissue to skin. In women, this connective tissue tends to run vertically, which lets the fat push up to the surface and bulge. In men, it runs in a horizontal, criss-cross pattern, which prevents the fat from bulging to the surface. "When the skin weakens on women, the effect is like a mattress, with the fat bulging like stuffing between the tethers," says Dr. Sklar. "Men's horizontal connective tissue prevents that from happening. Plus, their skin is thicker, so the fat underneath is less visible."

Smoothing Your Curves

A little cellulite is a perfectly natural thing. It's unlikely that you'll ever find a way to make it all disappear. But you can diminish its appearance and give your lower body a firmer, younger contour. Here's what experts recommend.

Burn fat. Regardless of any other factors that may be involved, the bottom line is that cellulite is fat, says Dr. Kling. "When you have less fat, you have less cellulite. When you put on weight, the cellulite becomes much more noticeable."

The best way to burn fat is by exercising, says Dr. Sklar. Working out 3 or 4 days a week burns calories, so you'll shed pounds and reduce those fat deposits. It also makes your muscles grow, eventually making your skin look more firm. Here are eight activities that burn a lot of calories—and that will help you reduce cellulite more quickly. (The number of calories each activity burns is based on a 150-pound person.)

ACTIVITY	CALORIES BURNED PER HOUR
Cardio kickboxing (like Tae-Bo)	680
Jogging (moderate pace)	612
Cross-country skiing	544
Swimming (sidestroke laps)	544
Stationary cycling (moderate pace)	476
Tennis	476
Racewalking	442
Stairclimbing	408

Tone your "zones." You probably already know that it's impossible to spot-reduce, or lose weight in one specific area. But you can benefit by paying special attention to your problem areas. Work out as you normally do. Then tack on a few additional exercises that target the areas that need extra attention, says Wayne Westcott, Ph.D., training consultant for the American Senior Fitness Association in New Smyrna Beach, Florida. These extra toning exercises will build up the muscles in your trouble spots while burning more calories. You'll lose fat a little more quickly and have shapely, toned muscles besides.

Here are two exercises that can help tone your outer thighs and butt, says Amy Goldwater, a certified fitness specialist and fitness advisor to the TOPS (Take Off Pounds Sensibly) Club in Milwaukee. She recommends doing one to three sets of each exercise with 10 to 15 repetitions per set.

Straight-Leg Lifts

Lie on on your left side, with your legs together and the bottom leg slightly bent. Bend your left elbow and rest your head comfortably on your arm. Place your right hand on the floor in front of you for balance. Keeping your top leg slightly bent, slowly raise it as far as it will comfortably go. Your foot can be pointed or flexed. There should be no swinging or momentum. Hold, then lower. Complete a set, then roll over and do a set with your other leg. When the exercise becomes too easy, loop an exercise band around your ankles for extra resistance.

Muscles worked: Abductors (outer thighs) and gluteals (buttocks)

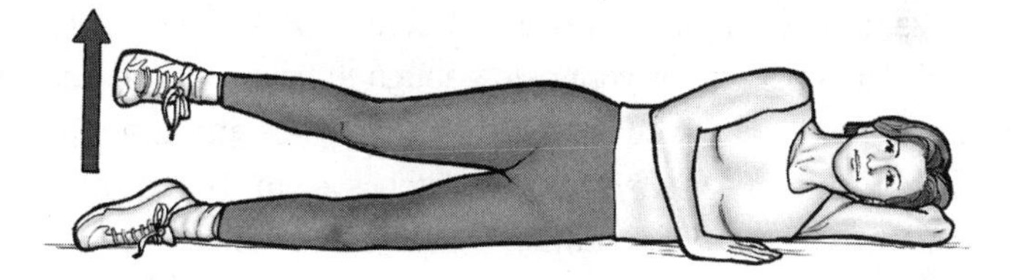

Standing Kickbacks

Stand behind a sturdy chair, with your hands on the back for support. Lean forward from the waist, keeping your back flat. Bend your right knee so that your calf and thigh are at a 90-degree angle. Then tighten your gluteal (buttocks) muscles and move your right heel up toward the ceiling until your back and thigh are in line. Maintain the 90-degree angle between your calf and thigh. Hold, then lower. Complete a full set with your right leg, then do a set with your left.

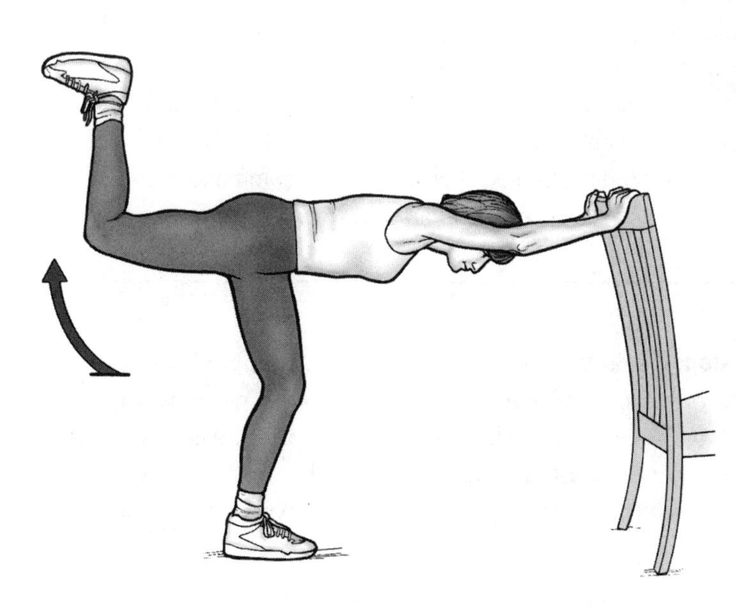

Muscles worked: Hamstrings (back of thighs) and gluteals (buttocks)

Fat Chance

Some women would pay anything to rid themselves of cellulite. And, unfortunately, many do—with little, if any, success. There are countless creams, machines, supplements, and treatments that will remove the bulges from your weekly paycheck but won't help your legs a lick. Here's what to watch for.

Creams. In theory, thigh creams work by inhibiting a body enzyme that stimulates your body to store and conserve fat. In fact, the creams don't do much more than moisturize, says Dr. Jeffrey Sklar of the Center for Aesthetic Dermatology. "No cream available penetrates your skin enough to have any real benefit," he says. In order for any cream to be effective, it must also be able to remain in your body without being swept away by your circulatory system. This is an impossible demand for an over-the-counter product. "Save your money," he adds.

Supplements. "There is no pill you can take to get rid of cellulite," says Dr. Sklar. A supplement must be able to target cellulite areas without being toxic. Manufacturers of herbal products claim that their supplements can strengthen the connective tissue around fat, increase circulation, and remove fluids from the area. "There's no proof to back these claims," says Dr. Sklar. "And the products may be dangerous."

Wraps. Manufacturers of cellulite body wraps tout them as fat burners, but all they really do is sap fluid from your body. Those lost inches are all water weight. They'll return as soon as you eat and drink normally, says Dr. Sklar.

Surgery. Liposuction is currently one of the most popular cosmetic surgeries in the country, but it can't remove cellulite. In fact, it can make it look worse, says Dr. Alan Kling of Mount Sinai Medical Center. "I would never recommend liposuction for cellulite. The skin may look even more dimpled when you're done."

Darken your complexion. If you have naturally dark skin, cellulite is not as much of a problem. For one thing, African-American and other women with dark complexions tend to have thicker skin and less dimpling. Also, dark skin camouflages cellulite better. Though suntanning is unhealthy and out of vogue, self-tanners are useful for camouflage. Pale-skinned women who are very concerned about the appearance of cellulite may benefit from darkening their skin tone a bit, says Dr. Kling.

"Cellulite often has a yellowish, orangy, or paler tone than the surrounding skin, which makes it more noticeable," he says. "A little tanning can cover that up and make it blend." Instead of lying out and baking under the sun's harmful rays, you can get the same effect from a liquid self-tanner.

Deep massage it . . . maybe. While some experts frown on anticellulite potions and devices, one recent invention designed to smooth bumpy hips and thighs may get a small thumbs-up from your doctor. The machine is called Endermologie. Originally developed in France, it's a suction-massage device that gently pulls cellulite-affected tissue into a pair of rolling balls that act as rollers. The manufacturers claim that Endermologie works by stretching the connective fibers that give cellulite its uneven appearance as well as by increasing bloodflow and lymph drainage from the area.

The American Society of Plastic and Reconstructive Surgeons doesn't agree. The society has stated that reports of the benefit of Endermologie do not meet accepted scientific standards and that until someone presents clinical proof, the society considers the technique of "unproven medical value."

Dr. Sklar warns that the effect is temporary and does not completely resolve the problem. Some patients have seen positive improvements, while others have not. "You need to continue with follow-up treatments to maintain the results," he says. Each treatment lasts about 45 minutes, and you need about 15 sessions to see benefits. The cost is about $100 per treatment.

Keeping It Off for Good

GRAB A PIECE OF PAPER AND A PEN.

RIGHT THIS VERY MOMENT, WRITE DOWN THE HIGHEST WEIGHT YOU WILL TOLERATE. PERHAPS IT'S ABOUT 5 POUNDS HEAVIER THAN YOU ARE NOW. MAYBE IT'S A LITTLE MORE.

Now be practical and give yourself *some* breathing room. We all know that weight can fluctuate a few pounds from week to week.

For example, say that you met your goal of getting back down to 140 pounds. You figure that your upper limit is 145. You don't want to reach it, but it's your limit.

Now put that piece of paper somewhere where you'll see it. Maybe on the fridge. In your day planner. Near the scale in the bathroom.

That number is your emergency brake. It's your rip cord, your panic button. The day you step on the scale and see the needle bob and weave until it settles on those digits, you know it's time to get back to work.

"When you reach that point, it's time to put the brakes on. You have to decide in advance what the trigger will be to get you back on the program," says weight-loss expert Dr. Ross Andersen of Johns Hopkins University School of Medicine.

It's a tad unrealistic to think that you'll never gain a few pounds again. After all, consider holidays, menstrual periods, bad weeks at the office, and vacations. But what usually happens when people regain weight is that they start off with a simple 5 pounds. They don't think much of it, so it slowly and rather stealthily creeps up to 10 pounds. Frustrated and angry, they figure, why try? And that 10 becomes 20, then 30, and so on.

It doesn't have to be that way, Dr. Andersen says. Nowhere does it say that a 5-pound regain erases all your hard work. Consider it a wake-up call. It's telling you to stop what you're doing before you gain any more weight. After all, it's much easier to lose that 5 than it is to lose 10, 20, or 30 pounds, or more. So your first step in keeping off the weight for good is to settle on this very important number.

"Once people have lost a certain amount of weight, I think they need to get a very clear picture in mind of what their new upper limit of acceptance will be," Dr. Andersen says.

When You Reach Your Limit

Now that you've decided on your number, also jot down what you will do the very moment you see that number pop up. "What will you do when you hit that weight? That's the real secret to keeping off weight. What are you going to do right away to stop it?" Dr. Andersen says.

It's not good enough to say that when you reach that weight, you'll buckle down again. Just what does that mean? You need specifics. What will you do and how will you do it? The specifics got you to your goal weight, and the specifics will get you back to it again.

Based on what worked for you during The *Prevention* Get Thin, Get Young Plan, you know best what you need to do to lose weight. Think about what worked and what you enjoyed. Write it down. That's what you'll do the moment you see that number. If you need some ideas, Dr. Andersen recommends that you try one or two of these.

Pull out your weight-loss diary. Find out why you're gaining. To do that, write down everything in your diary: What are you eating, when, and why. How active you are.

You may find that you've changed your routine in some way that's adding the pounds. Think about the following: Are you eating bigger portions than you were before? Have you developed an afternoon snack habit? Are you walking a lot less lately? Have you stopped taking the stairs?

Call a friend. Perhaps you've lost touch with your walking buddy,

Living Proof
PANEL

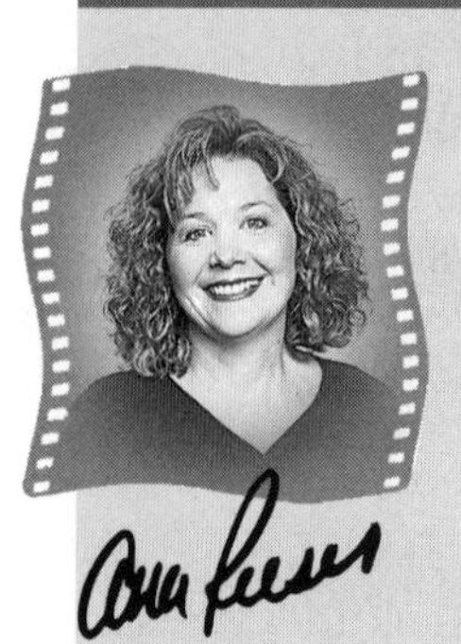

This Time, It's Different

My husband, John, and I have tried to lose weight a number of times before, but it never seemed to stick. Something would come up, and we'd fall off the wagon. We just weren't ready.

But this time, we both had events that motivated us. I started a new job, and I didn't want to wear my big and baggy clothes. John saw that his Naval Reserve fitness test scores were declining. So we both wanted to do something.

What made this time different from all our other endeavors? A few things. First, we had a program. We always had those specific food and exercise goals in our sights. Not that the program was too rigid, but at least we had something to go by. For previous times, we had just said that we would eat better or exercise more—ambiguous stuff.

Second, our program was based on healthy lifestyle changes—not extreme changes or crazy gimmicks. We could see ourselves making these changes and sticking with them. They didn't require major alterations in our daily lives.

Finally, we have learned from our past mistakes. One of our diet downfalls was that we would run out to Taco Bell when we got so tired and busy. Now when I feel that way, I just boil some water and toss in spaghetti. We have learned that you can still have quick and easy meals without running out to a fast-food joint.

or you have a friend or relative whom you know will be supportive. Call and tell that person what's happened and ask for help to get you back on track.

Take a walk. Don't think about getting more active, just do it. Maybe that number popping up is the impetus you need to get moving again.

A walk will help you feel that you are doing something about it right now.

Set new goals. As you followed the Get Thin, Get Young Plan, your goals provided you with inspiration and a road map to success. It's time to go back to them. If you aren't exercising enough, set a goal of walking 45 minutes every other day. If you aren't getting the fiber that you should, set a goal of eating 30 grams a day.

The Secrets of Success

What do the duck-billed platypus, the condor, the bald eagle, and people who have lost weight and kept it off have in common? They are rare breeds. And they have tons of experts spending lots of time and money trying to figure out what makes them so hard to find.

While plenty of people lose weight every year, very few keep it off. Studies of people in weight-loss programs have found that most people regain all their weight within 3 to 5 years. It's as if the land of getting thinner were just a vacation spot where people spend some quality time and then leave, always pining to go back.

Scientists and doctors scrutinize those who maintain their weight loss in order to learn the answer to one question: What do they do that the rest of us don't?

What they have found is that people who keep it off tend to follow the same basic principles: They exercise regularly, they keep track of their weight, they have the support of others, and they recognize that it's a lifetime change instead of a short-term program, says Dr. Andersen. Apply these principles now and for the rest of your life, and maybe you'll never need to use that emergency brake.

Keep Moving

What is the number one predictor of people who will keep off weight? They exercise regularly. No other measure so accurately predicts who will keep the weight off and who won't.

"We know that you can lose weight without exercise," Dr. Andersen says. "But we also know that you can't keep it off without exercise."

In one landmark study at the Kaiser Permanente Regional Health Education Center in Oakland, California, researchers found that 90 percent of women who lost and kept off 20 pounds exercised at least three times a week. Yet only 34 percent of the people who regained weight said that they exercised on a regular basis.

A review of the National Weight Control Registry—a long-term study of people who have lost weight and kept it off—shows that more than half of all weight maintainers engage in activities that make them sweat three or more times a week.

Why does exercise keep the weight off? Obviously, you burn more calories. But several other factors also contribute to weight-loss maintenance success, Dr. Andersen says.

- It increases your resting metabolic rate. In other words, you burn more calories even when you aren't active.
- It improves your overall fitness level, allowing you to be more active in your daily life and burn even more calories.
- It improves mood and general well-being, making you feel better about yourself and your weight-loss efforts.
- It gets you into a healthier state of mind. After exercising for an hour, you're less likely to pick up a candy bar. Just putting the effort into it makes you think, "After all the good I did today with my exercise, why ruin it for a lousy piece of candy?"

Here's how to keep exercise in your life after you've lost your weight.

Get at least 30 minutes. Strive for 30 minutes of some kind of activity each day. That can include walking, swimming, stairclimbing, jogging—whatever activity you enjoy.

Make being active a way of life. The best way to fit more exercise into your life is to pepper it throughout your day with lifestyle activities such as parking your car farther away from your office and taking the stairs instead of the elevator. If time is your mortal enemy, that's when lifestyle changes are your greatest asset. These seemingly small actions add up over time. "Look for those little ways that you can expend calories," Dr. Andersen says.

Break it up. If you have a bad day when you can't give up 30 minutes, break it into six 5-minute walks throughout the day, Dr. Andersen says. Take a lap around the office every hour.

Do whatever you can. Even if you can't exercise as much as you want to or know you should, do as much as you can. "We've seen that people who exercise only 50 percent of what they should can maintain full weight loss.

It is important to realize that something is better than nothing," Dr. Andersen says.

Use the Scale to Your Advantage

In your quest to keep the pounds off, the scale is your friend and not your enemy. About 75 percent of the people in the National Weight Control Registry weighed themselves at least once a week, says Mary Lou Klem, Ph.D., assistant professor of psychology at the University of Pittsburgh School of Medicine.

In order to not gain weight, you have to know what you weigh. All too often, people shun the scale, afraid that it will tell them something that they don't want to know: that they're gaining. They ignore it, until it's too late.

Or they go on their merry way, thinking that, yeah, maybe they've gained a *few* pounds. Then, while visiting a friend's house one day, they walk into the bathroom and on a whim decide to step on the scale. To their horror, those "few pounds" are really 10 to 20. Weighing in every week or so will stop a small gain from sliding into a large one, Dr. Andersen says.

Before you run screaming at the idea of stepping on the scale every week, relax. If you approach it the right way, it doesn't have to be an exercise in torture. Consider it a preventive measure: Don't get all upset when you see your weight creep up a bit. Read it as a sign that you have to make a few changes to stop it in its tracks.

Remember: You'd rather tackle a small gain than a big one. Here's how Dr. Andersen says to do it.

Make it a routine. Pick one night a week when you'll step on the scale. Do it every week on that night and at that time. Write down your weight and keep tabs on it.

Put the scale away. Do not step on the scale every day. Your weight fluctuates naturally, and you'll drive yourself crazy. Keep in mind that monthly weight changes could cause your weight to go up and down. Don't beat yourself up over that.

Keep your diary. Another way to keep tabs on yourself is your weight-loss diary. Don't throw it away once you've met your goals. Dr. Andersen says that of the people he's treated who lost and kept off the weight, the majority of them relied on using diaries for self-monitoring.

While you don't have to use it as religiously as you did before, it's a good idea to spot-check yourself once in a while to get a handle on how you're doing with your exercise and eating goals. If you find that you're not meeting your targets, set new goals for yourself.

Surround Yourself with Support

You've no doubt heard stories about people who made it to the top, only to forget all the people who helped them get there.

Don't do that.

You're going to need the help of friends and family as much now as you did when you were losing weight. "When you look at the number of people who succeed, what they all have in common is support from others," Dr. Andersen says. So keep the troops rallied around you. Here's how to do it.

Stick with your support group. Don't stop going to your support group meetings just because you've met your goal. These kindred spirits in weight loss can be sources of comfort and inspiration as you face maintaining your new weight. Just as you discussed and overcame the difficulties and obstacles of trying to lose weight, you can share the secrets and tips for keeping it off as well.

Keep your walking dates. You and your exercise/walking buddy should be on the same pace and schedule as you were when you were on the program. Whether you're trying to lose or maintain, an exercise buddy always makes it easier to stick to your routine.

Tell your family that it's not over. When you started this plan, you had a nice chat with your family. You told them what you needed, what you didn't want, and what you expected from them during your weight-loss period. Now it's time for another chat: Tell them that it's not back to the way it was before. Plainly explain what you need from them now and that you expect that they'll continue their support as you try to keep the weight off.

Motor Up Your Motivation

Those who are successful at long-term weight loss know one important thing: This is no short-term program.

"Here's the challenge: It's forever," says Cynthia G. Last, Ph.D., professor of psychology at Nova Southeastern University in Fort Lauderdale, Florida, and author of *The Five Reasons Why We Overeat.* "This isn't something you are going to do like a diet. This is how you live your life from now on."

And that's why the Get Thin, Get Young Plan will succeed where others failed. Fad diets or other gimmicks had you live one way during the program, then sent you back to your old ways once you finished. Before you knew it, those pesky pounds returned.

But the simple lifestyle changes you've made now aren't going anywhere: They're here to stay. So your maintenance phase isn't going to be much different from your weight-loss stage. This new attitude will help ensure that the pounds stay off.

If weight maintenance alone isn't enough motivation for you to continue with your healthier ways, think of the other benefits of your new lifestyle: more energy, better health, a more youthful look, and protection against heart disease and cancer.

Obviously, there are going to be times—like when a German chocolate cake calls your name—when you need a bit more motivation than this. If you feel your spirit dragging, try the following to keep you on track.

Set new goals. When you were losing weight, you set goals for yourself and put all your energy toward meeting those benchmarks. But now that you've met your goals, you might feel as though there's nothing to strive for. Nonsense.

Just because you are at your goal weight doesn't mean that you can't keep pushing yourself to the next level, Dr. Andersen says. Here are some maintenance goals: Increase how long you exercise by 5 minutes each week; increase your strength-training efforts by 5 to 10 percent; try a new low-fat recipe every week. Even maintaining your goal weight every week can be something to set your sights on.

Reward yourself. To truly stay motivated, you need your own reward system. For every month you stay at your goal weight, buy yourself a new compact disc. Or treat yourself to good pair of walking shoes once you achieve one of your personal exercise goals. "You need to give yourself pats on the back for all the good you do," Dr. Andersen says.

Accept setbacks. Two sisters who both lost 20 pounds go to their mother's house for Thanksgiving. The table overflows with turkey, gravy, sweet potatoes, and pumpkin pie. Both sisters dive mouthfirst into the wealth of food. Both feel as if they are about to burst open. And both feel guilty.

Why will one of these women regain her weight and the other won't? Because one sister will wake up Friday morning and say, "I totally blew it. I might as well go downstairs and raid the refrigerator for leftovers."

The other sister will wake up and say to herself, "I totally blew it. I need to go out for a brisk walk and then be extra careful how I eat today to make up for yesterday." The second sister realizes that one bad day doesn't negate months of success.

"The real secret is what you are going to do the next day. Those who get right back on the program are the ones who will keep off the weight," Dr. Andersen says.

Index

Underscored page references indicate boxes and tables. **Boldface** references indicate illustrations.

A

B

G

I

J

K

L

M

Q

R

S

U

V

W

Y